MRI in Sports Medicine

Editor

TIMOTHY G. SANDERS

CLINICS IN
SPORTS MEDICINE

www.sportsmed.theclinics.com

Consulting Editor
MARK D. MILLER

July 2013 • Volume 32 • Number 3

ELSEVIER

1600 John F. Kennedy Boulevard • Suite 1800 • Philadelphia, Pennsylvania, 19103-2899

http://www.theclinics.com

CLINICS IN SPORTS MEDICINE Volume 32, Number 3
July 2013 ISSN 0278-5919, ISBN-13: 978-1-4557-7612-2

Editor: Jennifer Flynn-Briggs

Clinics in Sports Medicine (ISSN 0278-5919) is published quarterly by Elsevier Inc., 360 Park Avenue South, New York, NY 10010-1710. Months of issue are January, April, July, and October. Business and Editorial Offices: 1600 John F. Kennedy Blvd., Ste. 1800, Philadelphia, PA 19103-2899. Customer Service Office: 3251 Riverport Lane, Maryland Heights, MO 63043. Periodicals postage paid at New York, NY and additional mailing offices. Subscription prices are $324.00 per year (US individuals), $523.00 per year (US institutions), $159.00 per year (US students), $367.00 per year (Canadian individuals), $631.00 per year (Canadian institutions), $222.00 (Canadian students), $446.00 per year (foreign individuals), $631.00 per year (foreign institutions), and $222.00 per year (foreign students). Foreign air speed delivery is included in all *Clinics* subscription prices. All prices are subject to change without notice. **POSTMASTER:** Send address changes to *Clinics in Sports Medicine*, Elsevier Health Sciences Division, Subscription Customer Service, 3251 Riverport Lane, Maryland Heights, MO 63043. Customer Service (orders, claims, online, change of address): Elsevier Health Sciences Division, Subscription Customer Service, 3251 Riverport Lane, Maryland Heights, MO 63043. Tel: 1-800-654-2452 (U.S. and Canada); 314-447-8871 (outside U.S. and Canada). Fax: 314-447-8029. E-mail: journalscustomerservice-usa@elsevier.com (for print support); journalsonlinesupport-usa@elsevier.com (for online support).

Reprints. For copies of 100 or more of articles in this publication, please contact the Commercial Reprints Department, Elsevier Inc., 360 Park Avenue South, New York, NY 10010-1710. Tel.: 212-633-3812; Fax: 212-462-1935; E-mail: reprints@elsevier.com.

Clinics in Sports Medicine is covered in *MEDLINE/PubMed (Index Medicus) Current Contents/Clinical Medicine, Excerpta Medica,* and *ISI/Biomed.*

Printed and bound by CPI Group (UK) Ltd, Croydon, CR0 4YY

Transferred to digital print 2012

Contributors

CONSULTING EDITOR

MARK D. MILLER, MD
S. Ward Casscells Professor of Orthopaedic Surgery, University of Virginia; Team Physician, JBJS Deputy Editor for Sports Medicine, Director, Miller Review Course, James Madison University, Charlottesville, Virginia

EDITOR

TIMOTHY G. SANDERS, MD
Medical Director, NationalRad, Weston, Florida

AUTHORS

CHRISTIAN N. ANDERSON, MD
Sports Medicine Fellow, Department of Orthopaedic Surgery, Stanford University Medical Center, Redwood City, California

ASHEESH BEDI, MD
Assistant Professor of Orthopedic Surgery, MedSport, Department of Orthopaedic Surgery, University of Michigan, Ann Arbor, Michigan

STEPHANIE A. BERNARD, MD
Associate Professor of Radiology, Penn State Milton S. Hershey Medical Center, Hershey, Pennsylvania

PAM BRIAN, MD
Department of Radiology, Penn State Milton S. Hershey Medical Center, Hershey, Pennsylvania

GEORGE D. CHLOROS, MD
Resident, Department of Radiology "Panagiotis and Aglaia Kyriakou" Children's Hospital, Athens, Greece; Research Associate Department of Radiology, Virginia Commonwealth University School of Medicine, Richmond, Virginia, USA

STEVEN COHEN, MD
Department of Orthopedics, Rothman Institute, Philadelphia, Pennsylvania

KIRKLAND W. DAVIS, MD
Associate Professor of Radiology, Department of Radiology, University of Wisconsin School of Medicine and Public Health, Madison, Wisconsin

DONALD J. FLEMMING, MD
Professor of Radiology and Orthopedics, Radiology, Penn State Milton S. Hershey Medical Center, Hershey, Pennsylvania

EDWARD J. FOX, MD
Penn State Hershey Bone and Joint Institute, Hershey, Pennsylvania

ELIZABETH E. FRAUENHOFFER, MD
Department of Pathology and Laboratory Medicine, Penn State Milton S. Hershey
Medical Center, Hershey, Pennsylvania

ROBERT A. GALLO, MD
Assistant Professor, Department of Orthopaedics, Penn State Milton S. Hershey Medical
Center, Hershey, Pennsylvania

MICHAEL GITHENS, MD
Resident, Department of Orthopaedics, Stanford University, Redwood City, California

GARRY E. GOLD, MD
Professor of Radiology and (by courtesy) Bioengineering and Orthopaedic Surgery,
Department of Radiology, Stanford University Medical Center, Stanford, California

BEN K. GRAF, MD
Associate Professor of Orthopedics, Department of Radiology, University of Wisconsin
School of Medicine and Public Health, Madison, Wisconsin

JUSTIN W. GRIFFIN, MD
Resident Physician, Department of Orthopaedic Surgery, University of Virginia Health
System, Charlottesville, Virginia

PETER J. HAAR, MD, PhD
Assistant Professor, Department of Radiology, Virginia Commonwealth University School
of Medicine, Richmond, Virginia

CURTIS W. HAYES, MD, FACR
Professor of Radiology and Orthopedic Surgery, Department of Radiology, Virginia
Commonwealth University Health Sciences, Virginia Commonwealth University School of
Medicine, Richmond, Virginia

KENNETH J. HUNT, MD
Assistant Professor, Department of Orthopaedics, Stanford University, Redwood City,
California

JON A. JACOBSON, MD
Professor of Radiology, Department of Radiology, University of Michigan, Ann Arbor,
Michigan

MICHAEL KIM, MD
Fellow, Department of Radiology, Stanford University, Stanford, California

VICTOR LONGO, DO
Department of Radiology, Penn State Milton S. Hershey Medical Center, Hershey,
Pennsylvania

THOMAS P. LOUGHRAN, MD
Professor of Orthopedic Surgery, Department of Orthopaedic Surgery, Virginia
Commonwealth University School of Medicine, Richmond, Virginia

WILLIAM C. MEYERS, MD
President, Vincera Institute; Professor of Surgery, Department of Surgery, Drexel University College of Medicine; Adjunct Professor, Department of Surgery, Thomas Jefferson University, Philadelphia, Pennsylvania; Consulting Professor, Department of Surgery, Duke University School of Medicine, Durham, North Carolina

MARK D. MILLER, MD
S. Ward Casscells Professor, Department of Orthopaedic Surgery, University of Virginia Health System, University of Virginia, Charlottesville, Virginia

YOAV MORAG, MD
Associate Professor of Radiology, Department of Radiology, University of Michigan, Ann Arbor, Michigan

WILLIAM B. MORRISON, MD
Professor of Radiology, Department of Radiology, Thomas Jefferson University Hospital, Philadelphia, Pennsylvania

TIMOTHY J. MOSHER, MD
Distinguished Professor, Departments of Orthopaedics and Radiology, Penn State Milton S. Hershey Medical Center, Hershey, Pennsylvania

MARK MURPHEY, MD
Chief of Musculoskeletal Imaging, American Institute for Radiologic Pathology, Silver Spring, Maryland; Department of Radiology, Walter Reed National Military Medical Center; Department of Radiology and Nuclear Medicine, Uniformed Services, University of the Health Sciences, Bethesda, Maryland

ANDREW PALISCH, MD
Clinical Musculoskeletal Radiology Fellow, Department of Radiology, Thomas Jefferson University Hospital, Philadelphia, Pennsylvania

GEOFFREY M. RILEY, MD
Clinical Associate Professor of Radiology, Department of Radiology, Stanford University Medical Center, Stanford, California

HUMBERTO G. ROSAS, MD
Assistant Professor of Radiology, Department of Radiology, University of Wisconsin School of Medicine and Public Health, Madison, Wisconsin

MARC R. SAFRAN, MD
Professor of Orthopaedic Surgery, Associate Director of Sports Medicine, Department of Orthopaedic Surgery, Stanford University Medical Center, Redwood City, California

PRANSHU SHARMA, MD
Department of Radiology, Thomas Jefferson University Hospital, Philadelphia, Pennsylvania

ERIC WALKER, MD
Department of Radiology, Penn State Milton S. Hershey Medical Center, Hershey, Pennsylvania; Department of Radiology and Nuclear Medicine, Uniformed Services, University of the Health Sciences, Bethesda, Maryland

CORRIE M. YABLON, MD
Assistant Professor of Radiology, Department of Radiology, University of Michigan, Ann Arbor, Michigan

ADAM C. ZOGA, MD
Associate Professor of Radiology, Director of Musculoskeletal MRI and Ambulatory Imaging Centers, Vice Chair for Clinical Practice, Department of Radiology, Thomas Jefferson University Hospital, Philadelphia, Pennsylvania

Contents

Foreward   xi

Mark D. Miller

Preface   xiii

Timothy G. Sanders

Imaging of the Shoulder with Arthroscopic Correlation   339

Pranshu Sharma, William B. Morrison, and Steven Cohen

> Shoulder pain with or without trauma is a common complaint. MRI is often
> the most useful imaging study for evaluating the shoulder. This review pro-
> vides an overview of various modalities and their role in evaluating various
> clinical issues in shoulder pathologies. Imaging and arthroscopic correla-
> tion of common conditions are provided.

Imaging of Glenoid Labrum Lesions   361

George D. Chloros, Peter J. Haar, Thomas P. Loughran, and Curtis W. Hayes

> This article reviews the current status of the imaging of the glenoid labrum
> and associated structures, including anatomic variants and the different
> types of labral disease.

Ultrasonography of the Shoulder with Arthroscopic Correlation   391

Corrie M. Yablon, Asheesh Bedi, Yoav Morag, and Jon A. Jacobson

> Ultrasonography is a well-established and widely accepted modality for
> the evaluation of rotator cuff tears and injury to the biceps brachii tendon.
> Ultrasonography and magnetic resonance imaging have comparable
> sensitivity and specificity for diagnosing both full-thickness and partial-
> thickness rotator cuff tears. This article addresses the ultrasonographic
> diagnosis of abnormalities of the rotator cuff, rotator interval, and biceps
> brachii, with magnetic resonance imaging and arthroscopic correlation.
> Characteristic ultrasonographic findings as well as imaging pitfalls are
> reviewed.

Hip-Femoral Acetabular Impingement   409

Christian N. Anderson, Geoffrey M. Riley, Garry E. Gold, and Marc R. Safran

> Magnetic resonance imaging (MRI) has become a valuable technology for
> the diagnosis and treatment of femoroacetabular impingement (FAI). This
> article reviews the basic pathophysiology of FAI, as well as the techniques
> and indications for MRI and magnetic resonance arthrography. Normal
> MRI anatomy of the hip and pathologic MRI anatomy associated with
> FAI are also discussed. Several case examples are presented demon-
> strating the diagnosis and treatment of FAI.

Imaging of Athletic Pubalgia and Core Muscle Injuries: Clinical and Therapeutic Correlations   427

Andrew Palisch, Adam C. Zoga, and William C. Meyers

Athletes frequently injure their hips and core muscles. Accurate diagnosis and proper treatment of groin pain in the athlete can be tricky, frequently posing vexing problem for trainers and physicians. Clinical presentations of the various hip problems overlap with respect to history and physical examination. This article reviews clinical presentations and magnetic resonance imaging findings specific to the various causes of groin pain in the athlete. The focus is on the core muscle injuries (athletic pubalgia or "sports hernia"). The goal is to raise awareness about the variety of injuries that occur and therapeutic options.

Magnetic Resonance Imaging and Arthroscopic Appearance of the Menisci of the Knee   449

Kirkland W. Davis, Humberto G. Rosas, and Ben K. Graf

 Videos of arthroscopic treatment of meniscal tears accompany this article

The menisci are critical for normal function of the knee, providing shock absorption and load transmission that reduce stress on the articular cartilage. When torn, a meniscus may require surgery to restore function, reduce pain, and eliminate mechanical symptoms. Patterns of meniscal tears include longitudinal and bucket-handle, which are often reparable; and horizontal, radial, vertical flap, horizontal flap, and complex. Root tears are usually radial and occur in the posterior roots. When reviewing magnetic resonance images, one must be aware of normal variants and imaging pitfalls that may simulate pathology.

Imaging of Cartilage and Osteochondral Injuries: A Case-Based Review   477

Robert A. Gallo and Timothy J. Mosher

Current high-field magnetic resonance imaging (MRI) techniques provide a sensitive and reliable diagnostic tool for the evaluation of cartilage and osteochondral injury. This article summarizes technical factors for optimal MRI evaluation of articular cartilage of the knee. There is emphasis on the important correlation of the MRI signal to the structure of the type II collagen matrix in normal cartilage, with an understanding that alterations in this signal pattern can be an important sign of cartilage injury. Finally, specific patterns of cartilage injury and application of MRI in evaluating cartilage repair are illustrated through a series of selected cases.

MRI of the Knee with Arthroscopic Correlation   507

Justin W. Griffin and Mark D. Miller

Major advances in MRI and arthroscopy have allowed for enhanced diagnosis and subsequent management of ligamentous and soft tissue injuries of the knee. Recognition of the appearance of acute ACL and PCL injuries on MRI can enhance arthroscopic reconstruction. PCL injuries are often more subtle and can present with indirect signs. T2-weighted MRI imaging can examine which structures have been damaged in the posterolateral corner which may manifest arthroscopically as a drive-through sign. Characterization of PLC, meniscus, MCL injuries and OCD lesions on MRI have remarkable correlation with arthroscopic findings. This article focuses on current understanding of how MRI and athroscopy can enhance treatment of ligamentous and soft tissue injuries of the knee.

Foot and Ankle Injuries in Sport: Imaging Correlation with Arthroscopic and Surgical Findings   525

Kenneth J. Hunt, Michael Githens, Geoffrey M. Riley, Michael Kim, and Garry E. Gold

Foot and ankle injuries are common in sport. Although many available imaging techniques can be useful in identifying and classifying injuries, magnetic resonance imaging (MRI) provides high levels of sensitivity and specificity for articular and soft-tissue injuries. Arthroscopic and minimally invasive treatment techniques for foot and ankle injuries are rapidly evolving, minimizing morbidity and improving postoperative rehabilitation and return to play. Correlation between MRI and surgical findings can aid in both accessing and treating pathologic processes and structures.

Dilemmas in Distinguishing Between Tumor and the Posttraumatic Lesion with Surgical or Pathologic Correlation   559

Eric Walker, Pam Brian, Victor Longo, Edward J. Fox, Elizabeth E. Frauenhoffer, and Mark Murphey

This article discusses the most common diagnostic dilemmas when trying to distinguish between tumor and sports injury or other trauma. Bone tumors frequently occur in the same young active patients who experience sports injuries. If the pain persists longer than expected, imaging studies should be obtained to prevent a delay in diagnosis or an inappropriate arthroscopy. A history of spontaneous fracture or a fracture after minor trauma should raise suspicion for underlying lesion as the cause. Occasionally necrosis and/or hemorrhage within a soft tissue sarcoma is so extensive that only a small cuff of viable tumor tissue is present.

Arthritis Mimicking Sports-Related Injuries   577

Donald J. Flemming and Stephanie A. Bernard

Arthritis, including inflammatory, crystal deposition, and synovial proliferative disorders, may mimic sports injury. The purpose of this article is to review the clinical and radiologic findings of arthropathies that can present in athletes and be confused with internal derangement.

Index   599

CLINICS IN SPORTS MEDICINE

FORTHCOMING ISSUES

October 2013
Unicompartmental Knee Arthroplasty
Kevin Plancher, MD, *Editor*

January 2014
Shoulder Instability in the Athlete
Stephen Thompson, MD, *Editor*

RECENT ISSUES

April 2013
Blunt Trauma Injuries in the Athlete
Thomas M. DeBerardino, MD, *Editor*

January 2013
Anatomic ACL Reconstruction
Freddie H. Fu, MD, and
Volker Musahl, MD, *Editors*

October 2012
Rotator Cuff Surgery
Stephen F. Brockmeier, MD, *Editor*

July 2012
Leg Pain in the Running Athlete
Alexander K. Meininger, MD, *Editor*

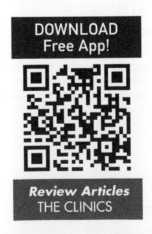

Foreword

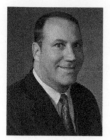

Mark D. Miller, MD
Consulting Editor

MRI-Arthroscopy Correlation has been an interesting pet-project of mine that has really gone the distance! Twenty years ago, when I was at the Air Force Academy, I would routinely meet with a musculoskeletal radiologist and go over cases with him preoperatively and postoperatively. This eventually led to the publication of the textbook *MRI-Arthroscopy Correlative Atlas* (W.B. Saunders, 1997). Dr Timothy Sanders, who I met in my second job in the Air Force shortly after this book was published, embraced this concept and we met regularly with other surgeons and musculoskeletal radiologists to correlate cases. Tim and I successfully adapted this concept for a stand-alone course sponsored by the American Orthopaedic Society for Sports Medicine (AOSSM), a "standing-room only" Symposium at the American Academy of Orthopaedic Surgeons (AAOS), and successful Instructional Course Lectures at the AOSSM and the AAOS that are still popular to this day. Dr Sanders and I recently published a sequel of sorts to the *Atlas* entitled *Presentation, Imaging and Treatment of Common Musculoskeletal Conditions* (Elsevier, 2012) that continues this tradition.

So, who better to spearhead this edition of *Clinics in Sports Medicine*? As usual, Dr Sanders has done an excellent job. This edition covers imaging and arthroscopic correlation from head to toe (well, OK, shoulder to foot). Like sports medicine itself, the focus is on the shoulder (cuff, labrum, and ultrasound) and knee (ligaments, cartilage, and menisci), but this treatise provides a comprehensive update on imaging in sports medicine. Dr Sanders and I have been working together for a long time, and I am honored to be his colleague! This should be a popular edition, especially for orthopedic surgeons, because there are a lot of pictures!

Mark D. Miller, MD
University of Virginia
James Madison University
Miller Review Course
400 Ray C. Hunt Dr, Suite 330
Charlottesville, VA 22908-0159, USA

E-mail address:
MDM3P@hscmail.mcc.virginia.edu

Clin Sports Med 32 (2013) xi
http://dx.doi.org/10.1016/j.csm.2013.05.002
0278-5919/13/$ – see front matter © 2013 Published by Elsevier Inc.

sportsmed.theclinics.com

Preface

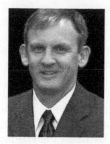

Timothy G. Sanders, MD
Editor

In 2006, I was given the opportunity to guest edit 2 volumes in *The Clinics in Sports Medicine* dealing with imaging of the upper and lower extremities in sports-related injuries. Those articles were authored solely by radiologists and dealt primarily with the use of advanced imaging modalities in the evaluation of the inured athlete. Once again, I have been given the honor of guest editing a volume on imaging of the injured athlete. In this updated issue however we have taken a different approach. Each article is coauthored by a radiologist and a clinician who are experts in their respective areas of sports medicine. The focus of this issue is to correlate advanced imaging findings with surgical and arthroscopic findings in an attempt to foster better communication and a greater understanding between the medical imager and the clinician who care for the injured athlete.

The first 2 articles in this issue deal with MRI-arthroscopic correlation of the rotator cuff and glenoid labrum. These articles give a clear framework for evaluating the complex anatomy of the shoulder with ample case material presenting direct correlation between the imaging and arthroscopic findings. The next article deals specifically with the use of ultrasound in the evaluation of the shoulder. Ultrasound continues to gain popularity with both clinicians and radiologists as a cost-effective method to evaluate the shoulder. Direct correlation between ultrasound and arthroscopic findings helps us to understand the value and limitations of ultrasound in the evaluation of the athletic shoulder. An article is dedicated to MRI-arthroscopic correlation of the hip with regard to femoral acetabular impingement. Our understanding of this entity and recommended treatment options continue to evolve and this article does an excellent job of reviewing the pertinent imaging findings and correlating them with arthroscopic findings of the hip. An article is also dedicated to imaging and surgical correlation of athletic pubalgia. This is another area in which our understanding of imaging findings and appropriate treatment options have evolved significantly since the previous imaging issue published in 2006. The authors do an excellent job of defining the role of imaging in the evaluation of the complex and sometimes difficult diagnosis of hip and groin pain in the athlete. There are 3 articles that focus on MRI-arthroscopic correlation of the knee. These include imaging of ligaments, menisci, and cartilage. The authors review the various imaging findings of normal anatomy, anatomic variants, and

Clin Sports Med 32 (2013) xiii–xiv
http://dx.doi.org/10.1016/j.csm.2013.05.001
0278-5919/13/$ – see front matter © 2013 Published by Elsevier Inc.

pathology in the knee. A single article deals with MRI-arthroscopic correlation of the foot and ankle and the authors use excellent surgical correlation images to review the normal anatomy and common sports-related foot and ankle injuries. The final 2 articles deal with imaging of tumors and arthritis specifically because these entities can mimic sports-related injuries or confound the diagnosis in the injured athlete. Both articles provide an outstanding review with surgical and imaging correlation as a reminder to the reader that underlying conditions can sometimes complicate diagnosis in the injured athlete.

I would like to thank each of the authors for their time and expertise in the preparation of these articles. I fully understand that a collaborative writing between a clinician and a radiologist can be a difficult and sometimes trying task, but in each case, these authors have done a superb job. Promoting collaboration between the imager and the clinician will result in enhanced diagnostic accuracy, optimized treatment, and improved outcomes for the injured athlete and that is the true goal of this issue.

Timothy G. Sanders, MD
Medical Director
NationalRad, Weston, FL, USA

E-mail address:
radmantgs@cs.com

Imaging of the Shoulder with Arthroscopic Correlation

Pranshu Sharma, MD[a], William B. Morrison, MD[a,*],
Steven Cohen, MD[b]

KEYWORDS

- Shoulder pain • Shoulder pathology • Arthroscopic correlation • Imaging studies

KEY POINTS

- A thorough history and physical examination are essential to determine which imaging examination is appropriate.
- Radiographs are generally the beginning of any imaging evaluation.
- Ultrasound of the shoulder requires operator expertise; however, it is an excellent method for targeted evaluation of pathology, such as rotator cuff disease.
- MRI gives the best overall evaluation of the shoulder for several pathologic entities and is usually the test of choice.
- Direct magnetic resonance (MR) arthrography (ie, injection of gadolinium contrast directly into the shoulder joint) is the test of choice for evaluation of suspected labral tear.

INTRODUCTION

Shoulder pain with or without trauma is a common complaint. For acute fractures and dislocations, radiography is often sufficient. In patients with protracted shoulder pain, however, further evaluation is often required. Such patients often present with nonspecific signs and symptoms, and accurate clinical diagnosis is often difficult. Multiple imaging tests are available for evaluation of these patients and can be daunting for shoulder physicians to fully comprehend. MRI is often the most useful imaging study for evaluating the shoulder. This review provides an overview of various modalities and their role in evaluating various clinical issues in shoulder pathologies. Imaging and arthroscopic correlation are provided.

[a] Department of Radiology, Thomas Jefferson University Hospital, 132 South 10th Street, Suite 1079a, Philadelphia, PA 19107, USA; [b] Department of Orthopedics, Rothman Institute, 925 Chestnut Street, Philadelphia, PA 19107, USA
* Corresponding author.
E-mail address: William.morrison@jefferson.edu

Clin Sports Med 32 (2013) 339–359
http://dx.doi.org/10.1016/j.csm.2013.03.009
0278-5919/13/$ – see front matter © 2013 Elsevier Inc. All rights reserved.

MODALITIES FOR EVALUATING PATIENTS WITH SHOULDER COMPLAINTS
Radiography

Radiographs are often the first imaging study obtained in patients presenting with the chief complaint of shoulder pain. The complex anatomy of the shoulder has led to the development of numerous radiographic views, each designed to optimize the evaluation of a specific feature of the shoulder girdle.

Radiographic shoulder series
1. Anteroposterior (AP) view: obtained in an AP direction relative to the body rather than the glenohumeral joint (tilted 40° anteriorly in relation to the body). The humeral head overlaps the glenoid rim. It can be obtained in neutral, internal, or external rotation and provides the best overall survey of the shoulder girdle. Hill-Sachs lesion may be well seen on the radiographs.
2. Glenohumeral true AP (Grashey) view: obtained by rotating the patient 35° to 40° posteriorly. The x-ray beam parallels the glenohumeral joint, eliminating the overlap of the AP view. It is particularly helpful for evaluation of glenohumeral joint space and demonstrating loss of articular cartilage and subtle subluxation, indicating possible glenohumeral instability.
3. Axillary view: provides a tangential view of the glenohumeral joint from superior to inferior. It is helpful in the evaluation of possible glenohumeral dislocation and anterior/posterior subluxation. It requires patients to abduct the arm, which can be difficult after acute trauma.
4. Scapular Y view: provides a lateral view of the glenohumeral joint and can be obtained with the arm down by the side and is, thus, more useful in the setting of acute trauma.

CT

CT is most commonly used after trauma to the shoulder to evaluate the full extent of osseous abnormalities. Multidetector CT examination with sagittal and coronal reconstructions is often used to evaluate the extent of humeral head and neck fractures. The precise number of fracture fragments, amount of articular surface step-off, displacement, and angulation of fracture fragments can be accurately determined with CT examination. Each of these variables is important in relation to treatment choice and in determining prognosis for recovery.

CT examination is also the study of choice in suspected sternoclavicular joint injuries and accurately depicts subtle fractures and dislocations. The scapula is a complex anatomic structure composed of the body, coracoid, and acromion processes and the glenohumeral articular surface. Suspected scapular fractures are typically evaluated with CT examination, which shows the full extent of injury. Fractures limited to the body of the scapula are usually treated conservatively, whereas fractures of the coracoid or acromion processes or the glenoid may require surgical intervention. After glenohumeral dislocation, CT examination is useful to depict the size and position of the glenoid rim fracture fragment.

Ultrasound

Ultrasound is most extensively studied and more frequently used in the evaluation of the shoulder than any other joint. Ultrasound accurately depicts rotator cuff pathology and in experienced hands can accurately detect and differentiate a normal cuff from tendinosis or partial-thickness or full-thickness tear. Ultrasound can also be used to dynamically assess for impingement and other pathology through range of motion. The major disadvantages of ultrasound, however, include its limited field of view, inability to assess the deep soft tissue structures and bones, limited evaluation of labrum and articular surfaces, and operator dependence. Therefore, ultrasound is best reserved for evaluation of rotator cuff tear in patients with primary impingement.

MRI

MRI is, in most instances, the study of choice for evaluating the shoulder. It accurately depicts abnormalities of the rotator cuff and can demonstrate subtle abnormalities of the capsule and labrum that are associated with glenohumeral instability. The use of intravenous gadolinium (indirect MR arthrography) or intra-articular gadolinium contrast (direct MR arthrography) often increases the conspicuity of these subtle labral lesions. The osseous structures are nicely depicted, including osseous Bankart and Hill-Sachs lesions (**Fig. 1**). Finally, MRI is the only modality that can assess the composition of bone marrow for edema related to trauma and other conditions.

High field (ie, 1.0 T or higher) is recommended to achieve the best image quality. In older patients with concern for rotator cuff tear, a standard noncontrast MRI is the

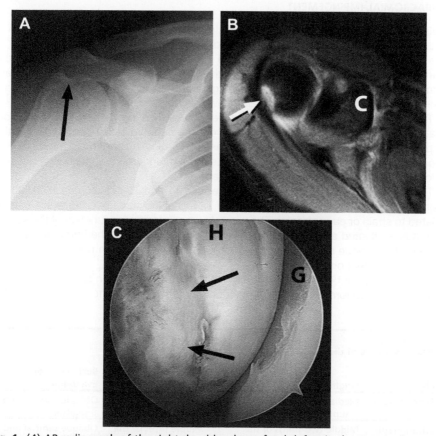

Fig. 1. (A) AP radiograph of the right shoulder shows focal defect in the superior humeral head typical for Hill-Sachs lesion (arrow). (B) Axial fat-suppressed MRI at the level of superior aspect of coracoid (C) shows an impaction fracture of the posterolateral humeral head (arrow). (C) Arthroscopic view of the shoulder shows Hill-Sachs lesion (arrow). Humerus (H) and glenoid (G).

study of choice. In younger patients with instability and concern for labral/capsular pathology, an MR arthrogram is the best test.

Standard shoulder imaging protocol
1. T2-weighted sequences with fat suppression in the oblique sagittal, oblique coronal, and axial imaging planes
2. Proton density or gradient-echo sequences in the axial imaging plane for evaluation of the labral/capsular structures
3. T1-weighted images in the oblique coronal and oblique sagittal imaging planes to aid in the evaluation of marrow abnormalities and to evaluate for fatty atrophy of the cuff musculature

MR Arthrography
   T1-weighted sequences with fat suppression in multiple planes combined with fluid-sensitive sequences are employed to increase conspicuity of labral, ligamentous, and intra-articular pathology.

SUBACROMIAL IMPINGEMENT

Painful impingement of the shoulder is a clinical entity that results from compression of the rotator cuff and subacromial-subdeltoid bursa between the greater tuberosity of the humeral head and the acromion (**Table 1**). Over time, this process may lead to a partial-thickness or full-thickness tear of the cuff. A diagnosis of the impingement cannot be established from imaging findings alone but rather physical examination, which elicits pain during abduction and elevation of the arm.

   The role of imaging in impingement is to identify and define the extent of the abnormalities of the cuff and bursa. Additionally, osseous abnormalities contributing to the impingement should be noted. To be successful, surgical management must not only repair injured soft tissue structures (cuff repair and débridement of the bursa) but also address the underlying cause of impingement.

   The muscles should demonstrate intermediate T1 and T2 signal intensity. High T1 signal indicates fatty atrophy whereas high T2 signal indicates edema, which can be related to strain or early atrophy. The normal musculotendinous junction of the supraspinatus is situated at approximately the 1-o'clock position of the humeral head, as seen on the oblique sagittal plane, with the infraspinatus tendon posteriorly and the subscapularis tendon anteriorly.

   Tendons arise out of the 4 separate muscles and then broaden and flatten peripherally, merging to form a single watertight unit that inserts onto the tuberosities of the

Table 1
MRI appearance of the normal rotator cuff

Muscle	Origin	Tendon Insertion on Humeral Head	Best Plane for Evaluation
Supraspinatus	Medial two-thirds of the supraspinatus fossa	Highest facet of the greater tuberosity	Oblique coronal and sagittal
Infraspinatus	Middle two-thirds of the infraspinatus fossa	Middle facet of the greater tuberosity	Oblique sagittal and oblique coronal
Teres minor	Dorsal aspect of the lateral margin of the scapula	Lowest facet of the greater tuberosity	Oblique sagittal
Subscapularis	Anterior border of the scapula	Lesser tuberosity	Axial

humeral head. The normal tendon demonstrates low signal intensity on all MR pulse sequences (**Fig. 2**).

Ultrasound Appearance of the Rotator Cuff

From superficial to deep, ultrasound of the normal rotator cuff demonstrates (1) hypoechoic (dark) deltoid muscle, (2) a stripe of bright echoes representing the subacromial subdeltoid bursa, (3) a bandlike appearance of medium-level echoes representing the rotator cuff, (4) a thin layer of hypoechoic cartilage, and (5) a rim of bright echoes from the osseous interface of the humeral head (see **Fig. 2**). The biceps tendon is seen as an oval-appearing area of bright echoes located within the bicipital groove.

Tendinosis may manifest as focal or diffuse areas of tendon thickening with altered echogenicity, either increased or decreased. Partial-thickness tear appears as an anechoic area within the bright tendon whereas full-thickness tear demonstrates focal

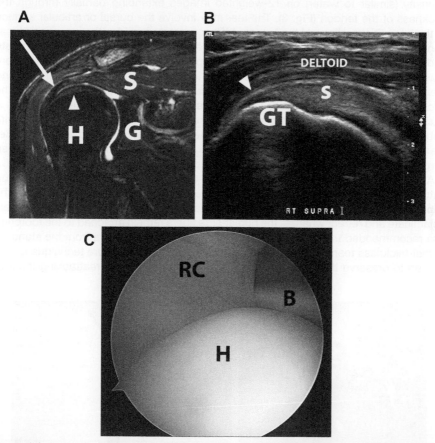

Fig. 2. (*A*) Coronal oblique T2-weighted fat-suppressed MRI of normal shoulder shows supraspinatus muscle (S) and markedly hypointense supraspinatus tendon (*arrow*) inserting on the greater tuberosity of the humerus (H). Also, note intermediate intensity articular cartilage at the humeral head (*arrowhead*). (*B*) Coronal oblique ultrasound image of normal shoulder shows mildly hypoechoic deltoid muscle, thin hyperechoic subacromial-subdeltoid bursa (*arrowhead*), and mildly hyperechoic supraspinatus tendon (S) inserting on the greater tuberosity (GT). (*C*) Arthroscopic view of normal shoulder showing rotator cuff (RC), humeral head (H), and intra-articular portion of the long head of biceps tendon (B).

defect or even complete absence. A secondary sign of rotator cuff pathology may include fluid within the subdeltoid bursa. In the hands of the experts, the sensitivity and specificity of ultrasound for rotator cuff tears is identical to that of MRI.

MRI Appearance of Rotator Cuff Pathology

The sensitivity of MRI in the detection of rotator cuff tears ranges from 88% to 100%. On MRI, tendinopathy appears as intermediate signal intensity within the substance of the tendon on both T1-weighted and T2-weighted images (bright, but less than water, on T2 images). The tendon may also demonstrate thickening or thinning (attritional wear). Histologically, the increased signal represents mucoid degeneration of the tendon.

A partial-thickness tear of the rotator cuff is defined as a tear that extends partially through the superior-inferior thickness of the tendon. MRI demonstrates fluid signal intensity (similar to water) on T2-weighted images extending partially through the thickness of the tendon (**Fig. 3**). The tear may involve the bursal or articular surface or the interstitial portions of the tendon. MRI accurately provides the extent and location of a partial-thickness tear, which may have an impact on the decision to operate and influence the surgical approach and the type of surgery. A tear that extends more than 70% through the thickness of the tendon is usually completed by a surgeon and then treated as a full-thickness tear. A tear that extends less than 30% through the thickness of the tendon is usually treated conservatively or by débridement alone. A tear that extends 30% to 70% through the thickness of the tendon is treated with débridement followed by suturing to shorten the bridge that is created by the débridement. In all cases, the cause of impingement (ie, subacromial spur) must be addressed surgically to prevent recurrence of the rotator cuff pathology.

A partial articular-side supraspinatus tendon avulsion lesion is a subset of supraspinatus tears that represents a partial-thickness articular-side (undersurface) tear of the supraspinatus tendon at its most anterior attachment site. The deeper, torn fibers delaminate and retract whereas the bursal-side fibers remain attached to the footprint. The recommended treatment of this subset of tendon tears differs from the standard partial-thickness tears (discussed previously). A transtendon suture technique is performed to preserve the intact portion of the tendon while firmly reattaching the torn

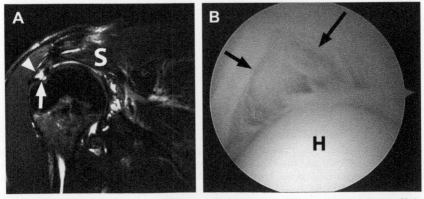

Fig. 3. (*A*) T2-weighted fat-suppressed coronal oblique MRI through the rotator cuff shows a high-grade partial tear of the supraspinatus tendon involving the articular surface (*arrow*). The bursal surface is intact (*arrowhead*). Supraspinatus muscle (S). (*B*) Arthroscopic view shows partially torn rotator cuff (*arrows*). Humeral head (H).

portion of the tendon to the humeral footprint. On MRI, fluid signal is seen extending into articular surface of the supraspinatus tendon.

A full-thickness tear of the rotator cuff is defined as a tear that extends completely through the thickness of the tendon from superior to inferior. MRI demonstrates bright fluid on T2-weighted images extending through the entire thickness of the tendon **(Fig. 4)**. There may be retraction of the torn tendon end. Sagittal and axial images can be helpful in differentiating a partial-thickness tear from a full-thickness tear, especially when the tear is located at the level of attachment to the humeral head. Small full-thickness tears often involve the most anterior aspect of the supraspinatus tendon immediately adjacent to its attachment to the greater tuberosity. It is important to evaluate the supraspinatus tendon on the most anterior coronal image to avoid missing a small full-thickness tear at the most anterior bone tendon interface. The extent of tear should be measured and reported in both AP and medial-lateral directions. A tear that is larger in the AP direction is often repaired using a tendon-to-bone suture technique, whereas a tear that is greater in the medial-lateral direction may be amenable to repair using a mattress-type tendon-to-tendon repair technique.

Tears of the subscapularis tendon are best depicted on axial and sagittal images and are often associated with subluxation or dislocation of the biceps tendon out of the intertubercular groove. The subscapularis tendon is typically seen covering the anterior portion of the humeral head on the sagittal imaging plane. Fluid within the expected location of the subscapularis tendon anterior to the humeral head indicates a complete tear with retraction of the torn tendon end.

A complete tear of a rotator cuff tendon is defined as tear that disrupts the entire thickness of the tendon from anterior to posterior. MRI demonstrates complete discontinuity of the tendon, resulting in retraction of the musculotendinous junction. A high-riding humeral head is usually associated with an extensive tear of the rotator cuff, involving at least the supraspinatus and infraspinatus tendons. The high-riding humeral head is best depicted on coronal images and may be seen abutting the undersurface of the acromion on coronal or sagittal images.

After evaluation of the type and extent of rotator cuff tear, the cuff should also be evaluated for the presence of musculotendinous retraction and fatty atrophy. The extent of musculotendinous retraction should be described in all patients with a full-thickness rotator cuff tear. The extent of retraction is best described as the

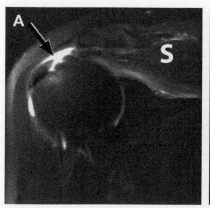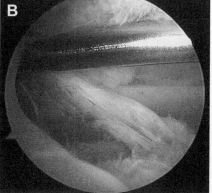

Fig. 4. (*A*) T2-weighted coronal oblique MRI of the right shoulder shows full-thickness tear (*arrow*) of the rotator cuff with retraction. Supraspinatus muscle (S). (*B*) Arthroscopic view of the shoulder shows probe going through full-thickness rotator cuff tear.

medial-to-lateral gap between the torn ends of the tendon. More than 3 cm of tendinous retraction indicates a poor prognosis for cuff repair and is useful information for surgeons during treatment planning.

In the early phase of atrophy, there is loss of the normal muscle bulk. The supraspinatus muscle should completely fill the suprascapular fossa, and the circumference of the supraspinatus and infraspinatus muscles should be similar. Asymmetric loss of bulk of 1 or more of the cuff muscles is described as "decreased size" and is reversible. Fatty atrophy is characterized by high T1 signal within the substance of the muscle. This represents irreversible change; repair of the tendon at this point has an increased chance of failure. Fatty atrophy is graded using the Goutallier scale: grade 1 = fatty streaks; grade 2 = increased fat but less fat than muscle; grade 3 = equal fat and muscle; and grade 4 = more fat than muscle. Increasing grades of fatty atrophy worsen the prognosis for repair and are useful information for surgeons during surgical planning.

In addition to depicting changes to the rotator cuff, MRI evaluates presence of a subacromial spur, which is an important cause of impingement. It appears as an osseous excrescence along the undersurface of the acromion anterolaterally or at the attachment of the coracoacromial ligament anteriorly.

Another cause of shoulder pain due to rotator cuff pathology is calcium hydroxyapatite deposition disease, which can occur within the rotator cuff tendon (calcific tendinosis) (**Fig. 5**) or other periarticular soft tissues, including the glenohumeral ligaments and adjacent bursa (calcific bursitis). These calcifications are best detected on radiographs but may also be identified on MRI as focal areas of globular black signal on both TI-weighted and T2-weighted images (**Table 2**). Calcific tendinosis is often associated with intense inflammatory changes of the adjacent soft tissues, resulting in surrounding increased signal on T2-weighted images. On MRI, it may be difficult in some cases to detect the calcification because the normal tendon is also low signal. Gradient-echo imaging can be helpful in this regard, because magnetic susceptibility artifact exaggerates the size and appearance of the calcification (known as blooming).

GLENOHUMERAL INSTABILITY

The topic of glenohumeral instability is complex, and knowledge and understanding of the synergistic role that the various anatomic structures play in maintaining normal shoulder mobility continue to evolve. The configuration of the glenohumeral joint, with a shallow glenoid fossa and the large articular surface of the humeral head, allows for an extensive range of motion of the upper extremity but high risk for instability. Numerous soft tissue structures contribute to the stability of the glenohumeral joint, including the static stabilizers (glenoid labrum, joint capsule, and glenohumeral ligaments) and the dynamic stabilizers (rotator cuff and long head of the biceps tendon [LHBT]).

Glenohumeral instability may range from mild static or dynamic subluxation (microinstability) to complete dislocation. Various descriptors can be used to further categorize shoulder instability, including the temporal relationship of the instability to the antecedent trauma (first time vs recurrent) and the degree (subluxation vs dislocation) and direction (anterior, posterior, inferior, or multidirectional) of instability. Glenohumeral instability can be divided into 2 broad categories. The first group of patients has a history of antecedent trauma followed by unidirectional subluxation or dislocation. The traumatic event results in a Bankart lesion or one of its variants and typically requires surgery to correct the instability. This group of patients is referred to as **T**raumatic **U**nilateral injury with **B**ankart lesion and usually [or often] requiring **S**urgery (TUBS). MRI

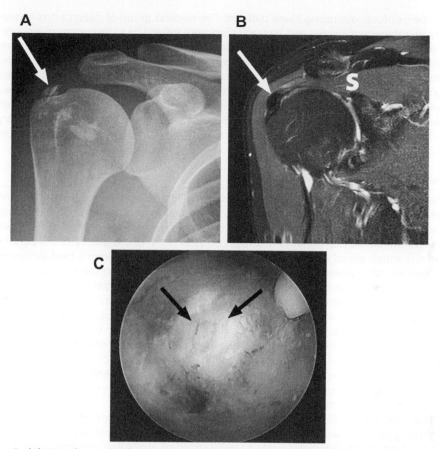

Fig. 5. (*A*) AP radiograph of the right shoulder in external rotation shows calcific tendinosis as globular foci of calcification in the rotator cuff including the supraspinatus (*arrow*). (*B*) T2-weighted fat-suppressed coronal MRI shows globular calcification within the supraspinatus tendon (*arrow*). Supraspinatus (S). (*C*) Arthroscopic view of severe calcific tendinosis of the rotator cuff (*arrow*) with surrounding hyperemia.

Table 2
Summary of MRI findings that should be described in all patients who present with the clinical signs and symptoms of impingement and rotator cuff pathology

Anatomic Structure	Potential Abnormalities
Acromion	Inferiorly directed osteophyte/spur Unfused os acromiale
Subacromial subdeltoid bursa	Fluid, surrounding edema Calcification
Rotator cuff	Tendinopathy (mild, moderate, or severe) Partial-thickness tear (articular, interstitial, or bursal) Full-thickness tear (size and location) Musculotendinous retraction (size of tendon gap) Fatty atrophy (mild, moderate, or severe)

can be helpful in evaluating these patients. The second group of patients has no history of antecedent trauma and typically displays bilateral multidirectional glenohumeral instability. The instability is evaluated by capsular laxity rather than labral pathology. These patients are treated first with rehabilitation (strengthening of the rotator cuff musculature) and, only after therapeutic failure, are offered a capsular-tightening procedure. This group of patients is referred to as atraumatic, multidirectional, bilateral, rehabilitation, and occasionally requiring an inferior capsular shift (AMBRI). The AMBRI type of instability can usually be diagnosed solely from history and clinical examination and imaging is not particularly helpful except to exclude a surgical lesion.

Normal Labrum and Capsular Anatomy

The glenoid labrum is a fibrocartilaginous structure that encircles the glenoid rim and serves to deepen the glenoid fossa. It is usually triangular in appearance, but it may also demonstrate a rounded or blunted appearance. Even when blunted or rounded, the labrum should demonstrate a smooth contour with no irregularity of the surface and no intrinsic signal abnormality. The anterior and posterior labrum is best evaluated on axial imaging, whereas the superior and inferior labrum is best seen on the oblique coronal images. Administering dilute gadolinium-based contrast material into the glenohumeral joint significantly improves detection of labral pathology.

The glenohumeral ligaments represent bandlike areas of capsular thickening that are best visualized from inside the joint capsule but can be seen with MRI, especially after intra-articular administration of dilute gadolinium-based contrast material. The superior glenohumeral ligament (SGHL) is best observed on axial MRI because it parallels the coracoid process. The middle glenohumeral ligament (MGHL) is located just superficial to the anterior labrum and sits just deep to the subscapularis muscle and is also best visualized on axial MRI.

The inferior glenohumeral ligament (IGHL) is the most important of the 3 ligaments regarding glenohumeral stability. It is best seen on the MRI by placing the arm in the fully abducted and externally rotated (ABER) position while it is stretched taut, thus improving visualization of the ligament.

Normal Anatomic Variants of the Labrum and Capsule

The glenoid labrum is composed of fibrocartilage and appears dark on all pulse sequences, and the articular surface of the glenoid fossa is covered with intermediate signal intensity hyaline articular cartilage. Any undermining or interruption of the dark signal of the labrum by higher signal intensity can be interpreted as a tear. There are several anatomic variants, however, that can mimic a tear, especially in the anterosuperior portion of the labrum:

1. The hyaline cartilage can occasionally undermine the fibrocartilage of the glenoid labrum in prominent fashion and mimic a tear on MRI. It can be easily differentiated from a tear because cartilage undermining is intermediate in signal, appears smooth and tapering, and does not extend completely beneath the labrum, whereas a tear is irregular in appearance, with fluid signal undermining the labrum, and may extend completely beneath the labrum, separating it from the adjacent osseous glenoid.
2. The sublabral foramen or hole is a normal anatomic variant in the anterosuperior quadrant of the glenoid in which the anterosuperior labrum is completely detached from the underlying osseous glenoid. The sublabral foramen variant can be misinterpreted as either an anterior labral tear or a superior labral from anterior to

posterior (SLAP) tear. The sublabral foramen occurs only in the anterosuperior quadrant of the glenoid, and the presence of a detached labrum in any other location is diagnostic of a tear. Extension of the labral detachment to involve the biceps anchor or posterior to the level of the biceps anchor represents a SLAP tear. Any extension of the labral detachment into the anteroinferior labrum also represents a tear.

3. The sublabral recess is defined as a tapering recess that extends beneath the free edge of the superior labrum, separating it from the osseous glenoid and creating a potential space between the 2 structures. It differs from the sublabral foreman in that although there is a recess deep to the labrum, the labrum remains firmly attached to the glenoid. At the time of arthroscopy, a probe can be placed into the recess and the labrum pulled back away from the glenoid, but the labrum remains firmly attached at its base. The undersurface of the labrum appears smooth with no fraying or irregularity. The recess smoothly tapers toward the osseous glenoid and never results in signal extending into the substance of the superior labrum. The superior labrum should demonstrate a dark triangular appearance with smooth surfaces, and any signal extending into the substance of the triangle represents a superior labral tear and not a superior labral recess.

4. The Buford complex is an anatomic variant that is composed of a cordlike thickened MGHL combined with an absent or diminutive anterosuperior labrum and can be easily misinterpreted as an avulsed anterior labrum. A thickened MGHL can be easily traced, however, on multiple serial axial sections because it arises from the superior glenoid tubercle and courses obliquely across the anterior glenohumeral joint to blend with the anterior capsule. The ligament is located just anterior to the expected position of the anterosuperior glenoid labrum.

Lesions of Instability

Traumatic glenohumeral dislocation usually results in a lesion of 1 or more of the static or dynamic stabilizers of the glenohumeral joint. The specific lesion that occurs depends on many factors:

1. Direction of dislocation—anterior dislocation results in disruption of the anterior stabilizers, whereas a posterior dislocation results in injury to the posterior capsule and posterior labrum.

2. Age of the patient—a first-time dislocation in an individual under 35 years of age usually results in a tear of the anterior labrum or capsule structures, whereas a first-time dislocation in a patient over the age of 35 usually results not in a labral tear but in a tear of the rotator cuff or in an avulsion of the greater tuberosity of the humeral head.

3. Mechanism of injury—acute trauma can cause anterior or posterior dislocation. Repetitive microtrauma, as occurs in throwers, weight lifters, and swimmers, can also result in labral pathology. Finally, trauma without dislocation, such as an impaction injury of the humeral head against the labrum and articular surface of the osseous glenoid, can lead to a tear of the labrum.

The term, Bankart lesion, was originally defined as a disruption of the anterior labroligamentous complex with disruption of the medial scapular periosteum. Over time, however, the phrase has come to be synonymous with any tear of the anteroinferior labrum, whereas the term, reverse Bankart lesion, describes a tear of the posteroinferior labrum. The term, SLAP tear, was first coined to describe a tear of the superior labrum extending from anterior to posterior, but SLAP tear is now commonly used to describe any tear involving the superior labrum and is usually associated with microinstability of glenohumeral joint. Although the terms, Bankart, reverse Bankart, and SLAP tear, describe 3 broad categories of labral pathology, there are many subtle variations of these lesions that can have significant implications regarding proper diagnosis and treatment of glenohumeral instability and need to be recognized on the MRI.

The Bankart Variants

The classic Bankart lesion is defined as a tear of the anterior labroligamentous complex with disruption of the medial scapular periosteum. On MRI, the labrum may lose its normal triangular appearance or become amorphous. Abnormal signal may be detected within the labrum, and the labrum may appear detached from the adjacent osseous glenoid (**Fig. 6**). The axial plane is the primary plane for evaluating anterior and posterior labral pathology; however, the coronal imaging plane is complementary and often helpful in detecting subtle lesions or in confirming the presence of a labral tear suspected on axial imaging. The double axillary pouch sign is defined as a small collection of fluid or contrast extending deep to or into the substance of the inferior labrum as seen on coronal images and can be helpful in detecting or confirming the presence of a suspected labral tear.

The osseous Bankart lesion is a tear of the anteroinferior glenoid labrum associated with a fracture of the adjacent glenoid rim. In addition to the labral abnormality, M|RI demonstrates a fracture and marrow edema involving the anteroinferior glenoid. It is critical to accurately describe the amount of bone loss of the anteroinferior glenoid rim because this information helps surgeons determine whether bone graft material is required at the time of Bankart repair. The extent of bone loss is usually best detected and described using the sagittal imaging plane. Although MRI is accurate in this regard, many surgeons prefer CT imaging with sagittal reconstructions to depict the extent of the osseous defect (**Fig. 7**).

Perthes lesion, referred to as a nondisplaced Bankart lesion, is a tear of the anterior glenoid labrum, but it differs from the classic Bankart lesion in that the medial scapular periosteum remains intact, holding the torn labrum in near anatomic position. Because the labrum is not displaced, the MRI signs and arthroscopic findings are both subtle, the labrum is unstable, and patients continue to demonstrate the clinical signs and symptoms of glenohumeral instability.

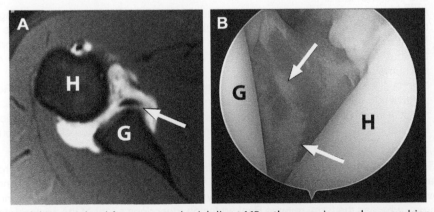

Fig. 6. (*A*) T1-weighted fat-suppressed axial direct MR arthrogram image shows avulsion of the anteroinferior labrum (*arrow*) with contrast-material undermining the labrum suggesting Bankart lesion. Humerus (H) and glenoid (G). (*B*) Arthroscopic view of the shoulder shows Bankart lesion (*arrows*). Glenoid (G) and humerus (H).

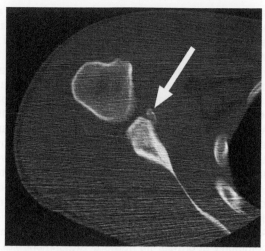

Fig. 7. Axial CT of the right shoulder shows osseous Bankart lesion with fracture at the anterior glenoid margin (*arrow*).

When a person demonstrates clinical evidence of glenohumeral instability in the face of a normal conventional MRI examination, further evaluation with direct MR arthrography and ABER imaging should be considered. Direct MR arthrography results in distention of the joint, which helps outline and accentuate the subtle MR findings of a nondisplaced labral tear. Next, by adding ABER imaging, the anterior band of the IGHL is stretched taut, placing tension on the anterior labrum. This results in subtle displacement of the anterior labrum and allows pooling of contrast deep to the anterior labrum. The presence of this tiny triangular fluid/contrast collection on the ABER image is diagnostic of Perthes lesion and is often the only abnormally that can be detected on MR arthrography.

The anterior labroligamentous periosteal sleeve avulsion (ALPSA) lesion is also referred to as medialized Bankart. The ALPSA lesion is similar to Perthes lesion in that although the labrum is torn, the medial scapular periosteum remains intact. With the ALPSA lesion, the labrum, however, rather than remaining in its normal position, is pulled in a medial direction as the scapular periosteum contracts. On MRI, the labrum may demonstrate abnormal morphology and is medially displaced along the anterior aspect of the osseous glenoid. Synovial tissue may cover the anteroinferior glenoid simulating an intact labrum.

The glenolabral articular disruption (GLAD) lesion is described as a nondisplaced tear of the anteroinferior labrum combined with an injury of the adjacent articular cartilage. There is some controversy as to whether this lesion exists as a separate clinical entity or whether it simply represents a Bankart lesion with an adjacent chondral abnormality. Patients typically present with the history of a fall and subsequent shoulder pain but have no history of dislocation and demonstrate no evidence of instability on physical examination. The absence of clinical findings of instability may delay the use of MRI in the evaluation of patients with a GLAD lesion.

MRI findings seen with GLAD lesions are often subtle and difficult to detect using only conventional MRI. MR arthrography with stress view ABER imaging is an optional method for visualizing the nondisplaced labral tear and the associated articular cartilage injury. The articular cartilage injury is located in the anteroinferior quadrant of the glenoid and may appear as an osteochondral defect or an articular cartilage flap tear

(Fig. 8). The nondisplaced labral tear is best seen on ABER imaging as a small collection of contrast material filling a triangular-shaped gap between the anteroinferior labrum and the osseous glenoid. The anterior band of the IGHL and the medial scapular periosteum remain intact.

Humeral avulsion of the glenohumeral ligament (HAGL) describes a disruption of the IGHL. The anterior labroligamentous complex is the most important structure with regard to anterior shoulder stability and comprises the anterior band of the IGHL and the anteroinferior labrum. The term, Bankart lesion, and its many variants describe injuries involving the labral portion of the anterior labroligament complex. A disruption of the anterior labroligamentous complex, however, anywhere along its course also results in anterior instability of the glenohumeral joint similar to that from a Bankart lesion. The term, HAGL lesion, was originally used to describe a tear of the anterior band of the IGHL at its humeral attachment site. A tear can occur anywhere along the course of the ligament, however, including the humeral attachment, midsubstance, or labral attachment site.

On MRI, the HAGL lesion is seen as disruption of the IGHL anywhere along its course but most commonly at or near its humeral attachment site. In the setting of acute trauma, edema is present within the soft tissues immediately adjacent to the disrupted ligament. MR arthrography can help with the detection of the lesion because extravasation of contrast can be seen extending through the defect in the ligament **(Fig. 9)**. It is critical to alert the arthroscopist to the presence of a HAGL lesion because it can be difficult to detect through standard arthroscopic portals. It has been suggested that many of the cases of recurrent shoulder instability after arthroscopy may be secondary to a missed HAGL lesion. A miniarthrotomy is typically required to identify and repair a HAGL lesion, and surgical repair is mandatory to reestablish shoulder stability.

Reverse Bankart is a tear of the posterior labrum. Such lesions are less common than the anterior labral lesions and can result from either a single traumatic event or, more commonly, from repetitive microtrauma to the posterior capsule and labrum, as occurs in weight lifting, throwing sports, and swimming. The mechanism for traumatic posterior dislocation is a fall on an outstretched hand with the arm in adduction and external rotation. In this position, the posterior capsule is taut, and the posteriorly

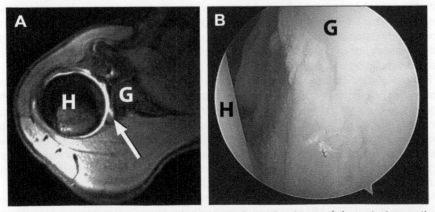

Fig. 8. (A) T2-weighted fat-suppressed axial MRI shows focal tear of the articular cartilage along posterior glenoid (*arrow*) suggesting GLAD lesion. Humerus (H) and glenoid (G). (B) Arthroscopic view shows fraying and tear of the articular cartilage of the glenoid (G). Humerus (H).

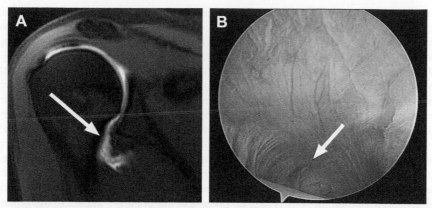

Fig. 9. (*A*) T1-weighted fat-suppressed coronal direct MR arthrogram image shows disruption of humeral attachment of IGHL (*arrow*) with extravasation of contrast material into the axillary soft tissues (HAGL). (*B*) Arthroscopic view shows defect at the humeral attachment of the IGHL (*arrow*).

directed force of the humeral head results in a disruption of the posterior stabilizers. Many of the Bankart variants that are seen in the anterior labrum can also occur in the posterior labrum. The term, *reverse*, is typically used to describe the posterior glenoid lesions (reverse Bankart or reverse Hill-Sachs lesion). The term, PHAGL, is used to describe a posterior HAGL lesion. Findings on MRI are similar to those seen with anterior labral/capsular injury and include abnormal morphology of the posterior labrum, a partially or completely detached posterior labrum, and an associated fracture of the posterior glenoid. Posterior labral lesions can be difficult to diagnose clinically and are more challenging to repair than the anterior labral lesions.

A SLAP lesion describes a tear that involves the superior labrum. The original classification scheme included 4 types of SLAP tears. The type I lesion is defined as fraying and degeneration of the surface of the superior labrum, but the labrum remains firmly attached to the glenoid with no displaced or unstable fragment. The type II lesion is defined as an avulsion of the labrum from the osseous glenoid, resulting in an unstable labral fragment and potentially an unstable biceps anchor. The type III lesion is defined as a displaced bucket handle tear of the superior labrum with an intact biceps anchor, whereas the type IV lesion is a displaced bucket handle tear of the superior labrum with involvement of the biceps anchor. Since the original description of the SLAP lesion, the classification scheme has been expanded to include 10 types. The additional types of SLAP tears primarily describe extension of the SLAP tear to involve adjacent structures, including the anteroinferior labrum, posterior labrum, MGHL, and rotator interval complex.

MRI is an excellent noninvasive means of evaluating the superior labrum. The coronal plane is the primary plane for the evaluation of the superior labrum, but a thorough evaluation in all 3 imaging planes is crucial to provide a thorough description of the SLAP tear and its involvement of adjacent structures. The normal superior labrum is triangular, arises from the superior glenoid, and demonstrates low signal intensity on all MR pulse sequences. The superior labrum demonstrates more variations than any other part of the labrum, and it is these anatomic variations that create the most difficulty with regard to correctly identifying and classifying the various SLAP lesions. These variations include the sublabral recess, the sublabral foramen, and the Buford complex and are described in detail previously.

It is not always possible to clearly distinguish among the 10 types of SLAP tear or accurately categorize a SLAP lesion with MRI. Direct or indirect MR arthography, however, may help better define the lesion and add a level of confidence when differentiating superior labral pathology from the normal variants (**Figs. 10** and **11**).

Posterior superior glenoid impingement (internal impingement) occurs primarily in athletes who participate in repetitive overhead activity, such as throwing and swimming. The injury occurs during maximum abduction and external rotation of the humeral head (late cocking phase of throwing) and results from impingement of the undersurface of the posterior aspect of the rotator cuff between the posterior superior labrum and the posterior aspect of the humeral head. MR findings include degenerative fraying of the posterior superior glenoid labrum and partial-thickness undersurface tearing of the posterior aspect of the rotator cuff, which may include the posterior fibers of the supraspinatus tendon or the infraspinatus tendon. Subchondral cystic change or marrow edema may be present in the posterior aspect of the greater tuberosity of the humeral head, but this is the most variable of the associated findings and is often absent. If ABER imaging is performed, entrapment of the undersurface of the posterior rotator cuff between the humeral head and the posterosuperior labrum may be visualized at the time of imaging. Other associated findings may include a lesion of the anterior labroligamentous complex leading to anterior instability and thickening and scarring of the posterior capsule. The findings of internal impingement are often subtle, but this combination of MR findings in young throwing athletes with shoulder pain is diagnostic of internal impingement.

BICEPS TENDON
Normal Anatomy

The LHBT demonstrates a broad triangular intra-articular origin, with fibers variably arising from the superior glenoid tubercle and the superior glenoid labrum. The short head of the biceps tendon has an extra-articular origin arising from the coracoid process along with the tendon of the coracobrachialis and pectoralis minor. The long and short heads of the biceps tendon are both accurately depicted on MRI of the shoulder but it is the LHBT that is most frequently affected by injury or disease. After its origin,

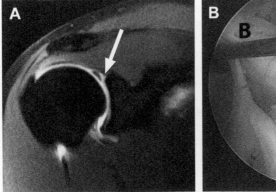
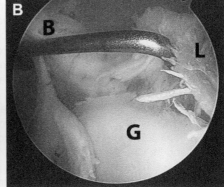

Fig. 10. (*A*) Coronal T1-weighted fat suppressed direct MR arthrogram image shows contrast material extending into the detached tear of the superior labrum (*arrow*). (*B*) Arthroscopic view of the shoulder shows probe passing through superior labral tear. Biceps tendon (B), torn labrum (L), and glenoid (G).

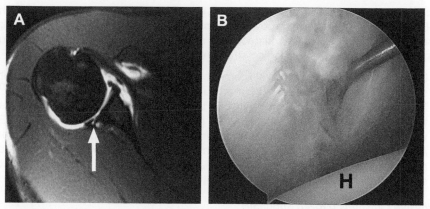

Fig. 11. (*A*) T1-weighted fat-suppressed axial direct MR arthrogram image shows tear of the posterior labrum (*arrow*). (*B*) Arthroscopic view shows probe passing through the posterior labral tear. Humerus (H).

the long head of the biceps follows an intra-articular course traversing the anterior joint space obliquely within the rotator cuff interval, covered by the coracohumeral and the SGHL. The LHBT exits the joint at the level of the intertubercular groove and enters the intertubercular sulcus anteriorly. At the transition level, the coracohumeral and SGHLs are the main stabilizers preventing medical subluxation of the tendon. As the LHBT courses more distally, it encounters secondary stabilizers, which include the transverse humeral ligament proximally and the pectoralis major tendon distally.

Pathology of the Long Head of the Biceps Tendon

Like any other tendon, the LHBT can be involved in a variety of injuries, including tenosynovitis, tendinopathy, partial-thickness or full-thickness tear, and entrapment. Because of its unique anatomic configuration, it can also undergo medial subluxation or dislocation if there is injury or disruption of its stabilizers. This usually occurs in association with a large rotator cuff tear or secondary to an isolated tear of the subscapularis tendon and coracohumeral ligament. Complete MR evaluation of the LHBT should include an evaluation of both the intra-articular and extra-articular (intertubercular groove) portions of the tendon. The oblique sagittal and oblique coronal imaging planes are the primary planes for evaluation the intra-articular portion of the tendon. The oblique sagittal plane allows visualization of the intra-articular portion of the tendon in cross-section from its origin to its exiting point at the level of the intertubercular groove. The normal tendon appears oval when viewed in the sagittal plane and dark on all pulse sequences. With tendinopathy, the tendon demonstrates thickness and intrinsic signal abnormality, whereas a partial-thickness tear demonstrates thinning or attenuation of the tendon or fluid signal within the substance of the tendon. With a complete tear, the tendon is nonvisualized and may demonstrate distal retraction. An empty intertubercular groove indicates disruption and distal retraction of the tendon extra-articular portion of the tendon.

Subluxation Patterns of the Long Head of the Biceps Tendon

The extra-articular portion of the LHBT is best evaluated using the axial imaging plane. The intertubercular groove portion of the LHBT should be evaluated for thickening, intrinsic signal abnormality, partial-thickness or full-thickness tear, adjacent fluid out of proportion to the joint fluid, loose bodies, and medial subluxation. Subluxation of the LHBT from the intertubercular groove can occur due to tears of the coracohumeral ligament, SGHL, subscapularis, and pectoralis major insertion. Direction of subluxation depends on which of the supporting structures are torn:

1. Disruption of the coracohumeral ligament in conjunction with avulsion of the subscapularis tendon results in an intra-articular dislocation of the LHBT (**Fig. 12**).
2. Tear of the coracohumeral ligament with a tear of the subscapularis tendon isolated to the transverse humeral ligament results in extra-articular dislocation of the LHBT with the tendon located superficial to the intact fibers of the subscapularis tendon.
3. An isolated tear of the coracohumeral ligament with an intact subscapularis tendon and transverse humeral ligament allows medial migration of the LHBT into the substance of the subscapularis tendon, resulting in interstitial tearing of the tendon.

Adhesive Capsulitis (Frozen Shoulder)

Adhesive capsulitis is a pathologic entity, unique to the shoulder that is characterized by inflammation and thickening of the synovium. The inflammatory changes are especially prominent in those areas of the shoulder that lack reinforcement by the rotator cuff tendons, primarily the rotator interval and axillary recess. Physical examination demonstrates a painful restriction of motion of the shoulder in all directions, but the most pronounced restriction of motion usually involves the external rotation of the humeral head.

The clinical presentation and age distribution of patients with adhesive capsulitis overlap those of rotator cuff pathology. Conventional arthrography demonstrates a small contracted joint capsule with a decreased joint volume of less than 10 mL. The axillary pouch appears small and contracted, and there is a lack of contrast filling the LHBT sheath.

Findings on MRI can be subtle and include abnormal soft tissue in the rotator interval, obliteration of the subcoracoid fat triangle, and thickening of the coracohumeral

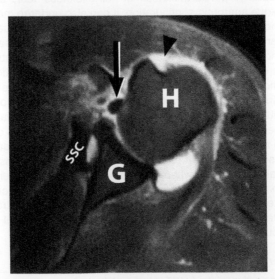

Fig. 12. T2-weighted fat-suppressed axial MRI shows empty bicipital groove (*arrowhead*) and dislocation of the biceps tendon into the glenohumeral joint (*arrow*). Torn and retracted subscapularis tendon (SSC), humerus (H), and glenoid (G).

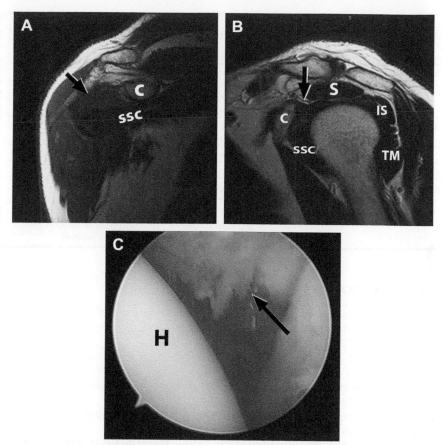

Fig. 13. Anterior coronal T1-weighted (*A*) and sagittal T2-weighted (*B*) images show replacement of fat within the rotator interval (*arrows*) in adhesive capsulitis. Coracoid process (C), subscapularis (SSC), supraspinatus (S), infraspinatus (IS), and teres major (TM). (*C*) Arthroscopic view shows synovial proliferation at the rotator interval (*arrow*) in a patient with adhesive capsulitis. Humerus (H).

ligament (**Fig. 13**). There may also be thickening of the joint capsule of more than 4 mm in the region of the axillary pouch. Inflammatory changes of the capsule may also be seen as increased T2 signal surrounding the capsule of the axillary pouch. Indirect MR arthrography, however, seems most specific for establishing the diagnosis of adhesive capsulitis. Findings specific for the diagnosis include enhancement of the abnormal soft tissues within the rotator interval combined with enhancement of the capsule and adjacent soft tissues in the region of the axillary pouch.

SUMMARY

Imaging is an essential tool for evaluation of patients with shoulder pain. This review should help practitioners understand the strengths and weaknesses of the different imaging modalities available and their indications for various presentations (**Table 3**). Understanding the extent of an injury with imaging is key to successful management.

Table 3 What a surgeon needs to know in patients with signs of impingement	
Anatomic Structure	**Potential Abnormalities**
Acromion	Types I–IV Anterior or lateral downsloping Inferiorly directed osteophyte Unfused os acromiale
Acromioclavicular joint	Osteoarthritis Mass effect on underlying cuff
Coracoacromial ligament	Thickening, nodularity, calcification
Subacromial subdeltoid bursa	Fluid, surrounding edema calcification
Rotator cuff	Tendinopathy (mild, moderate, or severe) Partial-thickness tear (articular, interstitial, or bursal) Full-thickness tear (size and location) Musculotendinous retraction (size of tendon gap) Fatty atrophy (mild, moderate, or severe)

RECOMMENDED READINGS

Bearcroft PW, Blanchard TK, Dixon AK, et al. An assessment of the effectiveness of magnetic resonance imaging of the shoulder: literature review. Skeletal Radiol 2000;29(12):673–9.

Beltran J, Kim DH. MR imaging of shoulder instability in the athlete. Magn Reson Imaging Clin N Am 2003;11:221–38.

Bencardino JT, Beltran J. MR imaging of the glenohumeral ligaments. Radiol Clin North Am 2006;44:489–502.

Bencardino JT, Garcia AI, Palmer WE. Magnetic resonance imaging of the shoulder: rotator cuff. Top Magn Reson Imaging 2003;14(1):51–67.

Bergin D. Imaging shoulder instability in the athlete. Magn Reson Imaging Clin N Am 2009;17(4):595–615.

Carrino JA, Chandnanni VP, Mitchell DB, et al. Pectoralis major muscle and tendon tears: diagnosis and grading using magnetic resonance imaging. Skeletal Radiol 2000;29:305–13.

Chaipat L, Palmer WE. Shoulder magnetic resonance imaging. Clin Sports Med 2006; 25(3):371–86.

De Maeseneer M, Van Roy P, Shahabpour M. Normal MR imaging anatomy of the rotator cuff tendons, glenoid fossa, labrum, and ligaments of the shoulder. Radiol Clin North Am 2006;44(4):479–87.

Farber A, Fayad L, Johnson T, et al. Magnetic resonance imaging of the shoulder: current techniques and spectrum of disease. J Bone Joint Surg Am 2006; 88(Suppl 4):64–79.

Fitzpatrick D, Walz DM. Shoulder MR imaging normal variants and imaging artifacts. Magn Reson Imaging Clin N Am 2010;18(4):615–32.

Fritz RC. Magnetic resonance imaging of sports-related injuries to the shoulder: impingement and rotator cuff. Radiol Clin North Am 2002;40(2):217–34.

Gordon BH, Chew FS. Isolated acromiclavicular joint pathology in the symptomatic shoulder on magnetic resonance imaging: a pictorial essay. J Comput Assist Tomogr 2004;28:215–22.

Jost B, Gerber C. What the shoulder surgeon would like to know from MR imaging. Magn Reson Imaging Clin N Am 2004;12(1):161–8.

Jung JY, Jee WH, Chun, et al. Adhesive capsulitis of the shoulder evaluation with MR arthrography. Eur Radiol 2006;16:791–6.

Kassarijian A, Bencardino JT, Palmer WE. MR imaging of the rotator cuff. Magn Reson Imaging Clin N Am 2004;12:39–60.

Kijowski R, De Smet AA. The role of ultrasound in the evaluation of sports medicine injuries of the upper extremity. Clin Sports Med 2006;25:569–90.

Mohana-Borges AV, Chung CB, Resnick D. MR imaging and MR arthrography of the postoperative shoulder; spectrum of normal and abnormal findings. Radiographics 2004;24:69–85.

Mohana-Borges AV, Chung CB, Resnick D. Superior labral antero-posterior tear: classification and diagnosis with MRI and MR arthrography. AJR Am J Roentgenol 2003;181:1449–62.

Moosikasuwan JB, Miller TT, Dines DM. Imaging of the painful shoulder in throwing athletes. Clin Sports Med 2006;25(3):433–43.

Morag Y, Jacobson JA, Shields G, et al. MR arthrography of rotator interval, long head of the biceps brachii, and biceps pulley of the shoulder. Radiology 2005;235:21–30.

Murray PJ, Shaffer BS. Clinical update: MR imaging of the shoulder. Sports Med Arthrosc 2009;17(1):40–8.

Sanders TG, Jersy SL. Conventional radiology of the shoulder. Semin Roentgenol 2005;40:207–22.

Steinbach LS. Magnetic resonance imaging of glenohumeral joint instability. Semin Musculoskelet Radiol 2006;9:44–55.

Wu J, Covey A, Katz LD. MRI of the postoperative shoulder. Clin Sports Med 2006;25:445–64.

Zlatkin MB. MRI of the postoperative shoulder. Skeletal Radiol 2002;31:63–80.

Imaging of Glenoid Labrum Lesions

George D. Chloros, MD[a,b,]*, Peter J. Haar, MD, PhD[a],
Thomas P. Loughran, MD[c], Curtis W. Hayes, MD, FACR[a]

KEYWORDS

- MRI arthrography • Glenoid • Labrum

KEY POINTS

- Diseases of the glenoid labrum are increasingly being recognized as a significant source of shoulder morbidity, especially in the high-demand athlete.
- The mainstay of diagnosis lies primarily on the imaging findings, because the signs and symptoms of labral disease are nonspecific.
- It is imperative for the radiologist to be familiar not only with the pathologic findings but also with the normal variants that are frequently encountered in imaging studies.
- The radiologist must effectively and precisely communicate normal variant and pathologic findings to the orthopedic surgeon to optimize preoperative diagnosis, assist the preoperative planning and avoid unnecessary procedures.

INTRODUCTION

Injuries to the glenoid labrum are a significant source of shoulder pain in athletes, especially during overhead activities. High physical demands imposed on the shoulder combined with repetitive strain result in abnormal shoulder joint kinematics that predispose to injury.[1,2] Although their incidence is unknown, labral tears are increasingly being recognized, and each year, an increasing number of arthroscopic surgeries are performed to repair them.[3,4] A variety of disorders coexist with labral tears, which render history and physical examination findings nonspecific, and therefore, clinical diagnosis of labral injuries is problematic and remains a challenge.[1,5–12] For example, Kim and colleagues[6] found 88% coexisting shoulder disease in 136 of 544 shoulder arthroscopies that revealed a labral tear. Therefore, imaging modalities, especially direct magnetic resonance (MR) arthrography, play a crucial role in the diagnosis of labral disease.[1,5,13–27]

[a] Department of Radiology, Virginia Commonwealth University School of Medicine, Richmond, VA 23298, USA; [b] Department of Radiology "Panagiotis and Aglaia Kyriakou" Children's Hospital, Athens, 15773, Greece; [c] Department of Orthopaedic Surgery, Virginia Commonwealth University School of Medicine, Richmond, VA 23298, USA
* Corresponding author.
E-mail address: gchlorosdoc@gmail.com

Clin Sports Med 32 (2013) 361–390
http://dx.doi.org/10.1016/j.csm.2013.04.001
0278-5919/13/$ – see front matter © 2013 Elsevier Inc. All rights reserved.

This article reviews the normal anatomy of the glenoid labrum, including anatomic variants and associated structures, and the different types of labral disease and provides insights, with some arthroscopic correlation to avoid potential pitfalls in interpretation.

RELEVANT ANATOMY AND NORMAL VARIANTS
Anatomy of the Glenoid Labrum

The labrum is a fibrocartilaginous ring that attaches to and encircles the glenoid rim.[28,29] It increases the concavity of the glenoid fossa by 9 mm in the superoinferior plane and 5 mm in the anteroposterior plane, to accommodate the larger humeral head.[28,30] Elimination of the labrum reduces the glenoid depth by more than 50% in both directions.[30] In addition, the labrum increases the surface area of contact between the humeral head and the glenoid and may share some of the load, similar to the meniscus in the knee.[31]

The labrum serves as the attachment site for the capsule and the glenohumeral ligaments and its superior portion anchors the long head of the biceps tendon (LHBT).[29,32] The labrum attaches more firmly at the posterior and inferior aspects of the glenoid, where it attaches to the glenoid articular cartilage by transferring its fibrous portion into fibrocartilage.[18,27,29,33] There are 2 different variations of the central attachment between the labrum and the cartilage: in a type A chondrolabral junction, there is an abrupt, narrow zone of transition between the 2 structures, whereas in type B chondrolabral junctions, the fibrous labrum blends with the hyaline cartilage.[18] In contrast to its inferior counterpart, the superior portion is more loosely attached, with several anatomic variations, which may frequently pose diagnostic dilemmas. The superior and the posterior portions of the labrum are thicker than their inferior and anterior counterparts, respectively.[32,34] In cross section, the shape of the glenoid labrum is typically triangular or rounded; however, other morphologies have been observed as well. Park and colleagues[35] looked at 108 MR arthrograms of asymptomatic individuals and determined the triangular shape to be the most common (anterior, 64%; posterior, 47%), followed by the rounded shape (anterior, 17%; posterior, 33%). Flat, absent, cleaved, or notched variants have also been reported.[35,36] The labrum is approximately 3 mm thick and 4 mm wide; however, the variation is considerable (from 2 to 14 mm in normal individuals), thus limiting the value of size as a diagnostic tool.[37]

For the purposes of orientation and reference, the labral circumference is superimposed on a clock. By convention, the 12 o'clock position is at the superior aspect, the 3 o'clock at the anterior aspect, the 6 o'clock at the inferior aspect, and the 9 o'clock at the posterior aspect (Fig. 1).[15,27,38,39] Knowledge of the considerable anatomic variability of the labrum is critical to image interpretation.

Variants and Pitfalls

Cartilage undercutting
Glenoid hyaline cartilage may sometimes undermine the superior labrum. Glenoid hyaline cartilage may resemble a superior-labrum-anterior-to-posterior (SLAP) lesion at first, but the cartilage signal is intermediate compared with the high-signal gadolinium. In addition, the cartilage signal follows the glenoid contour, whereas an SLAP lesion is oriented away from the contour (Fig. 2).[18,27,40,41]

Buford complex
Found in 1.5%[42] to 7.4%[43] of patients, the Buford complex consists of absence of the anterosuperior labrum and thickening of the middle glenohumeral ligament (MGHL), which may sometimes be mistaken for a labral tear, especially on axial MR

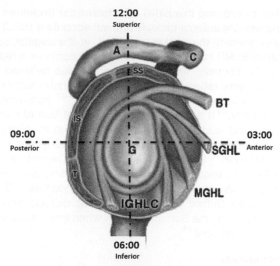

Fig. 1. Sagittal view of the glenoid, showing the labrum, the biceps tendon, the glenohumeral ligaments and their relations with the glenoid clock positions. A, acromion; BT, biceps tendon; C, coracoid process; G, glenoid; IGHLC, inferior glenohumeral ligament complex; IS, infraspinatus muscle; SGHL, superior glenohumeral ligament; SS, supraspinatus muscle; T, teres minor. (*Modified from* Modarresi S, Motamedi D, Jude CM. Superior labral anteroposterior lesions of the shoulder: part 1, anatomy and anatomic variants. AJR Am J Roentgenol 2011;197(3):600; with permission.)

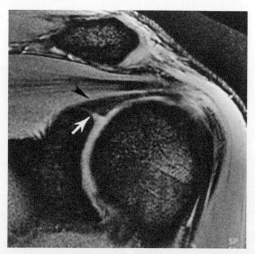

Fig. 2. T2-weighted coronal oblique image showing normal glenoid labrum. Deep to the labrum, the hyaline cartilage on the glenoid undercuts the superior labrum (*arrowhead*), which creates a linear high signal (*arrow*). In this normal variant, the cartilage follows the contour of the glenoid, which is not the case for an SLAP lesion. (*From* Helms CA. Shoulder. In: Helms CA, editor. Musculoskeletal MRI. Philadelphia: Saunders/Elsevier; 2009; with permission.)

images.[34,42] The key to avoiding this pitfall is to follow the thickened MGHL from its origin to its blending with the anterior capsule and subscapularis (SSC) tendon on axial MR cuts and to also identify the thickened MGHL in the sagittal oblique MR cuts **(Fig. 3)**.[23,44] In contrast to MR imaging (MRI), the Buford complex is readily recognized during arthroscopy. Traditionally, the Buford complex was believed to be a normal variant of the labrum. More recent literature has found increased correlation of the Buford complex with disease, including SLAP tears,[45–47] intra-articular abnormalities,[48] and even instability.[49] It is believed that in cases of Buford complex, the presence of an anterior and superior area devoid of labrum disrupts the normal biomechanics, with resultant increased forces on the labral-biceps anchor, thus predisposing to an SLAP lesion.[50] Based on these findings, a recent case series showed that in cases of SLAP tears associated with Buford complex, addressing the latter in addition to the SLAP repair may result in improved outcomes.[47] The investigators recommend that isolated Buford complexes without disease should not be addressed; however, addressing the Buford complex when there is concomitant disease may decrease the risk of reinjury.[47]

Mobility of superior labrum
During arthroscopy, the superior labrum is mobile, which is considered a normal variant.[51]

Meniscoidlike superior labrum
Meniscoidlike superior labrum is another normal variant, which does not require intervention.[52,53]

Sublabral (superior) recess (sulcus or cleft)
Sublabral (superior) recess (sulcus or cleft) is the commonest labrum variant and may be present in up to 73% of cases.[54–56] It is located at the 11-o'clock to 1-o'clock position and represents a sulcus between the labral-biceps complex and the glenoid cartilage, where the LHBT inserts on the glenoid.[13,15,55,56] The biceps-labral complex has been classified into 3 variants, based on the absence/presence and depth of the sublabral recess: in type I, there is a firm attachment of the labrum to the glenoid (ie, no

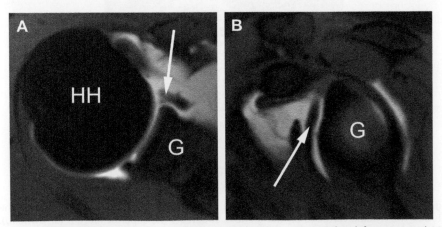

Fig. 3. Buford complex. (A) Axial and (B) sagittal oblique T1-weighted fat-saturated MR arthrogram images show absence of the anterior labrum and a thickened MGHL (*arrows*). G, glenoid; HH, humeral head. (*Courtesy of* the Department of Radiology, Virginia Commonwealth University; with permission.)

recess); types II and III represent a sulcus between the labrum and the glenoid cartilage, which is shallow in type II and deeper, even up to 5 mm, in type III.[55] This third type may sometimes be difficult to differentiate from a type II SLAP lesion.[13,57]

There are several helpful hints to avoid this potential pitfall:

1. Signal: the high signal is irregular in SLAP tears, but smooth in the sublabral recess.[41,57,58]
2. Orientation: the sublabral recess follows the glenoid curvature medially with a normal adjacent labrum, whereas the SLAP lesion is oriented laterally.[41,57–59]
3. Signal width: a width of more than 2 mm and more than 2.5 mm on MRI and MR arthrography is moderately specific for an SLAP lesion.[60] However, a cadaveric study has shown recesses deeper than 2 mm in 39% of cadavers.[55] Signal widths greater than 5 mm are most likely to represent an SLAP lesion, because gaps this wide are considered abnormal during arthroscopy.[61]
4. Presence of 2 signal lines: both a sublabral recess and an SLAP lesion may coexist, because the former may lead to the latter with overuse. In this case, there are 2 high-signal intensity lines, each corresponding to 1 of the entities, and this has been called the Oreo cookie sign.[39,41]
5. Patient age: sublabral recesses are not present at birth and their prevalence increases with age.[54,56,62] This finding suggests that the origin of the recess may be degenerative; hence, in a younger patient, the presence of an SLAP tear is more likely than a recess.[41]
6. Presence of concomitant anterosuperior labral tear or anteroposterior extension of signal on axial images.[59]
7. Anteriorly flared configuration of signal on axial images.[39]
8. Associated disease: rotator cuff tears, either partial or complete, and Bankart lesions are the commonest diseases associated with SLAP lesions. A large review by Snyder and colleagues[63] showed that only 28% of SLAP tears are isolated.

In previous literature, it was suggested that if the signal extends posterior to the LHBT insertion, an SLAP lesion should be suspected.[55] Several studies have now shown extension of a sublabral recess posterior to the LHBT insertion, ranging from 31% to 91%, and therefore the presence of high signal posterior to the LHBT is no longer considered a reliable indicator of a type II SLAP tear.[56,59] The presence of joint effusion or of intra-articular contrast agent enhances identification of the recess.[55] Several studies have reported that MR arthrography has sensitivities ranging from 81% to 92% and specificities of 100% in the detection of sublabral recesses.[55,56,59] Furthermore, MR arthrography is accurate in discerning a sublabral recess from an SLAP tear.[55,59] In patients with MRI contraindications, computed tomography (CT) arthrography performed on a 16-multidetector CT (MDCT) unit detects a sublabral recess effectively, with a sensitivity of 84% and a specificity of 100%.[56] A sublabral recess may coexist and be connected to a sublabral foramen.[13,18,23]

Other labral recesses
In addition to the sublabral (superior) recess at the 11-o'clock to the 1-o'clock position, there may exist recesses at different positions of the labrum, as reported in recent literature.[64,65] Lee and colleagues[64] reported clefts at all posterior hourly clock face positions (6 o'clock to 12 o'clock) in 16% to 19% of 127 shoulders. Most clefts (67%–71%) were at either the 7-o'clock or 8-o'clock position. In addition, the mean depth of the posterior clefts was 1.5 mm (range, 0.8–3 mm).

In a recent publication, Tuite and colleagues[65] examined 106 shoulders that underwent MR arthrography followed by arthroscopy to determine the prevalence of these variants in arthroscopically proved normal individuals. The most common variant was clefts, in about 38% to 61% of the normal labral segments, with a mean depth of 1 mm, especially in the anterior, anteroinferior, and posterosuperior segments. However, there were several limitations in this study, most notably the lack of correlation of each cleft with its corresponding arthroscopic image, the difficulty in differentiating true clefts from folds, the slight to moderate radiologist interobserver agreement, and the fact that surgeons were not blinded to the results of the MRI. Further investigations are warranted to more precisely characterize those potential normal variants.

Sublabral foramen

This normal variant represents a focal detachment of the labrum from the anterior and superior glenoid quadrant and may be confused with an anterior labral tear (**Fig. 4**).[42,48,57,66,67] It has not been determined whether the origin of this variant is developmental or acquired.[68] The reported incidence of sublabral foramen is variable,[42,46,48,57,66,67] ranging from 2.46%[67] to 18.5%.[46] In cadaveric studies, the reported incidence varies considerably, from 0% in a series of 84 cadaver specimens[69] to 26% in 19 specimens.[70] The sublabral foramen typically extends between the 1-o'clock and 3-o'clock positions, and several reports have stated that it should not extend below the level of the midglenoid notch, or junction of the superior and middle thirds of the glenoid.[18,71] Tuite and colleagues[50] showed that a sublabral foramen may extend below the midglenoid notch, so this statement is not to be taken as a hard-and-fast rule. Additional helpful features that point to the diagnosis of sublabral foramen instead of an SLAP tear include the presence of smooth margins of the foramen, displacement of less than 1 to 2 mm of the labrum, and lack of traumatic injury to adjacent capsule-ligamentous structures.[18] As pointed out in the discussion regarding the Buford complex, there is also an association between sublabral foramen and type II SLAP lesions.[6,46,48,67] In the largest series to date, Ilahi and colleagues[43] reported the findings in 334 shoulder arthroscopies and found a significant association between labral variants with SLAP tears compared with patients with more normal anatomy. A potential explanation for this association is that the presence of those variants may put higher stresses in the area, thus predisposing to injury. However, it is unclear whether

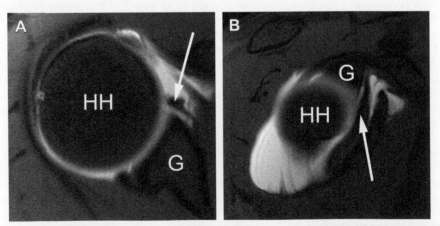

Fig. 4. Sublabral foramen. (*A*) Axial and (*B*) sagittal oblique T1-weighted fat-saturated MR arthrogram images show focal detachment of the labrum (*arrows*) from the anterior glenoid. G, glenoid; HH, humeral head. (*Courtesy of* the Department of Radiology, Virginia Commonwealth University; with permission.)

concomitant sublabral foramens should be addressed in addition to a type II SLAP lesion, as may seem the case in the Buford complex.[47] An isolated sublabral foramen should be left alone during arthroscopy, because its inadvertent closure may cause loss of external rotation.[72,73]

Potential pitfalls (sublabral foramen)
- The anterior band of the inferior glenohumeral ligament (IGHL) may be thickened or prominent, and this has been associated with hypoplastic or absent labrum. It is possible that some cases diagnosed as sublabral foramen may represent this variant.[23]
- Differentiation between a sublabral foramen and a Buford complex may sometimes be challenging: in the latter case, the thick MGHL is seen to converge and blend to the anterior capsule distally. In contrast, the labrum attaches to the glenoid distally, rather than the anterior capsule.[27]
- There is a communicating path between the sublabral foramen and the SSC recess, and loose bodies may dislodge from the joint into the recess via the foramen.[74]
- Sublabral foramen and recess may coexist and communicate with each other.[13,18,23]
- The presence of high origin of the anterior band of the IGHL may be confused with a sublabral foramen.[75]

Anatomy of the Glenohumeral Ligaments

The 3 glenohumeral ligaments consist of the superior glenohumeral ligament (SGHL), the MGHL, and the IGHL. They represent focal thickenings of the anterior joint capsule, and form a Z configuration when viewed from the front.[27] **Fig. 1** shows a classic depiction of a sagittal view of the glenoid, showing the glenohumeral ligaments and their relations to the glenoid clock (see **Fig. 1**).

SGHL

The SGHL is composed of parallel bundles of collagen fibers[76] and originates from the supraglenoid tubercle[77,78] or from the glenoid margin anterior and adjacent to the origin of the LHBT (1-o'clock position).[34,69,79] It then courses just superior to the lesser tuberosity before blending with the coracohumeral ligament (CHL) to insert in the fovea capitis of the humerus.[28,34,44,80] Its presence is generally constant,[13,44,76] and it is found in more than 94% of patients.[28,69,81,82] A recent anatomic study showed that the SGHL is composed of a direct and oblique component.[76] In addition to the classically described direct part, the investigators describe an oblique part, which inserts into the semicircular humeral ligament underneath the CHL.

Axial MR images clearly show the SGHL as a low-signal intensity thick linear structure arising from the supraglenoid tubercle, coursing parallel to the coracoid process.[18,27,34,44,83] The oblique MR sagittal image shows the course of the SGHL, which is intimate and inferior to the CHL and the coracoid.[84] The most crucial role of the SGHL, in concert with the remaining components of the rotator interval (RI), is to stabilize the LHBT in the groove, thus preventing subluxation[15,20,44,76,80,85]; it also limits inferior translation of the humerus in the abducted position.[27,86]

Variants of the SGHL
- The origin of the SGHL may be either with the LHBT alone or with the MGHL.[87]
- In 1 case, the SGHL originated from the posterior labrum instead of the antero-superior labrum or the MGHL, subsequently overriding the LHBT origin.[88]

- The SGHL is thin, but may thicken in patients with a hypoplastic or absent MGHL.[18,44,87]

MGHL

The MGHL is the most variable of all glenohumeral ligaments, and may be absent in 30% of cadaveric dissections[89] and in up to 21% on MR arthrography.[35] It originates at the anterior margin of the glenoid, just below the SGHL, courses inferiorly and later-ally and attaches to the medial aspect lesser tuberosity, deep to the tendon of the SSC.[27] On axial MR cuts, the MGHL is localized adjacent to the anterior labrum, from which it is separated by a small cleft, and is found just inferior to the tip of the coracoid process and deep to the SSC tendon.[27,44,90] This entity may mimic a labral tear. Oblique sagittal MR cuts show the MGHL on top of the anterior capsule from its labral attachment proximally to its capsular merge distally.[90] Unless the MGHL is redundant and thick, it is rarely seen on coronal MR images.[44,90]

The absence of MGHL is frequently accompanied by a prominent anterior capsular (SSC) recess,[34,90,91] as well as hypertrophy of the SGHL, as stated earlier.[18,44,87] In addition, the position of the MGHL varies in the degree of rotation of the arm during scanning. With external rotation, the MGHL stretches and opposes itself on the capsule even more, whereas with internal rotation, it becomes redundant and more medial, anterior to the scapular neck.[92] In the latter case, the MGHL may become mistaken for a loose body or stripped anterior capsule.[44] The MGHL, in concert with the SSC tendon, contributes to anterior stability.[27]

Variants of the MGHL

- Common origin of the MGHL with either (1) the SGHL, or (2) the SGHL and the LHBT, or (3) the LHBT. In this third case, the SGHL is absent.[44,90]
- Reported cases of longitudinally split or duplicate ligament[28] may represent either a normal variant or an old longitudinal tear of the MGHL.[44,90]
- As described earlier, thickening of the MGHL with absent anterosuperior labrum is called the Buford complex,[42] which may be found in up to 6.5% of patients.[46]

IGHL

The IGHL consists of 2 portions (anterior and posterior), separated by an intervening axillary recess (pouch). Both components arise from the labrum and attach to the sur-gical neck of the humerus.[18,27,28,93–95] The classic description of the origin of the ante-rior IGHL is around the 4-o'clock (2-o'clock to 4-o'clock) position, whereas the posterior IGHL originates at the posterior-inferior glenoid quadrant (7-o'clock to 9-o'clock).[94] The IGHL complex inserts just inferior to the anatomic neck of the hu-merus in 2 distinct patterns: a V-shaped attachment, in which both bands of the IGHL attach close to the articular edge of the humeral head, and a collarlike attach-ment, in which the entire IGHL complex inserts just distal to the articular edge of the humeral head.[44,94]

With the arm held in the abduction and external rotation (ABER) position, the anterior IGHL tightens and may be appreciated in its entirety,[89] which also may make labral tears more discernible.[96] We do not routinely use the ABER position, because it signif-icantly increases the examination time because the patient has to be repositioned and the surface coils changed. The IGHL is the most important structure in preventing dislocation when the arm is at 90° of ABER.[97] More specifically, the anterior IGHL acts as an anteroinferior stabilizer and primary restraint to anterior shoulder disloca-tion, whereas the posterior IGHL is the one that limits ABER.[27] The most frequently injured capsuloligamentous structure, especially in anterior shoulder dislocations, is the anterior part of the IGHL.[44,81,98]

Variants and pitfalls of the IGHL

- The anterior IGHL is thicker than the posterior IGHL in 75% of individuals.[94]
- The insertion of the IGHL complex may frequently have a jagged appearance on axial MR images, and this may be misinterpreted as fraying or tearing. In addition, at the axillary recess, the synovial folds may be prominent, which can be mistaken for debris or loose bodies.[87]
- Recent literature has shown that the anterior portion sometimes may also arise from the anterior or anterosuperior labrum (1–3 o'clock position) instead of the anteroinferior labrum, which may be confused with a labral tear.[75] In addition, in more than 85% of cases, the anterior IGHL attaches to both cartilage and bone instead of only bone.[95]
- Spiral ligament (fasciculus obliquus): this lesser-known ligament, initially described in classic anatomy texts, is also known as fasciculus obliquus or longitudinal oblique system.[99,100] In 2001, Kolts and colleagues[78] refined its description and named it spiral ligament secondary to its spiral course. More recent arthroscopic cadaveric studies have further characterized the spiral ligament and showed its consistency in all 22 cadavers examined.[101] The ligament originates in the axillary component of the IGHL and the infraglenoid tubercle, then crosses the anterior capsule upward and laterally, and ends up fusing with the MGHL. Superiorly, it blends with the superior portion of the SSC, with both structures inserting into the lesser tuberosity.[101,102] The biomechanical role of this ligament has not yet been elucidated.[18,101]
- The anterior IGHL may also, in some cases, arise from the MGHL.[53]
- A band of connective tissue may connect the IGHL to the SGHL and has been named as the periarticular fiber system,[103] but it has not yet been fully characterized.[18]

Anatomy of the RI, Long Head of the Biceps, and Biceps Pulley

The RI is a space between the supraspinatus (SST) and SSC tendons at the anterosuperior part of the glenohumeral joint. It is represented by a triangle; the base (medially) is the coracoid process and the apex (laterally) is at the transverse humeral ligament, forming the roof of the bicipital groove. The sides of the triangle are formed anteriorly by the capsule and CHL, and superiorly and inferiorly by the SST and SSC tendons.[20,79,85,104] The contents of the RI are the anterior capsule, CHL, SGHL, MGHL, and the LHBT, which crosses the RI toward the bicipital groove.[20,79,85,104,105] Although there is consensus on the contents of the RI, there is variability and debate on its various fine descriptions. As has been pointed out by Morag and colleagues,[20] a possible explanation for those discrepancies may be the great variability of the anterior capsule and ligaments.[106] In addition, Gaskill and colleagues[104] noted the different approach in studies that emphasize the intra-articular or extra-articular portion of the ligaments, the quality of cadavers used (fresh vs frozen), and the close association between the CHL and SGHL laterally.[107] To add to the complexity, there is debate as to the function of the RI; the visualization of its complex anatomy is challenging from both the imaging and arthroscopy perspectives, and the treatment of its disease remains controversial.[20,79,85,104,105]

CHL

The CHL originates on the lateral part of the base of the coracoid process and is a broad, thin structure with an irregular trapezoidal shape. Merged to the anterior capsule, it courses laterally through the RI superficial to the SGHL and inserts on both the lesser and greater tubercles, spanning the bicipital groove. In doing so, it fuses with the anterior fibers of SST and superior fibers of SSC insertions. Distally, this ligament divides into 2 major bands: a smaller medial band (medial CHL) and a lateral band (lateral CHL), which are believed to contribute to different components of the ligamentous sling encompassing the LHBT. The medial CHL blends with the SGHL to surround the medial and inferior aspect of the intra-articular portion of the LHBT, whereas the lateral CHL surrounds the remaining lateral and superior aspects of the LHBT. There is controversy as to whether the CHL histologically resembles more capsule than ligament and its biomechanical role.[20,85,104,105]

SGHL, CHL, and biceps pulley

The anatomy of the SGHL has already been described. Relative to the RI, the CHL and SGHL are separate medially, but the medial CHL and SGHL are closely opposed (or merged) laterally at the opening of the bicipital groove, forming a slinglike band surrounding the LHBT at the apex of the RI, which is called the biceps pulley or reflective biceps pulley or sling. This biceps pulley, along with the SSC and the transverse ligament, are the major soft tissue restraints to dislocation or subluxation of the LHBT from the groove. The SSC and SST insert on the lesser and greater tubercles, respectively, and are thus intimately associated with the biceps pulley.[20,85,104]

LHBT

The LHBT is intra-articular but extrasynovial[28] and originates almost 50-50 from both the posterosuperior or posterior portion of the labrum and the supraglenoid tubercle, respectively.[108] It then passes through the RI (see later discussion) and descends inside the bicipital groove of the humerus.[15,28] The tendon is larger and flatter in its intra-articular portion, transferring to smaller and rounder in the extra-articular portion.[109] As stated earlier, the LHBT enters the bicipital groove and becomes extra-articular; it is stabilized by a sling of soft tissues consisting of the CHL, the SGHL, and parts of the SSC, which is referred to as the biceps pulley.[20,85] There can exist several variations of the biceps tendon,[110–116] including absence,[110,117–119] hypoplasia,[120] accessory heads,[111,112,114] and origin variations, including aberrant origins,[121,122] extra-articular origin,[123] intracapsular origin,[124] confluence with the rotator cuff,[112] and origin from the SST tendon.[125] The prevalence of variations in the intra-articular portion of the LHBT ranges from 1.9%[116] to 7.2%.[113] Both of these studies classified LHBT variants into 12[116] and 7[113] types, respectively, and found that certain types had a statistically significant association with labral disease.[113,116] The function of the biceps in the shoulder is controversial, with some investigators believing that it is a vestigial structure,[126,127] whereas others believe that it may have a role in shoulder stability, especially in cases of injury to the glenohumeral ligaments or rotator cuff.[128–131]

LABRAL DISEASE

Injuries to the labrum that may be associated with glenohumeral joint instability include the Bankart lesion[132] and its variants, most notably the reverse Bankart lesion, the anterior labroligamentous periosteal sleeve avulsion (ALPSA),[133] and Perthes lesions.[134] Noninstability labral lesions include the SLAP lesion,[63,71,135,136] labral cysts, and the glenolabral articular disruption (GLAD) lesion.[137]

Lesions Associated with Traumatic Glenohumeral Instability

Lesions associated with traumatic glenohumeral instability most commonly involve the anteroinferior part of the labrum, and occur secondary to dislocations or subluxations of the glenohumeral joint.

Bankart lesion

First described by Bankart in 1923,[132] a fibrous Bankart lesion involves a focal detachment (with or without labral tear) of the labroligamentous complex off the anteriorinferior part of the glenoid, typically between the 3-o'clock and 6-o'clock position, with disruption of the periosteum. If there is an associated glenoid rim fracture, the lesion is termed an osseous Bankart lesion (**Fig. 5**). These lesions commonly occur secondary to anterior shoulder dislocations (or subluxations), which appear in almost 95% of cases, versus the less common posterior shoulder dislocation; in the latter case, a reverse Bankart lesion can occur, with detachment of the posteroinferior part of the labrum, and again this may or may not be associated with fracture. The MRI appearance of the Bankart lesion shows these features, but the labrum remains continuous with the anterior IGHL.[138] The healing capacity of a Bankart lesion is minimal secondary to the displacement from the glenoid rim and, therefore, requires operative stabilization.[139,140]

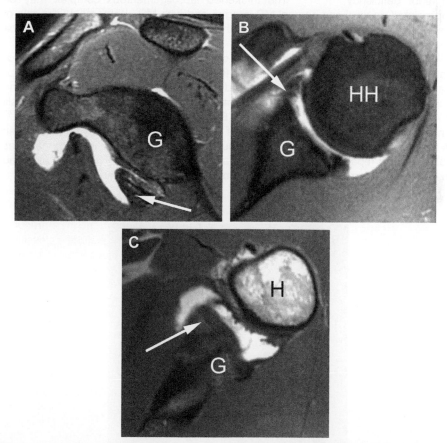

Fig. 5. Bony Bankart lesion with tear of the anterior labrum. (*A*) Sagittal oblique proton-density fast spin echo MR arthrogram image shows a fracture fragment (*arrow*) of the anteroinferior glenoid. (*B*) Axial T1-weighted fat-saturated MR arthrogram image shows an anterior labral tear (*arrow*). (*C*) Axial T1-weighted MR arthrogram image shows the anteroinferior glenoid fracture (*arrow*). G, glenoid; H, humerus. (*Courtesy of* the Department of Radiology, Virginia Commonwealth University; with permission.)

ALPSA lesion

This important Bankart-variant lesion was first described by Neviaser[133] and is defined as an avulsion of the anterior labrum from the anteroinferior part of the glenoid; however, with the periosteum intact and still attached to, but stripped from, the anterior scapula (periosteal sleeve avulsion) (**Fig. 6**). Although the ALPSA lesion may occur at the time of first dislocation,[141] it is usually the result of chronic injury and indicates a more severe trauma and recurrent dislocation.[139,142] There is controversy in the literature as to its origin, with some investigators believing that it may be a progressive (chronic) form of Bankart lesion, reflecting an advanced stage of Perthes lesion,[139,142] whereas others believe that it is a separate entity.[141,143] In any case, severe trauma displaces the labroligamentous complex medially, rotates it inferiorly, and positions it against the scapular neck.[139,142] With time, there is proliferation of fibrous tissue and synovium and resulting scarring of the lesion on the scapular neck, creating a pseudolabrum.[139,140,142] With subsequent repeated dislocations, the periosteal sleeve is stripped from the scapular neck and glenoid, which results in severe anteroinferior deficiency.[139,140,142] The thickened labroligamentous complex may be appreciated on axial and coronal MR images and with MR arthrography; the role of preoperative imaging is critical, because the thickened complex may commonly be missed during arthroscopy.[68]

ALPSA is a severe chronic lesion, which, compared with the Bankart lesion, is associated with higher incidence of associated factors, including cartilage erosion, preoperative number of dislocations, larger and more engaging Hill-Sachs defects, and increased synovitis, as well as higher extent of capsulolabral lesion.[142] The prognosis of ALPSA lesions is worse compared with Bankart lesions. Two recent studies[139,142] have shown that the arthroscopic repair of ALPSA lesions fails nearly twice as often as the Bankart lesion, which may be attributed to the result of the initial damage, as well as that of repairing a scarred, low-quality tissue.[139] The ALPSA lesion also had an increased recurrence of dislocation compared with the Bankart lesion.[142]

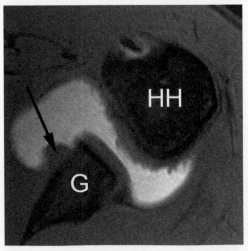

Fig. 6. ALPSA lesion. Axial T1-weighted fat-saturated MR arthrogram image shows avulsion of the anterior labrum, periosteal sleeve avulsion, and chronic medial displacement of the anterior labrum (*arrow*). G, glenoid; HH, humeral head. (*Courtesy of* the Department of Radiology, Virginia Commonwealth University; with permission.)

A less common posterior counterpart of the ALPSA lesion, termed the posterior labrocapsular periosteal sleeve avulsion lesion, has been described. It is similar to a nondisplaced ALPSA lesion, involving the detachment of an intact posterior labrum with periosteal stripping.[144]

Perthes lesion

The Perthes lesion is another Bankart-variant lesion, in which the periosteum also remains intact but is stripped medially (**Fig. 7**).[134] Imaging diagnosis of this entity is critical, because the pitfall that surgeons face with this lesion is that it may be difficult to diagnose during arthroscopy, because the anterior labrum is still in its correct anatomic position.[134] For this same reason, even MR arthrography in the neutral position, which has been widely accepted in clinical practice, may fail to detect this lesion.[134,145] The ABER position[146] stretches the anterior IGHL, and the resulting tension on the labrum separates the labrum from the glenoid, allowing better visualization. This situation is confirmed by recent studies that have shown that MR arthrography in the ABER position may significantly improve the sensitivity of anteroinferior lesions of the labroligamentous complex, especially in the case of Perthes lesions.[134,145,147]

Lesions Not Associated with Glenohumeral Instability

SLAP lesions

SLAP tears are a significant source of debilitating shoulder pain in athletes, especially during overhead activities.[1,15] An SLAP lesion is defined as a lesion of the superior labrum, which typically originates at the site of attachment of the LHBT (biceps anchor) and may extend to the anterior or posterior portions of the labrum and adjacent structures. A variety of disorders coexist with labral tears, which renders history and physical examination findings nonspecific; therefore, clinical diagnosis of labral injuries is problematic and remains a challenge.[1,6–12,148,149] For example, Kim and colleagues[6] found 88% coexisting shoulder disease in 136 of 544 shoulder arthroscopies that

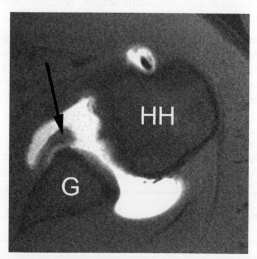

Fig. 7. Perthes lesion. Axial T1-weighted fat-saturated MR arthrogram image shows avulsion of the anterior labrum (*arrow*) with an intact medially stripped periosteum. The anterior labrum remains in its correct anatomic position. (*Courtesy of* the Department of Radiology, Virginia Commonwealth University; with permission.)

revealed a labral tear. Therefore, imaging modalities, especially direct MR arthrography, play a crucial role in the diagnosis of labral disease.[1,13–27] SLAP tears have been reported to have an incidence between 6%[71] and 26% in the general population.[6,63,150,151] Although their incidence is unknown, labral tears are increasingly being recognized, and each year, an increasing number of arthroscopic surgeries are performed to repair them.[3,4]

SLAP tears were first identified by Andrews and Carson in 1984[135]; however, the denomination SLAP was introduced by Snyder and colleagues in 1990,[71] who classified them into 4 main types (**Table 1**), with type II being the most frequent. At least 12 types of SLAP lesions have been identified in the literature.[27] We agree with other investigators that knowledge of the original 4-type Snyder classification is sufficient for the radiologist, and for practical purposes, an accurate descriptive analysis of a labral tear is critical regardless of classification.[27,41] Even for those 4 types, there is significant intraobserver and interobserver reliability among shoulder specialists.[152]

The gold imaging standard for the diagnosis of SLAP lesions is MR arthrography. The following points are helpful in describing a labral tear[27,41]:

- Localization of the tear by using the clock method reported previously
- Description of the detached component of the tear, including whether it is full or partial thickness; for example, a bucket-handle (type IV) tear should be described as a full-thickness, high-signal contrast line separating the superior labrum from the biceps anchor (see **Fig. 10**)
- Relationship of the lesion to the surrounding structures:
  ○ Extension and degree of involvement of the biceps anchor; it is crucial to report whether the biceps-labral anchor is either torn or not torn, because this influences treatment decisions
  ○ Extension into the MGHL, which requires repair of the MGHL
  ○ Extension into the RI structures
- Recognition of the presence of normal variants
- Description of concomitant lesions that occur in high frequency with labral lesions, including rotator cuff, Hill-Sachs lesions, articular cartilage, capsule, and bony structures

The normal labrum shows smooth and regular margins, and a dark signal on all MRI sequences. Potential pitfalls in interpretation of an SLAP lesion versus normal variants include undercutting of the normal cartilage, a sublabral recess, sublabral foramen, and Buford complex and have been already described previously in the corresponding normal variant sections. Examples of SLAP lesions are presented in (**Figs. 8–10**).

GLAD lesion

The GLAD lesion has recently been brought to clinical attention by Neviaser.[137] It is a rare lesion, with only a few patients reported,[83,153] and represents a nondisplaced tear

Table 1	
Snyder classification of SLAP lesions	
Type	**Description**
I	Degeneration and fraying of the superior labrum
II	Avulsion of the superior labrum and biceps anchor
III	Interiorly displaced bucket-handle tear of the superior labrum
IV	Extension of type III to involve the biceps anchor

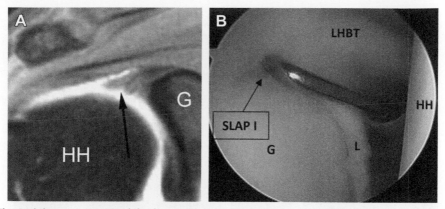

Fig. 8. (*A*) Type I superior labral anterior to posterior lesion. Coronal oblique T1-weighted fat-saturated MR arthrogram image shows fraying of the superior labrum (*arrow*). G, glenoid; HH, humeral head. (*B*) Corresponding arthroscopic image of the same patient, showing the type I SLAP tear. G, glenoid; HH, humeral head; L, labrum. (*Courtesy of* the Department of Radiology, Virginia Commonwealth University; with permission.)

of the anteroinferior labrum associated with a chondral injury (**Fig. 11**).[83,137,153] It is primarily a traumatic impaction injury with the arm in ABER and is not related to instability. Consequently, patients have complaints related to pain rather than instability, as seen, for example, in the case of Bankart-related lesions. A GLAD lesion may also result in chondral loose bodies.[154] MR arthrography shows the injury, because contrast material fills the cartilaginous defect; however, the nondisplaced small labral lesion may still not be discernible.

Paralabral Cysts

Paralabral cysts are uncommon,[155,156] but clinically relevant, because they are invariably associated with labral tears[27,155,156] and may extend to the spinoglenoid or

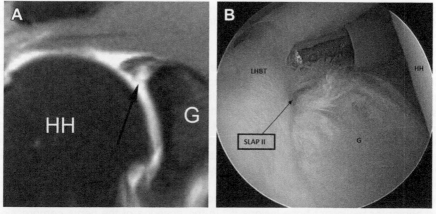

Fig. 9. (*A*) Type II SLAP lesion. Coronal oblique T1-weighted fat-saturated MR arthrogram image shows globular contrast-intensity signal of the articular surface of the superior labrum (*arrow*). (*B*) Corresponding arthroscopic image of the same patient, showing the type II SLAP tear. G, glenoid; HH, humeral head. (*Courtesy of* the Department of Radiology, Virginia Commonwealth University; with permission.)

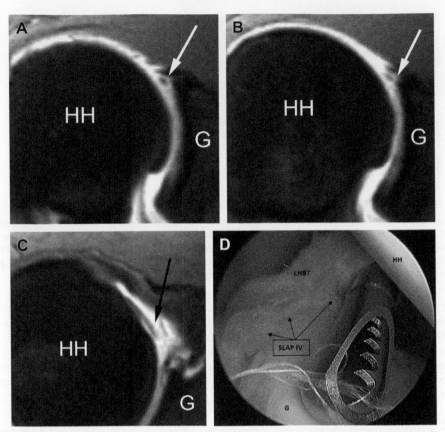

Fig. 10. Type IV SLAP lesion. (*A, B*) Coronal oblique T1-weighted fat-saturated MR arthrogram images show linear contrast-intensity signal extending from the superior labrum into the biceps anchor (*arrows*). (*C*) Axial T1-weighted fat-saturated MR arthrogram image shows a longitudinal tear of the LHBT (*arrow*). G, glenoid; HH, humeral head. (*D*) Corresponding arthroscopic image of the same patient, showing the type II SLAP tear. G, glenoid; HH, humeral head. (*Courtesy of* the Department of Radiology, Virginia Commonwealth University; with permission.)

suprascapular notches, leading to quadrilateral space syndrome, which is a rare presentation.[155,156] The mechanism of formation is similar to a ganglion: a labral tear extending through the joint capsule extrudes joint fluid via a 1-way valve mechanism.[155,156] Secondary to this mechanism, the cyst may sometimes be the most reliable sign of a labral tear. Although the most common location is the posterosuperior aspect of the labrum,[155,156] the cyst may occur anywhere.[27] The cysts are composed of thick protein-rich material, which remains after water has been reabsorbed from the cyst.[27] The diagnosis is challenging and may typically be delayed, because they present with nonspecific findings of history, physical examination, and pain, which prompt evaluation for other entities, including osteoarthritis, rheumatoid arthritis, and benign or malignant bone lesions.[156] In the absence of the nerve compression symptoms, which is the most frequent presentation, paralabral cysts have been low on the differential list of refractory shoulder pain.[156] In addition, concomitant shoulder disease may also delay the diagnosis,[156] and classically the symptoms are attributed to SLAP lesions or compression neuropathies.[156,157] T2-weighted MRI is the most

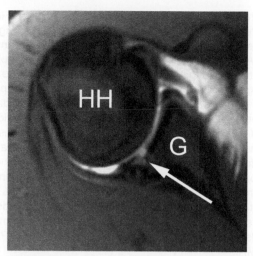

Fig. 11. Reverse Bankart lesion, with GLAD. Axial T1-weighted fat-saturated MR arthrogram image shows a fracture of the posterior glenoid with an articular cartilage lesion (*arrow*). G, glenoid; HH, humeral head. (*Courtesy of* the Department of Radiology, Virginia Commonwealth University; with permission.)

appropriate imaging for the diagnosis,[27,155,156] which may or may not show loculation (**Fig. 12**). Plain radiographs of the shoulder are usually negative, but in some instances, it has been shown that the presence of paralabral air on shoulder radiographs may give a clue for the presence of a paralabral cyst.[155,158]

Usefulness of the Various Imaging Techniques in the Detection of Labral Lesions, Including Anteroinferior Labral Lesions and SLAP Tears

Conventional MRI and MR arthrography
Although there are variations in the sensitivities and specificities reported in the literature for both techniques, most studies report that MR arthrography is superior to

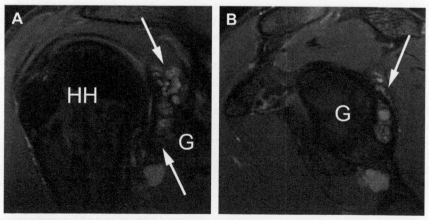

Fig. 12. Extensive paralabral cysts. (*A*) Coronal oblique and (*B*) sagittal oblique T2-weighted fat-saturated images show extensive loculated high signal structures adjacent to the posteroinferior labrum (*arrows*), in keeping with paralabral cysts. G, glenoid; HH, humeral head. (*Courtesy of* the Department of Radiology, Virginia Commonwealth University; with permission.)

conventional MRI in the diagnosis of labral lesions.[7,14,91,140,159] Recently, Amin and Youssef[160] compared conventional MR and MR arthrogram imaging studies in the diagnosis of SLAP tears. All patients underwent conventional MR and those with negative findings for SLAP were further investigated by MR arthrography. Twenty-two of the 34 patients with initial negative conventional MR were found to have an SLAP lesion by MR arthrography. Furthermore, even at 3 T, MR arthrography seems superior to conventional 3-T MRI.[161,162] With arthroscopy as the gold standard, MR arthrography has shown a sensitivity ranging from 82% to 89% and a specificity of 91% to 98% for the detection of SLAP lesions[14,159]; however, it has limitations in classifying the SLAP lesion.[14] In assessing MR arthrography in the anteroinferior labral lesions, Waldt and colleagues[138] found the accuracy of direct magnetic resonance angiography to be 89% in detection, and 84% in the classification of all anteroinferior labral tears. Overall, 80% of Bankart lesions, 77% of ALPSA lesions, and 50% of Perthes lesions were correctly identified. However, most of these studies involve dedicated musculoskeletal radiologists with a high-volume turnover. In the community setting, MR arthrography has also shown superior sensitivity in detecting SLAP lesions compared with conventional MRI.[163]

Positional maneuvers during MR arthrography

The importance of shoulder positioning is emphasized throughout the literature.[18,145,146,164,165] The routine arm position is the neutral/slight external rotation. However, the use of different positional maneuvers puts tension on different structures and increases diagnostic sensitivity and specificity, depending on what is the most desirable structure to be studied. External rotation results in tension/traction of the anterior structures and, therefore, better shows the anterior labral structures, whereas, by the same token, internal rotation is better for evaluating the posterior labral structures. Conversely, internal rotation is inadequate for visualization of the anterior structures, because it results in medial displacement of the joint capsule and contraction of the SSC tendon and may obscure the subjacent anteroinferior labrum.

ABER position The ABER position[146] stretches the anterior IGHL, and the resulting tension on the labrum separates the labrum from the glenoid, allowing better visualization. This situation is confirmed by recent studies that have shown that MR arthrography in the ABER position may significantly improve the sensitivity of anteroinferior lesions of the labroligamentous complex, especially in the case of Perthes lesions.[145,164] The only study in the literature that contradicts this finding is by Schreinemachers and colleagues.[164] These investigators reviewed 250 arthrograms in 92 patients with confirmed arthroscopic diagnosis and found no significant difference in the detection of anteroinferior labral tears. A recent study by Tian and colleagues[145] is the largest series to date comparing MR arthrography in the neutral versus the ABER position for proved lesions of the anteroinferior labrum. In concordance with previous studies,[164] the investigators found that the ABER position is better at classifying Perthes lesions, but worse in ALPSA lesions. They concluded that the ABER position increases significantly the sensitivity for anteroinferior labral lesions, especially for Perthes lesions, and recommended its use in equivocal cases when an anteroinferior labrum lesions is suspected.[145]

Flexion, adduction, and internal rotation position and adduction and internal rotation position In a preliminary investigation of 9 patients, Chiavaras and colleagues[166] found that flexion, adduction, and internal rotation positioning increased the diagnostic confidence of MR arthrography in patients with equivocal or subtle posteroinferior labral lesions.

In a retrospective review, Song and colleagues[167] introduced the MR arthrographic adduction and internal rotation (ADIR) position and compared it with the ABER and neutral positions. The investigators concluded that ADIR was superior to the other positions in discriminating between subtypes of Bankart injuries.

The major downsides of using positional maneuvers are the prolonged examination time (by approximately 25%)[146] and increased discomfort/sensation of instability and apprehension, particularly with the ABER position in recurrent dislocators.[18,146]

CT

MR arthrography is considered the reference standard for shoulder imaging. However, the development of high-resolution MDCT techniques has enhanced the capabilities of CT in the evaluation of the shoulder and has broadened its indications further than just the presence of absolute or relative contraindications to MR arthrography.[168] In a recent study, Acid and colleagues[168] examined the findings of MR arthrography and MDCT arthrography in 40 patients, using arthroscopy as the gold standard. MDCT arthrography had a higher sensitivity (100%) compared with MR arthrography (67%), especially in the case of glenoid rim fractures. In the diagnosis of ALPSA, MDCT arthrography was less sensitive (93%) versus MR arthrography (100%).[168]

In other recent studies, Kim and colleagues[169] found a 94% to 98% sensitivity of MDCT arthrography in the detection of SLAP lesions, whereas the specificity was 73% to 77% and overall accuracy was 86.3%. From the same group, Oh and colleagues[170] had a sensitivity of 86%, specificity of 90%, and overall accuracy of 88%. The corresponding results for MR arthrography were 72% and 95%, respectively.

To our best knowledge, the only CT arthrography study that has looked at positional maneuvers compared with MDCT arthrography in the neutral position versus external rotation and active supination is the recent study by Choi and colleagues,[171] which found that the last position is superior at detecting SLAP tears.

In selected cases, MDCT arthrography may provide reliable and accurate findings and may be preferable to MR arthrography, especially in the face of suspicion of glenoid rim fractures in the setting of preoperative planning of a Latarjet reconstruction or for the assessment of bone stock in recurrent dislocators.[140,168–170,172,173]

LHBT and RI Lesions

There is a spectrum of disease associated with the RI, including contractures on 1 end (eg, adhesive capsulitis) and laxity on the other (eg, instability), lesions involving the anterior aspect of the SST and superior SSC tendon, coracoid impingement, as well as LHBT and biceps pulley lesions and even rheumatologic and septic processes.[20,85,104] LHBT and biceps pulley lesions are reported in the following sections; a comprehensive analysis of RI disease is beyond the scope of this review.

Disease of the LHBT

Abnormalities of the LHBT are significant pain generators and include tendinosis, rupture, instability, pulley lesions, SLAP lesions, and commonly, a combination of these.[20,174] LHBT tendinopathy, pulley, SLAP, and rotator cuff disease are frequently associated.[174]

The working planes for visualizing the LHBT are the sagittal and axial planes imaged in T2-weighted sequences; localized changes proximal to the groove may also be appreciated in the coronal plane.[20] In LHBT tendinopathy, the tendon is swollen, with a high intratendinous signal, and often accompanied by synovitis and adhesions.[105] In tenosynovitis, the tendon sheath has an abnormal amount of fluid surrounding it, whereas in stenosing tenosynovitis, the fluid cannot go through past the stenosed

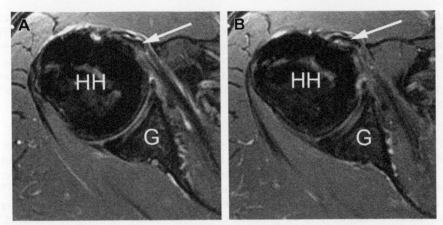

Fig. 13. Dislocation of the LHBT. (*A, B*) Axial T2-weighted fat-saturated images show medial dislocation of the LHBT (*arrows*) from the bicipital groove into a split tear of the SSC tendon, indirect indicators of a biceps pulley lesion. G, glenoid; HH, humeral head. (*Courtesy of* the Department of Radiology, Virginia Commonwealth University; with permission.)

region of the tendon sheath.[26] Partial tendon ruptures are seen as abrupt changes in tendon caliber; in high-T2-weighted images, intrasubstance clefts indicate longitudinal or circumferential tears.[105] Common MRI signs associated with tendinosis and partial tears include tendon thickening, attenuation, irregularity, and focal changes.[104] If the LHBT is completely ruptured, it is absent from the groove.[20,85,104,105]

Biceps pulley lesions

As described earlier, the biceps pulley is the major stabilizer of the LHBT in the bicipital groove, and therefore, pulley lesions result in instability of the LHBT.[20,85,104,105] The biceps pulley may suffer acute trauma, repetitive strain, degenerative changes, or injury associated with a rotator cuff tear.[85,175] Instability may occur in isolation; however, it is usually associated with an SSC and SST anterosuperior rotator cuff tear.[176] Pulley lesions cause significant morbidity, they are not infrequent, and the arthroscopic prevalence in 1007 patients has been reported at 7%,[177] and in a recent series of 229 patients, it was reported as high as 32.4%.[178] The diagnosis of biceps pulley lesions is not straightforward, and those lesions have been referred to as hidden lesions, because they can be missed during open or arthroscopic inspection.[79,85] MR arthrography has a central role in the diagnosis of biceps pulley lesions.[20,85,104,105] Injuries to the biceps pulley may be indirectly diagnosed when the LHBT is medially subluxed, dislocated, or perched on the lesser tubercle.[85] A subluxed LHBT is seen at the medial ridge of the groove, whereas a dislocated LHBT may be seen lying within or anterior to the SSC tendon (**Fig. 13**).[105] However, the direct diagnosis of pulley component lesion may sometimes be impossible.[179]

SUMMARY

More attention has been paid in recent years to disease of the glenoid labrum, and more procedures are performed every year,[3,4] especially in the high-demand athlete.[1,2] The mainstay of the preoperative diagnosis lies primarily in the imaging findings, because the signs and symptoms of labral disease are nonspecific.[1,5–12] It is imperative for the radiologist to be familiar not only with the pathologic findings but also with the normal variants that are frequently encountered in imaging studies and communicate those precisely to the orthopedic surgeon to optimize preoperative diagnosis, avoid unnecessary procedures, and provide vital hints to the surgeon, thereby assisting in preoperative planning.

REFERENCES

1. Knesek M, Skendzel JG, Dines JS, et al. Diagnosis and management of superior labral anterior posterior tears in throwing athletes. Am J Sports Med 2013;41(2):444–60.
2. Cohn RM, Jazrawi LM. The throwing shoulder: the orthopedist perspective. Magn Reson Imaging Clin North Am 2012;20(2):261.
3. Zhang AL, Kreulen C, Ngo SS, et al. Demographic trends in arthroscopic SLAP repair in the United States. Am J Sports Med 2012;40(5):1144–7.
4. Onyekwelu I, Khatib O, Zuckerman JD, et al. The rising incidence of arthroscopic superior labrum anterior and posterior (SLAP) repairs. J Shoulder Elbow Surg 2012;21(6):728–31.
5. Keener JD, Brophy RH. Superior labral tears of the shoulder: pathogenesis, evaluation, and treatment. J Am Acad Orthop Surg 2009;17(10):627–37.
6. Kim TK, Queale WS, Cosgarea AJ, et al. Clinical features of the different types of SLAP lesions: an analysis of one hundred and thirty-nine cases. J Bone Joint Surg Am 2003;85-A(1):66–71.
7. Phillips JC, Cook C, Beaty S, et al. Validity of noncontrast magnetic resonance imaging in diagnosing superior labrum anterior-posterior tears. J Shoulder Elbow Surg 2013;22(1):3–8.
8. Calvert E, Chambers GK, Regan W, et al. Special physical examination tests for superior labrum anterior posterior shoulder tears are clinically limited and invalid: a diagnostic systematic review. J Clin Epidemiol 2009;62(5):558–63.
9. Karlsson J. Physical examination tests are not valid for diagnosing SLAP tears: a review. Clin J Sport Med 2010;20(2):134–5.
10. Meserve BB, Cleland JA, Boucher TR. A meta-analysis examining clinical test utility for assessing superior labral anterior posterior lesions. Am J Sports Med 2009;37(11):2252–8.
11. Kemp K, Sheps DM. Clinical tests to identify SLAP lesions: a meta-analysis. Clin J Sport Med 2009;19(4):339–40.
12. Walton DM, Sadi J. Identifying SLAP lesions: a meta-analysis of clinical tests and exercise in clinical reasoning. Phys Ther Sport 2008;9(4):167–76.
13. De Maeseneer M, Van Roy F, Lenchik L, et al. CT and MR arthrography of the normal and pathologic anterosuperior labrum and labral-bicipital complex. Radiographics 2000;20(Spec No):S67–81.
14. Waldt S, Burkart A, Lange P, et al. Diagnostic performance of MR arthrography in the assessment of superior labral anteroposterior lesions of the shoulder. AJR Am J Roentgenol 2004;182(5):1271–8.
15. Modarresi S, Motamedi D, Jude CM. Superior labral anteroposterior lesions of the shoulder: part 1, anatomy and anatomic variants. AJR Am J Roentgenol 2011;197(3):596–603.
16. Smith TO, Drew BT, Toms AP. A meta-analysis of the diagnostic test accuracy of MRA and MRI for the detection of glenoid labral injury. Arch Orthop Trauma Surg 2012;132(7):905–19.
17. Jana M, Srivastava DN, Sharma R, et al. Magnetic resonance arthrography for assessing severity of glenohumeral labroligamentous lesions. J Orthop Surg 2012;20(2):230–5.

18. Dunham KS, Bencardino JT, Rokito AS. Anatomic variants and pitfalls of the labrum, glenoid cartilage, and glenohumeral ligaments. Magn Reson Imaging Clin North Am 2012;20(2):213.
19. Murray PJ, Shaffer BS. Clinical update: MR imaging of the shoulder. Sports Med Arthrosc Rev 2009;17(1):40–8.
20. Morag Y, Bedi A, Jamadar DA. The rotator interval and long head biceps tendon: anatomy, function, pathology, and magnetic resonance imaging. Magn Reson Imaging Clin North Am 2012;20(2):229–59.
21. Sandhu B, Sanghavi S, Lam F. Superior labrum anterior to posterior (SLAP) lesions of the shoulder. Orthop Trauma 2011;25(3):190–7.
22. Goh CK, Peh WC. Pictorial essay: pitfalls in magnetic resonance imaging of the shoulder. Can Assoc Radiol J 2012;63(4):247–59.
23. Cook TS, Stein JM, Simonson S, et al. Normal and variant anatomy of the shoulder on MRI. Magn Reson Imaging Clin North Am 2011;19(3):581.
24. Polster JM, Schickendantz MS. Shoulder MRI: what do we miss? AJR Am J Roentgenol 2010;195(3):577–84.
25. Farber AJ, Khanna AJ, Fayad LM, et al. The shoulder. In: Khanna AJ, editor. MRI for orthopaedic surgeons. New York: Thieme; 2010. p. 97–117.
26. Chung CB, Steinbach LS. Long bicipital tendon including superior labral anterior-posterior lesions. In: Chung CB, Steinbach LS, editors. MRI of the upper extremity: shoulder, elbow, wrist and hand. Philadelphia: Wolters Kluwer Health/Lippincott Williams & Wilkins; 2010. p. 320–45.
27. Helms CA. Shoulder. In: Helms CA, editor. Musculoskeletal MRI. Philadelphia: Saunders/Elsevier; 2009. p. 177–223.
28. Rockwood CA, Matsen FA, Wirth MA. The shoulder, vol. 1. Philadelphia: WB Saunders; 2009.
29. Cooper DE, Arnoczky SP, O'Brien SJ, et al. Anatomy, histology, and vascularity of the glenoid labrum. An anatomical study. J Bone Joint Surg Am 1992;74(1):46–52.
30. Howell SM, Galinat BJ. The glenoid-labral socket. A constrained articular surface. Clin Orthop Relat Res 1989;(243):122–5.
31. Soslowsky LJ, Flatow EL, Bigliani LU, et al. Quantitation of in situ contact areas at the glenohumeral joint: a biomechanical study. J Orthop Res 1992;10(4):524–34.
32. Smith C, Funk L. The glenoid labrum. Shoulder Elbow 2010;2(2):87–93.
33. Stoller DW. Magnetic resonance imaging in orthopaedics and sports medicine, vol. 1. Philadelphia: Lippincott Williams & Wilkins; 2006.
34. De Maeseneer M, Van Roy P, Shahabpour M. Normal MR imaging anatomy of the rotator cuff tendons, glenoid fossa, labrum, and ligaments of the shoulder. Radiol Clin North Am 2006;44(4):479–87, vii.
35. Park YH, Lee JY, Moon SH, et al. MR arthrography of the labral capsular ligamentous complex in the shoulder: imaging variations and pitfalls. AJR Am J Roentgenol 2000;175(3):667–72.
36. McCauley TR, Pope CF, Jokl P. Normal and abnormal glenoid labrum: assessment with multiplanar gradient-echo MR imaging. Radiology 1992;183(1):35–7.
37. Zanetti M, Carstensen T, Weishaupt D, et al. MR arthrographic variability of the arthroscopically normal glenoid labrum: qualitative and quantitative assessment. Eur Radiol 2001;11(4):559–66.
38. Chang D, Mohana-Borges A, Borso M, et al. SLAP lesions: anatomy, clinical presentation, MR imaging diagnosis and characterization. Eur J Radiol 2008;68(1):72–87.

39. Mohana-Borges AV, Chung CB, Resnick D. Superior labral anteroposterior tear: classification and diagnosis on MRI and MR arthrography. AJR Am J Roentgenol 2003;181(6):1449–62.
40. Chaipat L, Palmer WE. Shoulder magnetic resonance imaging. Clin Sports Med 2006;25(3):371–86, v.
41. Lin E. Magnetic resonance arthrography of superior labrum anterior-posterior lesions: a practical approach to interpretation. Curr Probl Diagn Radiol 2009; 38(2):91–7.
42. Williams MM, Snyder SJ, Buford D Jr. The Buford complex–the "cord-like" middle glenohumeral ligament and absent anterosuperior labrum complex: a normal anatomic capsulolabral variant. Arthroscopy 1994;10(3):241–7.
43. Ilahi OA, Cosculluela PE, Ho DM. Classification of anterosuperior glenoid labrum variants and their association with shoulder pathology. Orthopedics 2008;31(3): 226.
44. Bencardino JT, Beltran J. MR imaging of the glenohumeral ligaments. Radiol Clin North Am 2006;44(4):489–502, vii.
45. Bents RT, Skeete KD. The correlation of the Buford complex and SLAP lesions. J Shoulder Elbow Surg 2005;14(6):565–9.
46. Ilahi OA, Labbe MR, Cosculluela P. Variants of the anterosuperior glenoid labrum and associated pathology. Arthroscopy 2002;18(8):882–6.
47. Crockett HC, Wingert NC, Wright JM, et al. Repair of SLAP lesions associated with a Buford complex: a novel surgical technique. Arthroscopy 2011;27(3): 314–21.
48. Rao AG, Kim TK, Chronopoulos E, et al. Anatomical variants in the anterosuperior aspect of the glenoid labrum: a statistical analysis of seventy-three cases. J Bone Joint Surg Am 2003;85-A(4):653–9.
49. del Rey FC, Vazquez DG, Lopez DN. Glenohumeral instability associated with Buford complex. Knee Surg Sports Traumatol Arthrosc 2009;17(12):1489–92.
50. Tuite MJ, Blankenbaker DG, Seifert M, et al. Sublabral foramen and Buford complex: inferior extent of the unattached or absent labrum in 50 patients. Radiology 2002;223(1):137–42.
51. Davidson PA, Rivenburgh DW. Mobile superior glenoid labrum: a normal variant or pathologic condition? Am J Sports Med 2004;32(4):962–6.
52. Lee SB, Harryman DT 2nd. Superior detachment of a glenoid labrum variant resembling an incomplete discoid meniscus in a wheelchair ambulator. Arthroscopy 1997;13(4):511–4.
53. O'Brien SJ, Arnoczky SP, Warren RF. Developmental anatomy of the shoulder and anatomy of the glenohumeral joint. In: Rockwood CA, Matsen FA, editors. The shoulder. Philadelphia: Saunders; 1990. p. 1–33.
54. Kreitner KF, Botchen K, Rude J, et al. Superior labrum and labral-bicipital complex: MR imaging with pathologic-anatomic and histologic correlation. AJR Am J Roentgenol 1998;170(3):599–605.
55. Smith DK, Chopp TM, Aufdemorte TB, et al. Sublabral recess of the superior glenoid labrum: study of cadavers with conventional nonenhanced MR imaging, MR arthrography, anatomic dissection, and limited histologic examination. Radiology 1996;201(1):251–6.
56. Waldt S, Metz S, Burkart A, et al. Variants of the superior labrum and labrobicipital complex: a comparative study of shoulder specimens using MR arthrography, multi-slice CT arthrography and anatomical dissection. Eur Radiol 2006;16(2):451–8.

57. Tuite MJ, Orwin JF. Anterosuperior labral variants of the shoulder: appearance on gradient-recalled-echo and fast spin-echo MR images. Radiology 1996; 199(2):537–40.

58. Modarresi S, Motamedi D, Jude CM. Superior labral anteroposterior lesions of the shoulder: part 2, mechanisms and classification. AJR Am J Roentgenol 2011;197(3):604–11.

59. Jin W, Ryu KN, Kwon SH, et al. MR arthrography in the differential diagnosis of type II superior labral anteroposterior lesion and sublabral recess. AJR Am J Roentgenol 2006;187(4):887–93.

60. Tuite MJ, Rutkowski A, Enright T, et al. Width of high signal and extension posterior to biceps tendon as signs of superior labrum anterior to posterior tears on MRI and MR arthrography. AJR Am J Roentgenol 2005;185(6):1422–8.

61. Burkhart SS, Morgan CD, Kibler WB. The disabled throwing shoulder: spectrum of pathology. Part II: evaluation and treatment of SLAP lesions in throwers. Arthroscopy 2003;19(5):531–9.

62. Tena-Arregui J, Barrio-Asensio C, Puerta-Fonolla J, et al. Arthroscopic study of the shoulder joint in fetuses. Arthroscopy 2005;21(9):1114–9.

63. Snyder SJ, Banas MP, Karzel RP. An analysis of 140 injuries to the superior glenoid labrum. J Shoulder Elbow Surg 1995;4(4):243–8.

64. Lee GY, Choi JA, Oh JH, et al. Posteroinferior labral cleft at direct CT arthrography of the shoulder by using multidetector CT: is this a normal variant? Radiology 2009;253(3):765–70.

65. Tuite MJ, Currie JW, Orwin JF, et al. Sublabral clefts and recesses in the anterior, inferior, and posterior glenoid labrum at MR arthrography. Skeletal Radiol 2013; 42(3):353–62.

66. Stoller DW. MR arthrography of the glenohumeral joint. Radiol Clin North Am 1997;35(1):97–116.

67. Kanatli U, Ozturk BY, Bolukbasi S. Anatomical variations of the anterosuperior labrum: prevalence and association with type II superior labrum anterior-posterior (SLAP) lesions. J Shoulder Elbow Surg 2010;19(8):1199–203.

68. Yu D, Turmezei T, Kerslake R. FIESTA: an MR arthrography celebration of shoulder joint anatomy, variants, and their mimics. Clin Anat 2013;26(2):213–27.

69. Ide J, Maeda S, Takagi K. Normal variations of the glenohumeral ligament complex: an anatomic study for arthroscopic Bankart repair. Arthroscopy 2004; 20(2):164–8.

70. Bain GI, Galley IJ, Singh C, et al. Anatomic study of the superior glenoid labrum. Clin Anat 2013;26(3):367–76.

71. Snyder SJ, Karzel RP, Del Pizzo W, et al. SLAP lesions of the shoulder. Arthroscopy 1990;6(4):274–9.

72. Yoneda M, Nakagawa S, Mizuno N, et al. Arthroscopic capsular release for painful throwing shoulder with posterior capsular tightness. Arthroscopy 2006;22(7): 801.e1–5.

73. Burkhart SS, Sanders TG, Denard PJ, et al. MRI and arthroscopy correlations of the shoulder: a case-based approach. Instr Course Lect 2012;61:185–200.

74. Kaplan K, Sahajpal DT, Jazrawi L. Loose bodies in a sublabral recess: diagnosis and treatment. Bull Hosp Jt Dis 2006;63(3–4):161–5.

75. Ramirez Ruiz FA, Baranski Kaniak BC, Haghighi P, et al. High origin of the anterior band of the inferior glenohumeral ligament: MR arthrography with anatomic and histologic correlation in cadavers. Skeletal Radiol 2012;41(5):525–30.

76. Kask K, Poldoja E, Lont T, et al. Anatomy of the superior glenohumeral ligament. J Shoulder Elbow Surg 2010;19(6):908–16.

77. Burkart AC, Debski RE. Anatomy and function of the glenohumeral ligaments in anterior shoulder instability. Clin Orthop Relat Res 2002;(400):32–9.
78. Kolts I, Busch LC, Tomusk H, et al. Anatomical composition of the anterior shoulder joint capsule. A cadaver study on 12 glenohumeral joints. Ann Anat 2001; 183(1):53–9.
79. Hunt SA, Kwon YW, Zuckerman JD. The rotator interval: anatomy, pathology, and strategies for treatment. J Am Acad Orthop Surg 2007;15(4): 218–27.
80. Arai R, Mochizuki T, Yamaguchi K, et al. Functional anatomy of the superior glenohumeral and coracohumeral ligaments and the subscapularis tendon in view of stabilization of the long head of the biceps tendon. J Shoulder Elbow Surg 2010;19(1):58–64.
81. Palmer WE, Brown JH, Rosenthal DI. Labral-ligamentous complex of the shoulder: evaluation with MR arthrography. Radiology 1994;190(3):645–51.
82. Steinbeck J, Liljenqvist U, Jerosch J. The anatomy of the glenohumeral ligamentous complex and its contribution to anterior shoulder stability. J Shoulder Elbow Surg 1998;7(2):122–6.
83. Sanders TG, Tirman PF, Linares R, et al. The glenolabral articular disruption lesion: MR arthrography with arthroscopic correlation. AJR Am J Roentgenol 1999;172(1):171–5.
84. Yeh L, Kwak S, Kim YS, et al. Anterior labroligamentous structures of the glenohumeral joint: correlation of MR arthrography and anatomic dissection in cadavers. AJR Am J Roentgenol 1998;171(5):1229–36.
85. Petchprapa CN, Beltran LS, Jazrawi LM, et al. The rotator interval: a review of anatomy, function, and normal and abnormal MRI appearance. AJR Am J Roentgenol 2010;195(3):567–76.
86. O'Connell PW, Nuber GW, Mileski RA, et al. The contribution of the glenohumeral ligaments to anterior stability of the shoulder joint. Am J Sports Med 1990;18(6): 579–84.
87. Beltran J, Bencardino J, Mellado J, et al. MR arthrography of the shoulder: variants and pitfalls. Radiographics 1997;17(6):1403–12 [discussion: 1412–5].
88. Pradhan RL, Itoi E, Watanabe W, et al. A rare anatomic variant of the superior glenohumeral ligament. Arthroscopy 2001;17(1):E3.
89. Moseley HF, Overgaard B. The anterior capsular mechanism in recurrent anterior dislocation of the shoulder. J Bone Joint Surg Br 1962;44:913–27.
90. Beltran J, Bencardino J, Padron M, et al. The middle glenohumeral ligament: normal anatomy, variants and pathology. Skeletal Radiol 2002;31(5): 253–62.
91. Beltran J, Rosenberg ZS, Chandnani VP, et al. Glenohumeral instability: evaluation with MR arthrography. Radiographics 1997;17(3):657–73.
92. Kwak SM, Brown RR, Trudell D, et al. Glenohumeral joint: comparison of shoulder positions at MR arthrography. Radiology 1998;208(2):375–80.
93. Chandnani VP, Gagliardi JA, Murnane TG, et al. Glenohumeral ligaments and shoulder capsular mechanism: evaluation with MR arthrography. Radiology 1995;196(1):27–32.
94. O'Brien SJ, Neves MC, Arnoczky SP, et al. The anatomy and histology of the inferior glenohumeral ligament complex of the shoulder. Am J Sports Med 1990;18(5):449–56.
95. Itoigawa Y, Itoi E, Sakoma Y, et al. Attachment of the anteroinferior glenohumeral ligament-labrum complex to the glenoid: an anatomic study. Arthroscopy 2012; 28(11):1628–33.

96. Cvitanic O, Tirman PF, Feller JF, et al. Using abduction and external rotation of the shoulder to increase the sensitivity of MR arthrography in revealing tears of the anterior glenoid labrum. AJR Am J Roentgenol 1997;169(3):837–44.

97. Turkel SJ, Panio MW, Marshall JL, et al. Stabilizing mechanisms preventing anterior dislocation of the glenohumeral joint. J Bone Joint Surg Am 1981;63(8): 1208–17.

98. Yin B, Vella J, Levine WN. Arthroscopic alphabet soup: recognition of normal, normal variants, and pathology. Orthop Clin North Am 2010;41(3):297–308.

99. Delorme D. Die Hemmungsbänder des Schultergelenks und ihre Bedeutung für die Schulterluxationen. Archiv für Klin Chirurgie 1910;92:79–101 [in German].

100. Landsmeer JM, Meyers KA. The shoulder region exposed by anatomical dissection. Arch Chir Neerl 1959;11:274–96.

101. Merila M, Helio H, Busch LC, et al. The spiral glenohumeral ligament: an open and arthroscopic anatomy study. Arthroscopy 2008;24(11):1271–6.

102. Pouliart N, Somers K, Gagey O. Arthroscopic glenohumeral folds and microscopic glenohumeral ligaments: the fasciculus obliquus is the missing link. J Shoulder Elbow Surg 2008;17(3):418–30.

103. Huber WP, Putz RV. Periarticular fiber system of the shoulder joint. Arthroscopy 1997;13(6):680–91.

104. Gaskill TR, Braun S, Millett PJ. Multimedia article. The rotator interval: pathology and management. Arthroscopy 2011;27(4):556–67.

105. Lee JC, Guy S, Connell D, et al. MRI of the rotator interval of the shoulder. Clin Radiol 2007;62(5):416–23.

106. Cooper DE, O'Brien SJ, Warren RF. Supporting layers of the glenohumeral joint. An anatomic study. Clin Orthop Relat Res 1993;(289):144–55.

107. Yang HF, Tang KL, Chen W, et al. An anatomic and histologic study of the coracohumeral ligament. J Shoulder Elbow Surg 2009;18(2):305–10.

108. Arai R, Kobayashi M, Toda Y, et al. Fiber components of the shoulder superior labrum. Surg Radiol Anat 2012;34(1):49–56.

109. Ahrens PM, Boileau P. The long head of biceps and associated tendinopathy. J Bone Joint Surg Br 2007;89(8):1001–9.

110. Wahl CJ, MacGillivray JD. Three congenital variations in the long head of the biceps tendon: a review of pathoanatomic considerations and case reports. J Shoulder Elbow Surg 2007;16(6):e25–30.

111. Lee SE, Jung C, Ahn KY, et al. Bilateral asymmetric supernumerary heads of biceps brachii. Anat Cell Biol 2011;44(3):238–40.

112. Kim KC, Rhee KJ, Shin HD. A long head of the biceps tendon confluent with the intra-articular rotator cuff: arthroscopic and MR arthrographic findings. Arch Orthop Trauma Surg 2009;129(3):311–4.

113. Kanatli U, Ozturk BY, Esen E, et al. Intra-articular variations of the long head of the biceps tendon. Knee Surg Sports Traumatol Arthrosc 2011;19(9): 1576–81.

114. Gheno R, Zoner CS, Buck FM, et al. Accessory head of biceps brachii muscle: anatomy, histology, and MRI in cadavers. AJR Am J Roentgenol 2010;194(1): W80–3.

115. Gaskin CM, Golish SR, Blount KJ, et al. Anomalies of the long head of the biceps brachii tendon: clinical significance, MR arthrographic findings, and arthroscopic correlation in two patients. Skeletal Radiol 2007;36(8):785–9.

116. Dierickx C, Ceccarelli E, Conti M, et al. Variations of the intra-articular portion of the long head of the biceps tendon: a classification of embryologically explained variations. J Shoulder Elbow Surg 2009;18(4):556–65.

117. Franco JC, Knapp TP, Mandelbaum BR. Congenital absence of the long head of the biceps tendon. A case report. J Bone Joint Surg Am 2005;87(7): 1584–6.

118. Koplas MC, Winalski CS, Ulmer WH Jr, et al. Bilateral congenital absence of the long head of the biceps tendon. Skeletal Radiol 2009;38(7):715–9.

119. Kuhn KM, Carney J, Solomon D, et al. Bilateral absence of the long head of the biceps tendon. Mil Med 2009;174(5):548–50.

120. Georgiev GP, Jelev L. Bilateral hypoplasia of the long head of the biceps brachii muscle. Int J Shoulder Surg 2011;5(1):26–7.

121. Kim RS, Won MH, Lee TJ, et al. Aberrant branch of the long head of the biceps tendon. J Shoulder Elbow Surg 2011;20(4):e22–5.

122. Wittstein J, Lassiter T Jr, Taylor D. Aberrant origin of the long head of the biceps: a case series. J Shoulder Elbow Surg 2012;21(3):356–60.

123. Audenaert EA, Barbaix EJ, Van Hoonacker P, et al. Extraarticular variants of the long head of the biceps brachii: a reminder of embryology. J Shoulder Elbow Surg 2008;17(Suppl 1):114S–7S.

124. Parikh SN, Bonnaig N, Zbojniewicz A. Intracapsular origin of the long head of the biceps tendon with glenoid avulsion of the glenohumeral ligaments. Orthopedics 2011;34(11):e781–4.

125. Richards DP, Schwartz M. Anomalous intraarticular origin of the long head of biceps brachii. Clin J Sport Med 2003;13(2):122–4.

126. Giphart JE, Elser F, Dewing CB, et al. The long head of the biceps tendon has minimal effect on in vivo glenohumeral kinematics: a biplane fluoroscopy study. Am J Sports Med 2012;40(1):202–12.

127. Levy AS, Kelly BT, Lintner SA, et al. Function of the long head of the biceps at the shoulder: electromyographic analysis. J Shoulder Elbow Surg 2001;10(3): 250–5.

128. Pagnani MJ, Deng XH, Warren RF, et al. Effect of lesions of the superior portion of the glenoid labrum on glenohumeral translation. J Bone Joint Surg Am 1995; 77(7):1003–10.

129. Rodosky MW, Harner CD, Fu FH. The role of the long head of the biceps muscle and superior glenoid labrum in anterior stability of the shoulder. Am J Sports Med 1994;22(1):121–30.

130. Kido T, Itoi E, Konno N, et al. The depressor function of biceps on the head of the humerus in shoulders with tears of the rotator cuff. J Bone Joint Surg Br 2000;82(3):416–9.

131. Youm T, ElAttrache NS, Tibone JE, et al. The effect of the long head of the biceps on glenohumeral kinematics. J Shoulder Elbow Surg 2009;18(1):122–9.

132. Bankart AS. Recurrent or habitual dislocation of the shoulder joint. Br Med J 1923;2:1132–3.

133. Neviaser TJ. The anterior labroligamentous periosteal sleeve avulsion lesion: a cause of anterior instability of the shoulder. Arthroscopy 1993;9(1):17–21.

134. Wischer TK, Bredella MA, Genant HK, et al. Perthes lesion (a variant of the Bankart lesion): MR imaging and MR arthrographic findings with surgical correlation. AJR Am J Roentgenol 2002;178(1):233–7.

135. Andrews JR, Carson WG. The arthroscopic treatment of glenoid labrum tears in the throwing athlete. Orthopedic Transactions 1984;8:44.

136. Andrews JR, Carson WG Jr, McLeod WD. Glenoid labrum tears related to the long head of the biceps. Am J Sports Med 1985;13(5):337–41.

137. Neviaser TJ. The GLAD lesion: another cause of anterior shoulder pain. Arthroscopy 1993;9(1):22–3.

138. Waldt S, Burkart A, Imhoff AB, et al. Anterior shoulder instability: accuracy of MR arthrography in the classification of anteroinferior labroligamentous injuries. Radiology 2005;237(2):578–83.

139. Ozbaydar M, Elhassan B, Diller D, et al. Results of arthroscopic capsulolabral repair: Bankart lesion versus anterior labroligamentous periosteal sleeve avulsion lesion. Arthroscopy 2008;24(11):1277–83.

140. Macmahon PJ, Palmer WE. Magnetic resonance imaging in glenohumeral instability. Magn Reson Imaging Clin North Am 2012;20(2):295–312.

141. Law BK, Yung PS, Ho EP, et al. The surgical outcome of immediate arthroscopic Bankart repair for first time anterior shoulder dislocation in young active patients. Knee Surg Sports Traumatol Arthrosc 2008;16(2):188–93.

142. Lee BG, Cho NS, Rhee YG. Anterior labroligamentous periosteal sleeve avulsion lesion in arthroscopic capsulolabral repair for anterior shoulder instability. Knee Surg Sports Traumatol Arthrosc 2011;19(9):1563–9.

143. Antonio GE, Griffith JF, Yu AB, et al. First-time shoulder dislocation: high prevalence of labral injury and age-related differences revealed by MR arthrography. J Magn Reson Imaging 2007;26(4):983–91.

144. Yu JS, Ashman CJ, Jones G. The POLPSA lesion: MR imaging findings with arthroscopic correlation in patients with posterior instability. Skeletal Radiol 2002;31(7):396–9.

145. Tian CY, Cui GQ, Zheng ZZ, et al. The added value of ABER position for the detection and classification of anteroinferior labroligamentous lesions in MR arthrography of the shoulder. Eur J Radiol 2013;82(4):651–7.

146. Iyengar JJ, Burnett KR, Nottage WM, et al. The abduction external rotation (ABER) view for MRI of the shoulder. Orthopedics 2010;33(8):562–5.

147. Herold T, Hente R, Zorger N, et al. Indirect MR-arthrography of the shoulder– value in the detection of SLAP-lesions. Rofo 2003;175(11):1508–14 [in German].

148. Walsworth MK, Doukas WC, Murphy KP, et al. Reliability and diagnostic accuracy of history and physical examination for diagnosing glenoid labral tears. Am J Sports Med 2008;36(1):162–8.

149. Jones GL, Galluch DB. Clinical assessment of superior glenoid labral lesions: a systematic review. Clin Orthop Relat Res 2007;455:45–51.

150. Handelberg F, Willems S, Shahabpour M, et al. SLAP lesions: a retrospective multicenter study. Arthroscopy 1998;14(8):856–62.

151. Maffet MW, Gartsman GM, Moseley B. Superior labrum-biceps tendon complex lesions of the shoulder. Am J Sports Med 1995;23(1):93–8.

152. Gobezie R, Zurakowski D, Lavery K, et al. Analysis of interobserver and intraobserver variability in the diagnosis and treatment of SLAP tears using the Snyder classification. Am J Sports Med 2008;36(7):1373–9.

153. O'Brien J, Grebenyuk J, Leith J, et al. Frequency of glenoid chondral lesions on MR arthrography in patients with anterior shoulder instability. Eur J Radiol 2012; 81(11):3461–5.

154. Robinson G, Ho Y, Finlay K, et al. Normal anatomy and common labral lesions at MR arthrography of the shoulder. Clin Radiol 2006;61(10):805–21.

155. Lozano Calderon SA, Maldjian C, Magill RM. Paralabral "air" cyst of the shoulder. Am J Orthop (Belle Mead NJ) 2009;38(6):E107–9.

156. Ji JH, Shafi M, Lee YS, et al. Inferior paralabral ganglion cyst of the shoulder with labral tear–a rare cause of shoulder pain. Orthop Traumatol Surg Res 2012; 98(2):193–8.

157. Kessler MA, Stoffel K, Oswald A, et al. The SLAP lesion as a reason for glenolabral cysts: a report of five cases and review of the literature. Arch Orthop Trauma Surg 2007;127(4):287–92.

158. Demeter M, Vankan Y, Demeyere A, et al. Supralabral air on plain radiography of the shoulder: first sign of an air-containing paralabral cyst. JBR-BTR 2012;95(2):104.

159. Bencardino JT, Beltran J, Rosenberg ZS, et al. Superior labrum anterior-posterior lesions: diagnosis with MR arthrography of the shoulder. Radiology 2000;214(1):267–71.

160. Amin MF, Youssef AO. The diagnostic value of magnetic resonance arthrography of the shoulder in detection and grading of SLAP lesions: comparison with arthroscopic findings. Eur J Radiol 2012;81(9):2343–7.

161. Magee T. 3-T MRI of the shoulder: is MR arthrography necessary? AJR Am J Roentgenol 2009;192(1):86–92.

162. Major NM, Browne J, Domzalski T, et al. Evaluation of the glenoid labrum with 3-T MRI: is intraarticular contrast necessary? AJR Am J Roentgenol 2011;196(5):1139–44.

163. Reuss BL, Schwartzberg R, Zlatkin MB, et al. Magnetic resonance imaging accuracy for the diagnosis of superior labrum anterior-posterior lesions in the community setting: eighty-three arthroscopically confirmed cases. J Shoulder Elbow Surg 2006;15(5):580–5.

164. Schreinemachers SA, van der Hulst VP, Jaap Willems W, et al. Is a single direct MR arthrography series in ABER position as accurate in detecting anteroinferior labroligamentous lesions as conventional MR arthography? Skeletal Radiol 2009;38(7):675–83.

165. Jung JY, Ha DH, Lee SM, et al. Displaceability of SLAP lesion on shoulder MR arthrography with external rotation position. Skeletal Radiol 2011;40(8):1047–55.

166. Chiavaras MM, Harish S, Burr J. MR arthrographic assessment of suspected posteroinferior labral lesions using flexion, adduction, and internal rotation positioning of the arm: preliminary experience. Skeletal Radiol 2010;39(5):481–8.

167. Song HT, Huh YM, Kim S, et al. Anterior-inferior labral lesions of recurrent shoulder dislocation evaluated by MR arthrography in an adduction internal rotation (ADIR) position. J Magn Reson Imaging 2006;23(1):29–35.

168. Acid S, Le Corroller T, Aswad R, et al. Preoperative imaging of anterior shoulder instability: diagnostic effectiveness of MDCT arthrography and comparison with MR arthrography and arthroscopy. AJR Am J Roentgenol 2012;198(3):661–7.

169. Kim YJ, Choi JA, Oh JH, et al. Superior labral anteroposterior tears: accuracy and interobserver reliability of multidetector CT arthrography for diagnosis. Radiology 2011;260(1):207–15.

170. Oh JH, Kim JY, Choi JA, et al. Effectiveness of multidetector computed tomography arthrography for the diagnosis of shoulder pathology: comparison with magnetic resonance imaging with arthroscopic correlation. J Shoulder Elbow Surg 2010;19(1):14–20.

171. Choi JY, Kim SH, Yoo HJ, et al. Superior labral anterior-to-posterior lesions: comparison of external rotation and active supination CT arthrography with neutral CT arthrography. Radiology 2012;263(1):199–205.

172. Huijsmans PE, de Witte PB, de Villiers RV, et al. Recurrent anterior shoulder instability: accuracy of estimations of glenoid bone loss with computed tomography is insufficient for therapeutic decision-making. Skeletal Radiol 2011;40(10):1329–34.

173. Fritz J, Fishman EK, Small KM, et al. MDCT arthrography of the shoulder with datasets of isotropic resolution: indications, technique, and applications. AJR Am J Roentgenol 2012;198(3):635–46.
174. Elser F, Braun S, Dewing CB, et al. Anatomy, function, injuries, and treatment of the long head of the biceps brachii tendon. Arthroscopy 2011;27(4):581–92.
175. Nakata W, Katou S, Fujita A, et al. Biceps pulley: normal anatomy and associated lesions at MR arthrography. Radiographics 2011;31(3):791–810.
176. Bennett WF. Arthroscopic repair of anterosuperior (supraspinatus/subscapularis) rotator cuff tears: a prospective cohort with 2- to 4-year follow-up. Classification of biceps subluxation/instability. Arthroscopy 2003;19(1):21–33.
177. Baumann B, Genning K, Bohm D, et al. Arthroscopic prevalence of pulley lesions in 1007 consecutive patients. J Shoulder Elbow Surg 2008;17(1):14–20.
178. Braun S, Horan MP, Elser F, et al. Lesions of the biceps pulley. Am J Sports Med 2011;39(4):790–5.
179. Weishaupt D, Zanetti M, Tanner A, et al. Lesions of the reflection pulley of the long biceps tendon. MR arthrographic findings. Invest Radiol 1999;34(7):463–9.

Ultrasonography of the Shoulder with Arthroscopic Correlation

Corrie M. Yablon, MD[a],*, Asheesh Bedi, MD[b], Yoav Morag, MD[a],
Jon A. Jacobson, MD[a]

KEYWORDS

- Shoulder ultrasonography • Internal impingement • Rotator cuff tears
- Dynamic ultrasound imaging • Long head biceps brachii injury

KEY POINTS

- Ultrasonography and magnetic resonance imaging have equally high sensitivity and specificity for the diagnosis of both partial-thickness and full-thickness rotator cuff tears.
- Dynamic imaging is helpful for the confirmation of rotator cuff tears and for the diagnosis of impingement and biceps brachii tendon subluxation/dislocation.
- Ultrasonography has high accuracy for the diagnosis of biceps brachii tendon tears but is less sensitive for the detection of partial tendon tears.
- Familiarity with sonographic diagnostic pitfalls can improve the diagnostic accuracy of rotator cuff and biceps brachii injuries.

INTRODUCTION

Ultrasonography (US) of the shoulder has gained wide acceptance as a useful, versatile method of evaluating soft tissue injuries about the shoulder. The diagnostic accuracy of US in the evaluation of rotator cuff tears is comparable with magnetic resonance imaging (MRI) and yields a high correlation to arthroscopy, generating sensitivity and specificity up to 95% in the hands of experienced practitioners.[1-4]

The benefits of the US modality are manifest. Any patient may have a US examination. The modality is not limited by a patient's body habitus, as opposed to MRI. US is an excellent way to evaluate patients who are not candidates for MRI, including those patients who are claustrophobic, cannot lie flat, or who have implanted devices not compatible with the magnetized environment. Recently developed high-frequency transducers provide images of the rotator cuff with spatial resolution exceeding that of MRI.[5]

a Department of Radiology, University of Michigan, 1500 East Medical Center Drive, Ann Arbor, MI 48109, USA; b MedSport, Department of Orthopaedic Surgery, University of Michigan, 24 Frank Lloyd Wright Drive, Ann Arbor, MI 48109, USA
* Corresponding author.
E-mail address: cyablon@umich.edu

Clin Sports Med 32 (2013) 391–408
http://dx.doi.org/10.1016/j.csm.2013.03.001
0278-5919/13/$ – see front matter © 2013 Elsevier Inc. All rights reserved.

As US is performed in real time, the operator can receive direct feedback from the patient during scanning and on sonopalpation, allowing correlation of the site of pain to simultaneous imaging findings. The dynamic nature of US imaging offers versatility that is not at this time achievable with routine MRI. Using dynamic compression, the integrity of the rotator cuff can be assessed in great detail. Ranging the patient through motion either actively or passively can also provide valuable feedback regarding function and impingement. Comparison with the contralateral side is often used in US when pathology is in question. US is particularly helpful in the assessment of the post-operative rotator cuff, where metallic susceptibility artifact is not an issue, as it is with MRI.[6]

The major strength of US imaging of the shoulder is the ability to evaluate superficial tendons and soft tissues with a high degree of resolution, including the rotator cuff and muscles, and concomitant pathology of the biceps brachii tendon, acromioclavicular joint, and subacromial-subdeltoid (SASD) bursa. US should not be used for the evaluation of osseous structures, because of the inability of the sound beam to penetrate through the bone. In addition, US examination does not visualize deep structures such as the glenoid labrum in its entirety; the posterior labrum is the only aspect of the labrum that can be reliably seen on US. US should be viewed as complementary to MRI when the pathology being evaluated relates to the rotator cuff. MRI is preferred when labral and ligamentous injuries are suspected, or when underlying osseous pathology is a concern.

THE ROTATOR CUFF

Rotator cuff evaluation is the most common clinical indication for US of the shoulder. US has similar accuracy to MRI in diagnosing both full-thickness and partial-thickness tears of the rotator cuff compared with the gold standard of arthroscopy.[1,7,8] Many studies have been published regarding the accuracy of US versus MRI and its ability to detect full-thickness tears and partial-thickness tears. US has been reported to have a sensitivity of 57% to 100% and a specificity of 41% to 100% in the detection of full-thickness tears, and a sensitivity of 41% to 94% and specificity of 85% to 94% in the detection of partial-thickness tears.[1,4,7,9–13] Close inspection of the literature reveals that the studies with lower sensitivities and specificities used older equipment with low frequency transducers, or involved less experienced operators performing the US examinations. A meta-analysis of the literature in 2009 showed no significant difference in sensitivity or specificity between US and MRI in the diagnosis of partial-thickness or full-thickness rotator cuff tears.[14]

The rotator cuff tendon that most commonly shows degeneration or tear is the supraspinatus.[6,15] In an analysis of 360 shoulders to assess for the most common location of degenerative supraspinatus tears, Kim and colleagues[16] demonstrated that 93% of all full-thickness tears and 89% of all small full-thickness tears were found to involve the posterior aspect of the supraspinatus, 13 to 17 mm from the biceps tendon. In addition, small partial tears were found to involve this area as well, suggesting that this may be a common site for tear initiation.

Normal Rotator Cuff Appearance

The protocol for US examination of the shoulder has been previously described and validated.[1,4,12,13,17–23] With the advent of high-frequency transducers and improved US scanners, it is now standard practice to evaluate the rotator cuff with at least a 12 to 5 MHz linear phased array transducer. If a patient is very large, a lower frequency transducer may be used. The normal rotator cuff tendons scanned in long axis parallel to the orientation of the tendon are echogenic structures with a fibrillar internal structure (**Fig. 1**).[24] The fibrillar appearance reflects the parallel echogenic tendon fascicles due to tightly packed collagen fibers.

In the short axis image, perpendicular to the orientation of the rotator cuff, the long head biceps brachii tendon (LHBT) is seen in cross section anteriorly as a hyperechoic ovoid structure between the supraspinatus and subscapularis tendons. The supraspinatus tendon in short axis is seen as a hyperechoic linear soft tissue structure extending 2.0 to 2.5 cm posterior to the LHBT and rotator interval (see **Fig. 1**). When scanning in the long axis plane from anterior to posterior, the transition of the supraspinatus to the infraspinatus is seen as a subtle overlap and directional change of the overlapping tendon fibers.[25] In the short axis, the anterior 1.3 cm of the cuff footprint (superior facet) is composed solely of supraspinatus fibers and the posterior 1.3 cm (middle facet) is composed of the supraspinatus and infraspinatus.[26] Subjacent to the rotator cuff, the humeral head cartilage appears as a thin, 1-mm hypoechoic linear stripe, beneath which is the well-defined hyperechoic linear humeral head cortex.

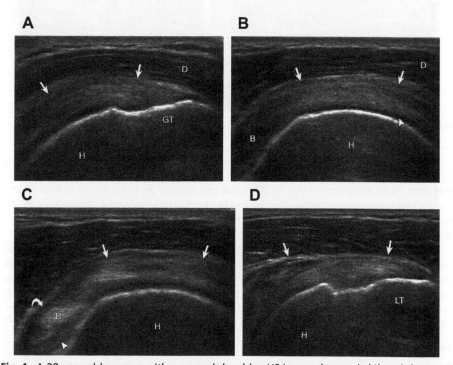

Fig. 1. A 38-year-old woman with a normal shoulder. US images long axis (*A*) and short axis (*B, C*) to the supraspinatus show the normal hyperechoic fibrillar appearance of supraspinatus tendon (*arrows*). Note the long head biceps brachii tendon (*B*) within the rotator interval, which is artifactually hypoechoic from anisotropy in (*B*) and corrected in (*C*) (D, deltoid muscle; H, humeral head; GT, greater tuberosity; *arrowhead* in (*B*), hyaline articular cartilage; *arrowhead* in (*C*), superior glenohumeral ligament; *curved arrow*, coracohumeral ligament). US images long axis (*D*) and short axis (*E*) to the subscapularis show hyperechoic multipennate tendon bundles (*arrows*) (H, humeral head; LT, lesser tuberosity). US images (*F, G*) show the long head biceps brachii tendon (*arrows*) in short axis (*F*) and long axis (*G*) (H, humerus; D, deltoid). US image (*H*) in the transverse plane over the posterior shoulder shows infraspinatus (I), humeral head (H), glenoid (G), deltoid (D), and posterior labrum (*curved arrow*).

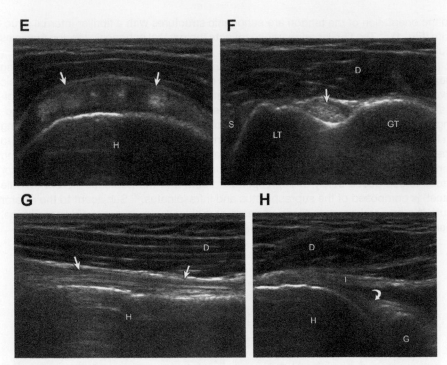

Fig. 1. (*continued*)

The normal SASD bursa appears as a linear hypoechoic structure surrounded by hyperechoic bursal walls and peribursal fat, which extends laterally beyond the tendon footprint. Fluid distention of the SASD bursa can appear as variable but with predominantly low echogenicity depending on the bursal fluid composition. Superficial to the SASD bursa, the normal hypoechoic deltoid muscle contains linear hyperechoic internal fibroadipose septations.

The normal rotator cable is seen sonographically in 99% of shoulders.[27] It has been described as the suspension bridge of the shoulder, and is believed to provide stress dispersal to the rotator cuff tendons and stability to the glenohumeral joint.[28] On long axis cuff images, the cable is seen in its short axis as a hyperechoic transversely oriented bundle of fibers running perpendicular and deep to the supraspinatus and infraspinatus tendons, located approximately 1 cm medial to the cuff footprint (**Fig. 2**).[27,29]

Tendinosis

Tendinosis or tendinopathy of the rotator cuff appears sonographically as hypoechoic heterogeneous thickening of the tendon, with loss of the normal fibrillar pattern[25,30] but without frank disruption of the tendon fibers (**Fig. 3**). Uncommonly, there may be increased color Doppler flow, representing hyperemia related to neovascularity and not true inflammation.[22,24] The use of the term tendinitis is therefore not appropriate as histologically there is tendon degeneration (mucoid, fibrillar, and eosinophilic) as well and chondroid metaplasia rather than active inflammation.[31,32] Tendinosis can be focal or diffuse. SASD bursal fluid may or may not be present in the case of tendinosis.

When a hypoechoic tendon is seen, it is important to assure that this appearance is not secondary to anisotropy, an artifact that is caused when the US beam hits a fibrillar

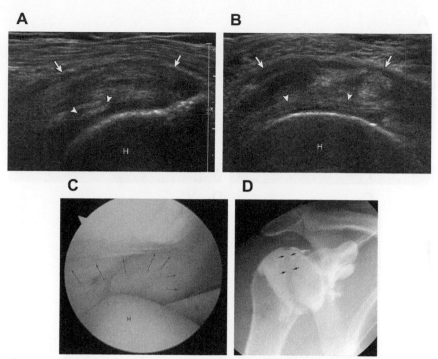

Fig. 2. A 70-year-old woman with a normal rotator cable. US images long axis (*A*) and short axis (*B*) to the supraspinatus tendon (*arrows*) show the rotator cable (*arrowheads*) (H, humeral head). Arthroscopy image (*C*) shows the contour of the rotator cable (*arrows*) (H, humeral head; B, long head biceps brachii tendon). Single contrast shoulder arthrogram image (*D*) shows a linear filling defect (*arrows*) representing impression of the rotator cable on the contrast column.

structure at an angle that is not perpendicular. Toggling the transducer from side to side to obtain a perpendicular angle eliminates anisotropy. If the hypoechoic appearance persists in 2 planes despite these maneuvers, then the finding is considered real. A tendon can demonstrate changes consistent with tendinosis, without concomitant tendon thickening.[30]

Full-Thickness Tears

Full-thickness tears extend through the substance of the tendon, from the articular to the bursal side, demonstrated by hypoechoic or anechoic fluid extending from the SASD bursa to the articular surface of the humerus. Full-thickness tears may involve only a portion of the tendon (partial width or focal), or the whole tendon (full width). Whatever the tendon tear morphology, it is important to document the size of the tendon defect in 2 planes or dimensions, which includes the degree of tendon retraction.

Focal full-thickness tears appear as hypoechoic or anechoic fluid-filled defects in the tendon. In the case of full-thickness, full-width, or complete tears of the supraspinatus and infraspinatus tendons, the tendon stump may retract proximally beneath the acromion, and thus the tendon stump may not be seen at all. In this instance, the degree of tendon retraction may be underestimated.[23] Cortical irregularity of the greater tuberosity at the supraspinatus tendon footprint and joint

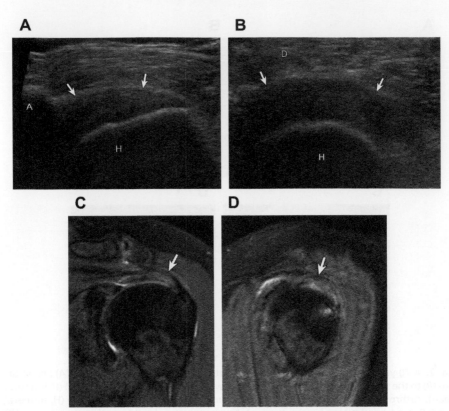

Fig. 3. A 66-year-old woman with supraspinatus tendinosis. US images (*A, B*) and fluid-sensitive MR images (*C, D*) long axis and short axis to the supraspinatus tendon, respectively, show diffuse hypoechoic tendon thickening on US (*arrows*) and mild increased signal on MRI (*arrows*) consistent with tendinosis (H, humeral head; A, acromion; D, deltoid).

effusion are often seen. Sonographically, joint effusion manifests as anechoic or hypoechoic fluid in the posterior recess, and fluid distending the biceps brachii tendon sheath.[12] The coincidental findings of cortical irregularity of the greater tuberosity and joint fluid together have been shown to have a 60% sensitivity and 100% specificity with 84% accuracy in the prediction of a full-thickness supraspinatus tendon tear.[12]

If a tear is acute, anechoic fluid is seen within the tendon defect (**Fig. 4**). There is volume loss at the site of the tear, and if the tear is large, the humeral head may migrate superiorly, abutting the undersurface of the deltoid muscle and acromion. If a tear is chronic, hyperechoic thickened synovial bursal tissue or granulation tissue may fill the tendon defect, obscure the tear, falsely giving the impression of preserved tendon volume. The use of dynamic graded compression can help to distinguish between intact tendon tissue and abnormal synovial or granulation tissue within the tendon defect.[33]

In the case of massive rotator cuff tendon tears, the acromiohumeral interval may be markedly diminished as a result of the loss of normal rotator cuff volume. The humeral head may be in contact with the acromion and deltoid and demonstrate subcortical cystic changes. In the short axis, the humeral head is devoid of overlying rotator

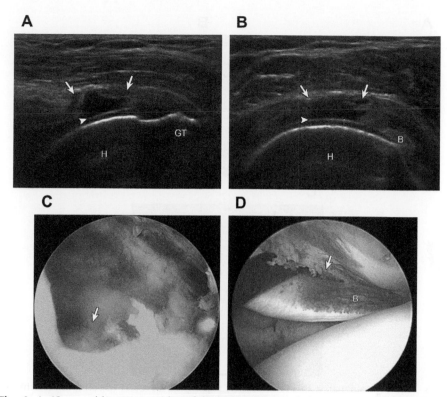

Fig. 4. A 48-year-old woman with a full-thickness tear of the supraspinatus (focal). US images short axis (*A*) and long axis (*B*) to the supraspinatus tendon show a focal full-thickness tendon tear (*arrows*). Note the linear echogenic line (*arrowhead*) over the surface of the humeral head articular hyaline cartilage (termed the cartilage interface sign) (H, humeral head; GT, greater tuberosity; B, long head biceps brachii tendon). Arthroscopy images (*C*) show the bursal side with a leading edge supraspinatus tendon tear (*arrow*) and the corresponding location from the articular side (*D*). Note the leading edge tear is associated with significant tenosynovitis of the biceps tendon (B).

cuff tendons and comes in direct contact with the SASD bursa and the deltoid muscle (**Fig. 5**). Chronic rotator cuff tears are often accompanied by fatty infiltration of the rotator cuff musculature and atrophy.

A frequent secondary sign of a rotator cuff tendon tear is the cartilage interface sign (see **Fig. 4**). This occurs when a fluid-filled tendon tear causes increased through transmission of the ultrasound beam, which causes the underlying cartilage surface to appear more hyperechoic than the adjacent cartilage.[25] Rotator cuff tendon tears exhibit focal volume loss and focal contour concavity. On dynamic compression, bursal fluid, the overlying deltoid muscle, and bursal fat can be displaced into the tendon gap.

Fatty atrophy may occur in the context of rotator cuff tears and the degree of fatty atrophy may be associated with the size and location of these tears.[34] US is effective for identifying fatty infiltration and atrophy of the rotator cuff musculature with an accuracy comparable with MRI.[35,36] Muscle atrophy is demonstrated on US as volume loss, increased echogenicity of the muscle, with an indistinct hazy border about the tendons.

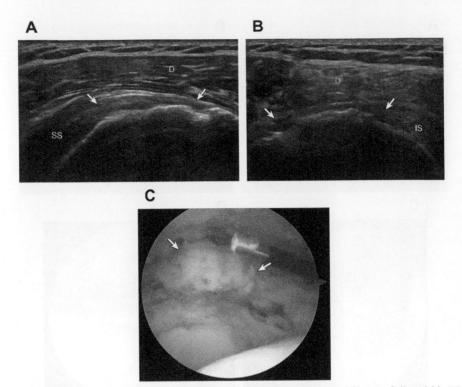

Fig. 5. A 49-year-old man with a full-thickness supraspinatus retear (chronic, full width). US images long axis (*A*) and short axis (*B*) to the supraspinatus (SS) show a retracted full-thickness tear (between *arrows*). Note the intact infraspinatus tendon (IST) (D, deltoid). Arthroscopy image (*C*) shows the retracted free edge of the supraspinatus tendon (*arrows*) resting medial to the glenoid. Note retained sutures from the previously failed repair.

Partial-Thickness Tears

The literature is discrepant with regard to the prevalence of partial tears of the rotator cuff. Partial tears occur in both older and young patients. In younger patients, tears are usually associated with trauma and overhead throwing sports. In patients more than 40 years of age, there is an age-related increased incidence of tendon degeneration, partial tears, and full-thickness tears.[37,38]

Cadaveric studies show a preponderance of partial-thickness tears arising within the supraspinatus tendon, the most dominant tear type being intrasubstance.[39,40] However, Payne and colleagues[41] demonstrated that in a patient cohort of young athletes, the most predominant partial tear type was articular-sided (91%).

US may be less accurate in the diagnosis of partial-thickness tears than of full-thickness tears.[21] However, both US and MRI are comparable for the diagnosis of partial-thickness tears with a sensitivity of greater than 97% and an accuracy of 87% compared with arthroscopy.[1] Other investigators have shown sensitivity of 93% to 94% and specificity of 94% to 95% in the diagnosis of partial-thickness rotator cuff tears.[4,42] In studies where partial tears were missed, most were found to be small grade I and grade II tears on arthroscopy for which the treatment is conservative management.[9,43] Difficulty has been reported in discriminating partial articular-sided tears from tendinosis, and differentiating high-grade partial tears from full-thickness tears on US.[23]

Partial tears are classified into several subtypes: articular-sided (**Fig. 6**), bursal-sided (**Fig. 7**), and intrasubstance or delaminating tears. Partial tears appear as a focal hypoechoic or anechoic gap, with focal disruption of the tendon architecture, either in direct contiguity with the SASD bursa in the case of partial bursal-sided tears, or with the articular cartilage in the case of partial articular-sided tears. Measurements of the tear should include both anteroposterior (measured in short axis) and transverse (measured in long axis) dimensions. The depth of tear conveyed as the percentage of the tendon thickness that is torn should also be reported. Subcortical cystic changes in the humeral head subjacent to partial articular-sided tears can also be seen on US.

A rim-rent tear is an articular-sided partial-thickness tear that specifically occurs at the undersurface of the supraspinatus immediately adjacent to its attachment on the greater tuberosity.[44,45] This type of tear is more frequently seen in younger patients and overhead or throwing athletes. The tear appears as an articular-sided anechoic or hypoechoic cleft within the distal aspect of the echogenic tendon at the tendon footprint on the greater tuberosity (see **Fig. 6**). There may be a small, linear echogenic focus area within the hypoechoic tear, believed to represent the underlying cartilage or torn tendon fiber. Similar to other supraspinatus tendon tears, a rim-rent tear may also

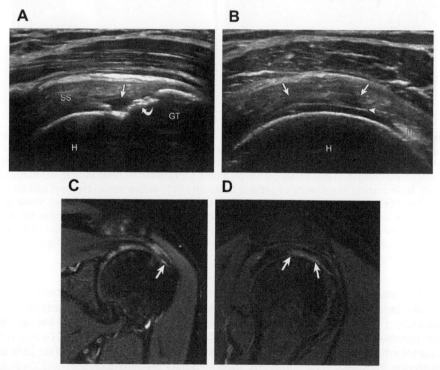

Fig. 6. A 46-year-old man with a partial-thickness supraspinatus tear (articular). US images (*A, B*) and fluid-sensitive MR images (*C, D*) long axis and short axis to the supraspinatus tendon (SS), respectively, show a diffuse anechoic tendon defect on US (*arrows*) and a fluid signal on MRI (*arrows*) consistent with an articular-sided partial-thickness (rim-rent) supraspinatus tear. There is adjacent supraspinatus tendinosis. Note (*A*) cortical irregularity at the supraspinatus tendon footprint (*curved arrow*) at the site of the tear most conspicuous on US, as well as (*B*) the cartilage interface sign (*arrowhead*) (H, humeral head; GT, greater tuberosity; B, long head biceps brachii tendon).

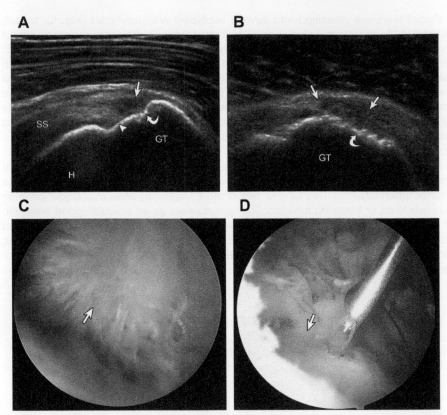

Fig. 7. A 62-year-old man with a partial-thickness supraspinatus tear (bursal). US images long axis (*A*) and short axis (*B*) to the supraspinatus tendon (SS) show an anechoic tendon defect (*arrow*) involving the bursal aspect of the tendon and partial uncovering of the footprint representing a bursal-sided partial-thickness supraspinatus tendon tear (H, humeral head). Note cortical irregularity of greater tuberosity (GT) at the site of the tear and intact articular fibers attaching to the footprint (*arrowhead*). Arthroscopy images show (*C*) abraded coracoacromial ligament (*arrow*) consistent with outlet impingement and secondary bursal-sided cuff injury, and (*D*) bursal-sided tear (*arrow*) secondary to outlet impingement with exposed lateral footprint. Spinal needle marks the location and trajectory for anchor placement for repair.

be associated with an underlying cortical irregularity of the greater tuberosity.[4,46] Articular-sided tears are sometimes accompanied by the cartilage interface sign, especially if fluid-filled.[12] A hypoechoic or anechoic cleft at the site of the tear is seen communicating with the articulating surface. Increasing attention has been given to partial articular-sided tears of the supraspinatus that are small, or less than 25% of the tendon thickness, as arthroscopic treatment may be beneficial.[41]

Intrasubstance tears can take several forms. The hallmark is that intrasubstance tears are concealed within the tendon without contacting either the bursal or articular tendon surface. An intrasubstance tear can be confined to the footprint of the tendon, appearing as a focal hypoechoic or anechoic defect within the footprint at the greater tuberosity, without contact with the articular surface or bursal surface. A delaminating intrasubstance tear appears as a linear, longitudinally oriented, anechoic or hypoechoic defect within the tendon itself. Delaminating tears may extend into the musculotendinous junction and may be associated with intratendinous or intramuscular cyst.[47]

Bursal-sided partial tears may become more conspicuous in that there will be bursal-sided volume loss, loss of definition of the bursal side of the cuff, and fluid filling the bursal defect. Bursal-sided tears may also appear as focal flattening or loss of convexity of the tendon. Cortical irregularity of the greater tuberosity is also common when the tear involves the distal tendon at its footprint (see **Fig. 7**). Bursal-sided tears can be more difficult to detect if the tear becomes filled with synovial tissue or granulation tissue. In this case, cuff volume may be artifactually maintained. These tears often reflect outlet impingement and may warrant evaluation and treatment of an associated acromial spur or prominent coracoacromial ligament.

INJURY PATTERNS
Posterosuperior Internal Impingement

Initially described by Walch and colleagues,[48] the mechanism for posterosuperior internal impingement is abduction and external rotation (ABER). When the shoulder is in this position, the undersurface of the rotator cuff may be compressed between the humeral head and the posterosuperior glenoid labrum. In athletes who participate in overhead throwing sports, this mechanism of impingement is exaggerated; partial articular-sided tears can be seen within both the anterior and posterior cuff.[49] The typical finding is a partial articular-sided tear, or a focal anechoic to hypoechoic articular-sided defect, in the posterior supraspinatus tendon extending into the undersurface of the anterior infraspinatus tendon; however, isolated infraspinatus tears can also occur. On US, the constellation of associated findings include cortical irregularity of the posterolateral humeral head subjacent to the posterior supraspinatus and anterior infraspinatus tears. Tearing of the posterior superior labrum may demonstrated as an anechoic or hypoechoic cleft within the labrum or labral detachment from the glenoid, which may be more conspicuous with dynamic US (**Fig. 8**).[50,51] Thickening of the posterior capsule is also associated with internal impingement.[52–54] Paralabral cysts can occur in the setting of posterosuperior capsulolabral tear (see **Fig. 8**). US imaging of the posterior aspect of the glenohumeral joint can reveal a paralabral cyst, which

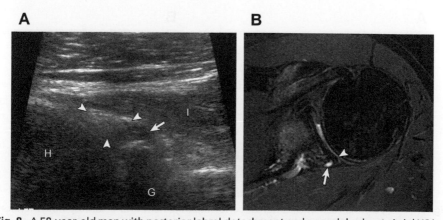

Fig. 8. A 58-year-old man with posterior labral detachment and a paralabral cyst. Axial US image over the posterior shoulder (*A*) and the corresponding fluid-sensitive MR image (*B*) show the paralabral cyst (*arrow*) between the labrum (*arrowheads*) and glenoid (G) (H, humeral head; I, infraspinatus).

appears as an anechoic to hypoechoic round mass within the spinoglenoid notch. Once diagnosed, US can also guide aspiration of the paralabral cyst.

Anterior Superior Internal Impingement

Athletes involved in overhead throwing sports are also prone to injury of the rotator interval and biceps pulley. The rotator interval structures include the intra-articular long head biceps tendon, the superior glenohumeral ligament and coracohumeral ligament (creating the biceps pulley or sling), and the superior margin of the subscapularis tendon.[55] On short axis imaging, the lateral aspect of the coracohumeral ligament is seen as a hyperechoic linear structure extending from the subscapularis to the supraspinatus (see **Fig. 1**C). The mechanism of injury is believed to occur during horizontal adduction and internal rotation where the subscapularis tendon and biceps pulley impinge on the anterosuperior glenoid rim.[56–61] Injury to these structures can be associated with microinstability.[62,63]

On US, anterior superior internal impingement is demonstrated by focal tearing of the anterior leading edge of the supraspinatus, a hypoechoic enlarged biceps tendon and/or biceps tendon subluxation, and partial articular-sided tears of the superior fibers of the subscapularis tendon (**Fig. 9**).[55] The short axis image is helpful to evaluate anterior leading edge supraspinatus tears, as the focal anechoic defect may be seen as an abnormally wide rotator interval. Evaluation of the subscapularis tendon should be performed in both the long axis and short axis. As the subscapularis tendon has a broad insertion on the lesser tuberosity, it is important to evaluate the full extent of the cranial and caudal fibers of the subscapularis tendon.

Subacromial Impingement

Dynamic imaging can aid in the diagnosis of subacromial impingement on the rotator cuff. As the patient abducts the arm under insonation, pooling of bursal fluid or bursal bulging can be observed and documented as the supraspinatus passes beneath the acromion.[64] Any bursal thickening at the acromion should be considered abnormal as the supraspinatus and the bursa should glide easily beneath the acromion. The patient's symptoms during the maneuver should be documented.[65]

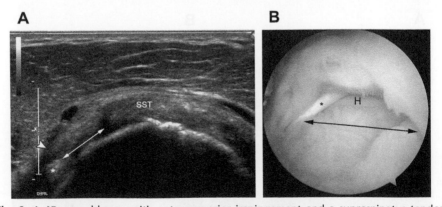

Fig. 9. A 45-year-old man with anterosuperior impingement and a supraspinatus tendon tear (full-thickness). US image (*A*) short axis to the supraspinatus tendon (SST) and arthroscopy image from the bursal surface (*B*) show an anterior leading edge supraspinatus tear (*double-headed arrow*) that extends into the rotator interval and involves the biceps brachii tendon (*asterisk*). Note thickening of the coracohumeral ligament (*arrowhead*).

LHBT

LHBT tears and subluxation/dislocation are well documented on US. However, US is less accurate in diagnosing partial tears and tendinosis of the LHBT compared with complete tears.[10,66,67] Injury of the LHBT is frequently associated with a rotator cuff injury, a rotator interval injury, or subacromial impingement. LHBT injuries range from tendinosis to a frank tear. As with the rotator cuff examination, the biceps tendon should be evaluated in both the short and long axes.

In younger patients, LHBT tears can be seen in the context of overhead throwing, acute trauma, as in a direct blow, or a fall on an outstretched hand. If the LHBT is completely torn, the LHBT is not seen in the bicipital groove or the rotator interval on short axis images and there may be fluid in the tendon sheath, depending on the age of the tear.[68,69] Once a full-thickness tear is identified, scanning should be performed along the expected course of the LHBT distally to the pectoralis major insertion on the humerus to search for the retracted tendon stump. The sonographic appearance may vary from an echogenic stump surrounded by hypoechoic fluid to hyperechoic hemorrhage at the musculotendinous junction.

Sonographic findings of tendinosis include decreased echogenicity, loss of the normal fibrillar pattern with possible tendon thickening, and variable increased flow on color Doppler imaging. Findings associated with a partial-thickness tear include surface irregularity of the LHBT, an associated bone spur, and tendon subluxation (**Fig. 10**).[66] On arthroscopy, these injuries appear as tendon swelling and hyperemia that progress to fraying and fibrillations, although tendons can also appear grossly normal. Longitudinal split thickness tears are diagnosed by a longitudinal hypoechoic cleft within the substance of the tendon on short and long axis images, with fluid in the tendon sheath. The tendon may be enlarged and hypoechoic, with effacement of the normal fibrillar pattern.

In the setting of concomitant rotator interval injury or tear of the subscapularis tendon, it is particularly useful to dynamically assess the LHBT for medial bicipital subluxation and dislocation.[67,69] The patient is scanned with the elbow flexed and palm up, with the elbow tight to the patient's side. As the arm is externally rotated with

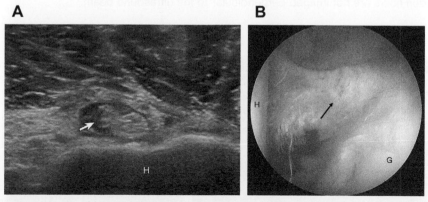

Fig. 10. A 59-year-old man with a partial-thickness tear of long head biceps brachii tendon. US image (*A*) short axis to long head biceps brachii tendon shows surface clefts (*arrow*) with surrounding heterogeneous tenosynovitis. Arthroscopic image (*B*) shows significant fraying in addition to hyperemia and tenosynovitis (*arrow*) (G, glenoid, H, humerus). (*Adapted from* Skendzel JG, Jacobson JA, Carpenter JE, et al. Long head of biceps brachii tendon evaluation: accuracy of preoperative ultrasound. AJR Am J Roentgenol 2011;197(4):942–8; with permission.)

the elbow tight to the side, the humeral head is seen to externally rotate. The LHBT should remain seated within the intertubercular groove during the range of motion. In the case of subluxation, the LHBT perches on the medial edge of the bicipital groove. With medial dislocation, the LHBT displaces medially superficial to, within, or deep to the subscapularis tendon depending on a concomitant subscapularis tendon tear and bicipital pulley injury. Medial dislocation may be static or dynamic, occurring only with external rotation maneuvers (**Fig. 11**).[70]

PITFALLS IN SONOGRAPHIC EVALUATION OF THE ROTATOR CUFF

The literature has reported some difficulty in diagnosing small partial tears less than 5 mm in size, particularly in the subscapularis tendon.[23] It is unclear whether these small tears are clinically significant. Diagnostic challenges can also be encountered when trying to determine between tendinosis and small partial-thickness tears, but this may not be clinically significant because of the similar management of both conditions.[23] Tears of the anterior leading edge of the supraspinatus abutting the rotator interval can be difficult to diagnose. In this case, the short axis view is extremely useful to diagnose these tears. In short axis, the supraspinatus should be immediately adjacent to the biceps tendon with a gap of no more than 1 to 2 mm. Extensive partial-thickness tears may also be mistaken for full-thickness tears, because of volume loss at the site of the tear. This distinction may also not be clinically significant because of similar clinical management of both conditions.

The SASD bursa is situated between the acromion/deltoid and the supraspinatus tendon. When scanning at the far distal edge of the supraspinatus in cases with tendinosis, it may be difficult to differentiate between abnormal tendon and adjacent thickened bursa.[71]

A pitfall occasionally encountered in the sonographic evaluation of the LHBT occurs when echogenic debris accompanying LHBT subluxation/dislocation fills the empty bicipital groove. Thus, one must always scan medial to the bicipital groove to exclude LHBT subluxation or dislocation. A normal LHBT may be misdiagnosed as pathologic due to anisotropy, which makes the tendon appear artifactually hypoechoic when tendon fibers are not imaged perpendicular to the ultrasound beam.[71]

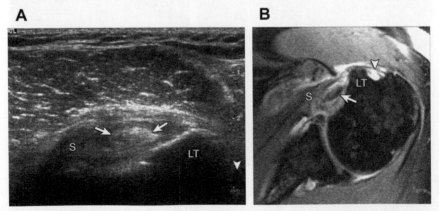

Fig. 11. A 57-year-old man with biceps brachii long head dislocation into a subscapularis tendon delaminating tear. US (*A*) and fluid-sensitive MR image (*B*) in the axial plane show the biceps brachii tendon (*arrows*) dislocated medial to the lesser tuberosity (GT) and within the subscapularis tendon (S) tear. Note the empty bicipital groove (*arrowhead*).

SUMMARY

US is a versatile and effective method for the evaluation of the rotator cuff with accuracy rivaling MRI. Recent work by experienced practitioners using high-resolution equipment has validated the observations that US and MRI are equally diagnostic for partial-thickness and full-thickness rotator cuff tears. As an imaging modality, US has several advantages over MRI, including portability, high resolution, dynamic assessment, and none of the limitations inherent with a magnetized environment.

REFERENCES

1. Teefey SA, Rubin DA, Middleton WD, et al. Detection and quantification of rotator cuff tears. Comparison of ultrasonographic, magnetic resonance imaging, and arthroscopic findings in seventy-one consecutive cases. J Bone Joint Surg Am 2004;86(4):708–16.
2. Iannotti JP, Ciccone J, Buss DD, et al. Accuracy of office-based ultrasonography of the shoulder for the diagnosis of rotator cuff tears. J Bone Joint Surg Am 2005;87(6):1305–11.
3. Al-Shawi A, Badge R, Bunker T. The detection of full thickness rotator cuff tears using ultrasound. J Bone Joint Surg Br 2008;90(7):889–92.
4. van Holsbeeck MT, Kolowich PA, Eyler WR, et al. US depiction of partial-thickness tear of the rotator cuff. Radiology 1995;197(2):443–6.
5. Nazarian LN. The top 10 reasons musculoskeletal sonography is an important complementary or alternative technique to MRI. AJR Am J Roentgenol 2008; 190(6):1621–6.
6. Jacobson JA, Miller B, Bedi A, et al. Imaging of the postoperative shoulder. Semin Musculoskelet Radiol 2011;15(4):320–39.
7. Rutten MJ, Spaargaren GJ, van Loon T, et al. Detection of rotator cuff tears: the value of MRI following ultrasound. Eur Radiol 2010;20(2):450–7.
8. Dinnes J, Loveman E, McIntyre L, et al. The effectiveness of diagnostic tests for the assessment of shoulder pain due to soft tissue disorders: a systematic review. Health Technol Assess 2003;7(29):iii1–166.
9. Bachmann GF, Melzer C, Heinrichs CM, et al. Diagnosis of rotator cuff lesions: comparison of US and MRI on 38 joint specimens. Eur Radiol 1997;7(2): 192–7.
10. Read JW, Perko M. Shoulder ultrasound: diagnostic accuracy for impingement syndrome, rotator cuff tear, and biceps tendon pathology. J Shoulder Elbow Surg 1998;7(3):264–71.
11. Milosavljevic J, Elvin A, Rahme H. Ultrasonography of the rotator cuff: a comparison with arthroscopy in one-hundred-and-ninety consecutive cases. Acta Radiol 2005;46(8):858–65.
12. Jacobson JA, Lancaster S, Prasad A, et al. Full-thickness and partial-thickness supraspinatus tendon tears: value of US signs in diagnosis. Radiology 2004; 230(1):234–42.
13. Rutten MJ, Maresch BJ, Jager GJ, et al. Ultrasound of the rotator cuff with MRI and anatomic correlation. Eur J Radiol 2007;62(3):427–36.
14. de Jesus JO, Parker L, Frangos AJ, et al. Accuracy of MRI, MR arthrography, and ultrasound in the diagnosis of rotator cuff tears: a meta-analysis. AJR Am J Roentgenol 2009;192(6):1701–7.
15. Millstein ES, Snyder SJ. Arthroscopic evaluation and management of rotator cuff tears. Orthop Clin North Am 2003;34(4):507–20.

16. Kim HM, Dahiya N, Teefey SA, et al. Location and initiation of degenerative rotator cuff tears: an analysis of three hundred and sixty shoulders. J Bone Joint Surg Am 2010;92(5):1088–96.

17. Crass JR. Current concepts in the radiographic evaluation of the rotator cuff. Crit Rev Diagn Imaging 1988;28(1):23–73.

18. Crass JR, Craig EV. Noninvasive imaging of the rotator cuff. Orthopedics 1988; 11(1):57–64.

19. Crass JR, Craig EV, Feinberg SB. Ultrasonography of rotator cuff tears: a review of 500 diagnostic studies. J Clin Ultrasound 1988;16(5):313–27.

20. Crass JR, Craig EV, Thompson RC, et al. Ultrasonography of the rotator cuff: surgical correlation. J Clin Ultrasound 1984;12(8):487–91.

21. Teefey SA, Hasan SA, Middleton WD, et al. Ultrasonography of the rotator cuff. A comparison of ultrasonographic and arthroscopic findings in one hundred consecutive cases. J Bone Joint Surg Am 2000;82(4):498–504.

22. Teefey SA, Middleton WD, Bauer GS, et al. Sonographic differences in the appearance of acute and chronic full-thickness rotator cuff tears. J Ultrasound Med 2000;19(6):377–8 [quiz: 83].

23. Teefey SA, Middleton WD, Payne WT, et al. Detection and measurement of rotator cuff tears with sonography: analysis of diagnostic errors. AJR Am J Roentgenol 2005;184(6):1768–73.

24. Martinoli C, Derchi LE, Pastorino C, et al. Analysis of echotexture of tendons with US. Radiology 1993;186(3):839–43.

25. Jacobson J. Fundamentals of musculoskeletal ultrasound. Philadelphia: Saunders Elsevier; 2007. p. 39–101.

26. Matava MJ, Purcell DB, Rudzki JR. Partial-thickness rotator cuff tears. Am J Sports Med 2005;33(9):1405–17.

27. Morag Y, Jamadar DA, Boon TA, et al. Ultrasound of the rotator cable: prevalence and morphology in asymptomatic shoulders. AJR Am J Roentgenol 2012;198(1):W27–30.

28. Burkhart SS, Esch JC, Jolson RS. The rotator crescent and rotator cable: an anatomic description of the shoulder's "suspension bridge". Arthroscopy 1993;9(6):611–6.

29. Morag Y, Jacobson JA, Lucas D, et al. US appearance of the rotator cable with histologic correlation: preliminary results. Radiology 2006;241(2):485–91.

30. Crass JR, Craig EV, Feinberg SB. Clinical significance of sonographic findings in the abnormal but intact rotator cuff: a preliminary report. J Clin Ultrasound 1988;16(9):625–34.

31. Buck FM, Grehn H, Hilbe M, et al. Magnetic resonance histologic correlation in rotator cuff tendons. J Magn Reson Imaging 2010;32(1):165–72.

32. Kjellin I, Ho CP, Cervilla V, et al. Alterations in the supraspinatus tendon at MR imaging: correlation with histopathologic findings in cadavers. Radiology 1991;181(3):837–41.

33. Finlay K, Friedman L. Common tendon and muscle injuries: upper extremities. Ultrasound Clin 2007;2(4):555–94.

34. Kim HM, Dahiya N, Teefey SA, et al. Relationship of tear size and location to fatty degeneration of the rotator cuff. J Bone Joint Surg Am 2010;92(4):829–39.

35. Khoury V, Cardinal E, Brassard P. Atrophy and fatty infiltration of the supraspinatus muscle: sonography versus MRI. AJR Am J Roentgenol 2008;190(4): 1105–11.

36. Sofka CM, Haddad ZK, Adler RS. Detection of muscle atrophy on routine sonography of the shoulder. J Ultrasound Med 2004;23(8):1031–4.

37. Iannotti JP, Zlatkin MB, Esterhai JL, et al. Magnetic resonance imaging of the shoulder. Sensitivity, specificity, and predictive value. J Bone Joint Surg Am 1991;73(1):17–29.
38. Seitz AL, McClure PW, Finucane S, et al. Mechanisms of rotator cuff tendinopathy: intrinsic, extrinsic, or both? Clin Biomech (Bristol, Avon) 2011;26(1):1–12.
39. Lohr JF, Uhthoff HK. Epidemiology and pathophysiology of rotator cuff tears. Orthopade 2007;36(9):788–95 [in German].
40. Fukuda H, Hamada K, Yamanaka K. Pathology and pathogenesis of bursal-side rotator cuff tears viewed from en bloc histologic sections. Clin Orthop Relat Res 1990;(254):75–80.
41. Payne LZ, Altchek DW, Craig EV, et al. Arthroscopic treatment of partial rotator cuff tears in young athletes. A preliminary report. Am J Sports Med 1997;25(3): 299–305.
42. Wiener SN, Seitz WH Jr. Sonography of the shoulder in patients with tears of the rotator cuff: accuracy and value for selecting surgical options. AJR Am J Roentgenol 1993;160(1):103–7 [discussion: 9–10].
43. Moosmayer S, Heir S, Smith HJ. Sonography of the rotator cuff in painful shoulders performed without knowledge of clinical information: results from 58 sonographic examinations with surgical correlation. J Clin Ultrasound 2007;35(1): 20–6.
44. Tuite MJ, Turnbull JR, Orwin JF. Anterior versus posterior, and rim-rent rotator cuff tears: prevalence and MR sensitivity. Skeletal Radiol 1998;27(5): 237–43.
45. Schaeffeler C, Mueller D, Kirchhoff C, et al. Tears at the rotator cuff footprint: prevalence and imaging characteristics in 305 MR arthrograms of the shoulder. Eur Radiol 2011;21(7):1477–84.
46. Wohlwend JR, van Holsbeeck M, Craig J, et al. The association between irregular greater tuberosities and rotator cuff tears: a sonographic study. AJR Am J Roentgenol 1998;171(1):229–33.
47. Manvar AM, Kamireddi A, Bhalani SM, et al. Clinical significance of intramuscular cysts in the rotator cuff and their relationship to full- and partial-thickness rotator cuff tears. AJR Am J Roentgenol 2009;192(3):719–24.
48. Walch G, Boileau P, Noel E, et al. Impingement of the deep surface of the supraspinatus tendon on the posterosuperior glenoid rim: an arthroscopic study. J Shoulder Elbow Surg 1992;1(5):238–45.
49. Nakagawa S, Yoneda M, Mizuno N, et al. Throwing shoulder injury involving the anterior rotator cuff: concealed tears not as uncommon as previously thought. Arthroscopy 2006;22(12):1298–303.
50. Giaroli EL, Major NM, Higgins LD. MRI of internal impingement of the shoulder. AJR Am J Roentgenol 2005;185(4):925–9.
51. Grainger AJ. Internal impingement syndromes of the shoulder. Semin Musculoskelet Radiol 2008;12(2):127–35.
52. Thomas SJ, Swanik CB, Higginson JS, et al. A bilateral comparison of posterior capsule thickness and its correlation with glenohumeral range of motion and scapular upward rotation in collegiate baseball players. J Shoulder Elbow Surg 2011;20(5):708–16.
53. Burkhart SS, Morgan CD, Kibler WB. Shoulder injuries in overhead athletes. The "dead arm" revisited. Clin Sports Med 2000;19(1):125–58.
54. Burkhart SS, Morgan CD, Kibler WB. The disabled throwing shoulder: spectrum of pathology Part I: pathoanatomy and biomechanics. Arthroscopy 2003;19(4): 404–20.

55. Parker BJ, Zlatkin MB, Newman JS, et al. Imaging of shoulder injuries in sports medicine: current protocols and concepts. Clin Sports Med 2008;27(4): 579–606.
56. Gerber C, Sebesta A. Impingement of the deep surface of the subscapularis tendon and the reflection pulley on the anterosuperior glenoid rim: a preliminary report. J Shoulder Elbow Surg 2000;9(6):483–90.
57. Morag Y, Jacobson JA, Miller B, et al. MR imaging of rotator cuff injury: what the clinician needs to know. Radiographics 2006;26(4):1045–65.
58. Morag Y, Bedi A, Jamadar DA. The rotator interval and long head biceps tendon: anatomy, function, pathology, and magnetic resonance imaging. Magn Reson Imaging Clin N Am 2012;20(2):229–59, x.
59. Morag Y, Jacobson JA, Shields G, et al. MR arthrography of rotator interval, long head of the biceps brachii, and biceps pulley of the shoulder. Radiology 2005; 235(1):21–30.
60. Barile A, Lanni G, Conti L, et al. Lesions of the biceps pulley as cause of anterosuperior impingement of the shoulder in the athlete: potentials and limits of MR arthrography compared with arthroscopy. Radiol Med 2013;118(1):112–22.
61. Habermeyer P, Magosch P, Pritsch M, et al. Anterosuperior impingement of the shoulder as a result of pulley lesions: a prospective arthroscopic study. J Shoulder Elbow Surg 2004;13(1):5–12.
62. Chang EY, Fliszar E, Chung CB. Superior labrum anterior and posterior lesions and microinstability. Magn Reson Imaging Clin N Am 2012;20(2):277–94, x–xi.
63. Woertler K, Waldt S. MR imaging in sports-related glenohumeral instability. Eur Radiol 2006;16(12):2622–36.
64. Farin PU, Jaroma H, Harju A, et al. Shoulder impingement syndrome: sonographic evaluation. Radiology 1990;176(3):845–9.
65. Khoury V, Cardinal E, Bureau NJ. Musculoskeletal sonography: a dynamic tool for usual and unusual disorders. AJR Am J Roentgenol 2007;188(1):W63–73.
66. Skendzel JG, Jacobson JA, Carpenter JE, et al. Long head of biceps brachii tendon evaluation: accuracy of preoperative ultrasound. AJR Am J Roentgenol 2011;197(4):942–8.
67. Armstrong A, Teefey SA, Wu T, et al. The efficacy of ultrasound in the diagnosis of long head of the biceps tendon pathology. J Shoulder Elbow Surg 2006;15(1): 7–11.
68. Farin PU. Sonography of the biceps tendon of the shoulder: normal and pathologic findings. J Clin Ultrasound 1996;24(6):309–16.
69. Farin PU, Jaroma H, Harju A, et al. Medial displacement of the biceps brachii tendon: evaluation with dynamic sonography during maximal external shoulder rotation. Radiology 1995;195(3):845–8.
70. Petchprapa CN, Beltran LS, Jazrawi LM, et al. The rotator interval: a review of anatomy, function, and normal and abnormal MRI appearance. AJR Am J Roentgenol 2010;195(3):567–76.
71. Jamadar DA, Robertson BL, Jacobson JA, et al. Musculoskeletal sonography: important imaging pitfalls. AJR Am J Roentgenol 2010;194(1):216–25.

Hip-Femoral Acetabular Impingement

Christian N. Anderson, MD[a], Geoffrey M. Riley, MD[b],
Garry E. Gold, MD[c], Marc R. Safran, MD[d],*

KEYWORDS

- Hip • Magnetic resonance imaging • Femoroacetabular impingement
- Magnetic resonance arthrography • Cam impingement • Pincer impingement
- Acetabular labral tears

KEY POINTS

- Femoroacetabular impingement is caused by repetitive abutment of a morphologically abnormal proximal femur and/or acetabulum during terminal range-of-motion of the hip.
- The abnormal pathomechanical impingement seen in femoroacetabular impingement results in damage to the labrum and acetabular cartilage.
- Magnetic resonance imaging of the hip requires high field imaging (1.5 or 3 T) and a dedicated hip protocol to ensure appropriate quality of images.
- Magnetic resonance arthrography increases contrast resolution and is important for evaluating the acetabular labrum and articular cartilage.
- Assessment of both normal and pathologic magnetic resonance imaging anatomy requires a systematic evaluation of bony structures, acetabular labrum, femoral and acetabular cartilage, chondrolabral junction, and other soft tissues including the ligamentum teres.

INTRODUCTION

Femoroacetabular impingement (FAI) was first described in the 1990s,[1,2] and since that time has been increasingly recognized as a source of hip pain and dysfunction.

Disclosures: None (C.N. Anderson, G.M. Riley); Paid consultant for Zimmer and ISTO, Inc (G. Gold); Consultant for Cradle Medical, Cool Systems Inc, Biomimedica, Eleven Blade Solutions (all stock options); Royalties: Lippincott Williams and Wilkins; Elsevier; Ross Creek/Stryker, Vista Publishing (M.R. Safran).
Funding Sources: None (C.N. Anderson, G.M. Riley); Research support from GE Healthcare (G. Gold); Research support from Ferring Pharmceuticals and Smith and Nephew. Fellowship funding from Smith and Nephew, ConMed Linvatec, and Ossur (M.R. Safran).
a Department of Orthopaedic Surgery, Stanford University Medical Center, 450 Broadway Street, Redwood City, CA 94063, USA; b Department of Radiology, Stanford University Medical Center, 300 Pasteur Drive, S-056, Stanford, CA 94305, USA; c Department of Radiology, Stanford University Medical Center, 1201 Welch Road, P271, Stanford, CA 94305, USA; d Department of Orthopaedic Surgery, Stanford University Medical Center, 450 Broadway Street, M/C 6342, Redwood City, CA 94063, USA
* Corresponding author.
E-mail address: msafran@stanford.edu

Extensive work by Ganz and colleagues[3] has demonstrated that FAI is caused by repetitive abutment of a morphologically abnormal proximal femur and/or acetabulum during terminal range-of-motion of the hip. This pathomechanical process eventually results in characteristic damage to the labrum and acetabular cartilage, depending on the location of the osseous abnormality.[3] The 2 most common osseous abnormalities that lead to FAI are a loss of the normal femoral head-neck offset, resulting in cam impingement, and acetabular overcoverage, resulting in pincer impingement.[3] A third type of FAI has components of both cam and pincer and is referred to as mixed or combined impingement.

Cam Impingement

- Most common form of isolated FAI (17% of all FAI types)[4]
- Typically seen in young adult men 20 to 30 years old[5]
- The loss of normal femoral head-neck contour can be due to an abnormal extension of the proximal femoral epiphysis,[6] short or long femoral neck, varus femoral neck, or residual deformity from femoral neck fracture, perthes, or slipped capital femoral epiphysis
- The nonspherical portion of the anterolateral femoral head produces a shear force at the chondrolabral junction as it enters the acetabulum during hip flexion[3]
- Over time, repetitive shearing results in chondrolabral separation, acetabular chondral delamination from the subchondral bone, and labral detachment (**Fig. 1**).[3,4,7,8]

Pincer Impingement

- Most commonly seen in women[9] 30 to 40 years old[10]
- Acetabular overcoverage can be caused from focal overcoverage at the anterosuperior acetabular rim, relative anterior overcoverage (acetabular retroversion), or global overcoverage (coxa profunda, protrusio acetabuli)
- Overcoverage of the acetabulum results in crushing the labrum against the normal femoral neck in hip flexion and internal rotation (**Fig. 2**).[3]

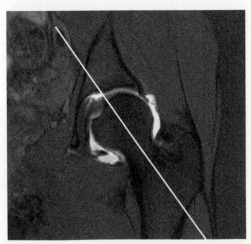

Fig. 1. Orientation to prescribe the oblique axial sequence. Coronal T1-weighted fat-suppressed MR arthrogram image demonstrates the plane used to obtain the oblique axial sequence.

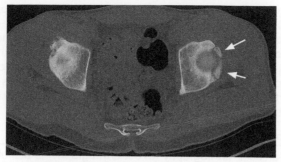

Fig. 2. Axial CT scan of the pelvis shows 2 bony fragments adjacent to the acetabulum (*arrows*).

- Continued abutment results in labral degeneration, with limited chondral injury, and possible ossification of the rim[3,11]
- Can result in damage to posterior femoral head and acetabulum as a result of contracoup mechanism of the femoral head levering on the acetabulum and shearing posteriorly.

Combined Impingement

- Most common form of FAI (72% of all FAI types)[4]
- Has components of both cam and pincer morphology; however, one type of intra-articular pathologic condition usually predominates

The diagnosis of FAI relies on patient history, physical examination, selective intra-articular anesthetic injection, and radiographic studies, including plain radiograph, magnetic resonance imaging (MRI), and computed tomography (CT). MRI and magnetic resonance arthrography (MRA) have been used with increasing frequency to identify the pathomorphologies associated with FAI and are important to a successful treatment and outcomes.

MRI TECHNICAL CONSIDERATIONS
MR Imaging Techniques for the Hip

- The hip remains one of the most challenging joints to image. This challenge is related to its unique orientation that does not conform to the standard planes of the body and the variation in orientation from person to person. In addition, the hip cannot be surrounded by a radiofrequency coil and is relatively deep from the skin surface. Because of these challenges, optimization of image quality is critical for the evaluation of hip pathologic condition related to femoroacetabular impingement.
- High field imaging is preferred (1.5 or 3.0 T). The use of 3.0 T systems offer a higher signal-to-noise ratio.
- A dedicated hip protocol should be used when there is a question of femoroacetabular impingement, optimizing images of the hip at the expense of excluding other areas of the pelvis and the contralateral hip. For this reason it is crucial to denote the side of interest in the imaging request.
- Imaging of the hip for the evaluation of femoroacetabular impingement typically includes 3 planes using a variety of MR sequences. For nonarthrographic imaging, a combination of T1-weighted, proton-density, and T2-weighted images with fat suppression is used. Because conventional anatomic planes (transverse, coronal, and sagittal) do not optimally demonstrate the pathologic condition,

particularly of the labrum, oblique sequences have been developed. These sequences include the following:

○ Axial oblique, obtained parallel to the long axis of the femoral neck (see **Fig. 1**).
○ Radial sequences, obtained perpendicular to the long axis of the femur. These radial sequences are helpful for determining the α angle, particularly when the osseous prominence is not evident on the oblique axial views.

• Other important factors include using a small field of view (16–20 cm) and a dedicated phased-array surface coil.

Use of Intra-articular Arthrography

The use of intra-articular arthrography (direct arthrography) is useful to distend the joint, separate the soft tissues, and increase contrast resolution, factors important to evaluating the labrum and cartilage structures. For MRA, a combination of fat-suppressed T1-weighted images and fluid-sensitive sequences is important to distinguish between fluid in the joint and extra-articular collections. The technique at the authors' institution consists of using a mixture of 5 mL Lidocaine 1%, 5 mL Ropivacaine 0.5%, 1 mL Omnipaque 240, and 0.1 mL Gd-DTPA (Magnevist) in a 20 mL syringe. A total of 5 to 10 mL is injected into the hip joint.

MRI NORMAL ANATOMY
Key Structures to Identify in the Assessment of Femoroacetabular Impingement

• Interpretation of a hip MRI for femoroacetabular impingement requires a through assessment of the following structures:
○ Bony structures, including acetabular morphology, femoral head morphology, head-neck junction morphology, and the presence of osseous bumps, osteophytes, and fibrocystic changes.
○ Acetabular labrum.
○ Acetabular articular cartilage and chondrolabral junction.
○ Femoral head articular cartilage.
○ Other soft tissues including the ligamentum teres.

Bony Structures

• Acetabular morphology: The acetabular version is best assessed on an anteroposterior radiograph of the pelvis (pelvic radiography is routinely used at the authors' institution as part of the workup for femoroacetabular impingement). On the MRI examination, the acetabulum is best assessed on the oblique axial images.
• The femoral head-neck junction can be assessed on the oblique axial images; however, the use of radial imaging can provide a more comprehensive assessment.[12]
• Bony fragments adjacent to the acetabular rim: The presence of bony fragments adjacent to the acetabular rim can be due to an ununited secondary acetabular ossification center. Other possible causes include ununited acetabular fractures (see **Fig. 2**), fragmentation of osteophytes, or labral ossification.[13]
• Juxta-articular fibrocystic changes at the anterosuperior femoral neck.
• Notching of the femoral neck in pincer FAI.

Cartilage

• Evaluation of cartilage is one of the most important reasons for imaging a patient with femoroacetabular impingement. The cartilage can be difficult to assess because it is thin and the articular surfaces are closely applied. The curvature of the acetabulum also contributes to the difficulty.

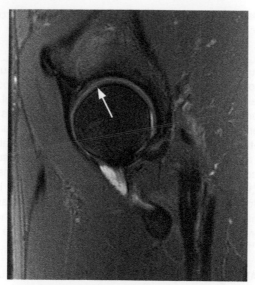

Fig. 3. Normal femoral head cartilage. Sagittal T1-weighted fat-suppressed MR arthrogram image shows the normal smooth femoral head cartilage (*arrow*).

- The femoral head articular cartilage should appear smooth and well defined (**Fig. 3**).

Labrum

- The labrum should appear as a dark, well-defined triangular structure. Although the anterior labrum generally appears sharp, the posterior can normally have a more rounded appearance (**Fig. 4**).
- The addition of a radial sequence to the standard planes can be helpful in the detection of labral pathologic condition.

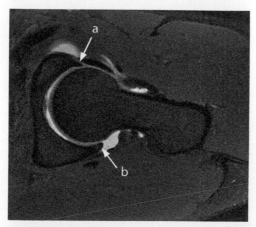

Fig. 4. Normal acetabular labrum. Oblique axial T1-weighted fat-suppressed MR arthrogram image shows the normal anterior (a *arrow*) and normal posterior (b *arrow*) acetabular labrum. Note the round appearance of the posterior labrum compared with the sharp well-defined anterior labrum.

- The chondral labral junction is also best evaluated on the coronal sequence and should appear smooth without defects (**Fig. 5**).

Normal Variants

- Supra-acetabular fossa represents a focal depression in the superior acetabulum that should not be mistaken for a cartilage defect. The absence of adjacent marrow signal and its characteristic location are helpful for identification (**Fig. 6**). Similarly, a stellate crease (stellate lesion) represents a normal focus of cartilage absence or thinning at the superomedial acetabulum, more medial to the supra-acetabular fossa, that is continuous with the acetabular notch.[13–15]
- The presence of a sublabral sulcus is much debated. These sublabral sulci have been described as representing variants in all labral locations.[16] Although it remains unclear which of these lesions is truly a normal variant, based on the locations of tears found at arthroscopy, it is more likely that a linear signal intensity at the base of the anterosuperior labrum represents a tear, whereas those in the posteroinferior labral cartilage junction more likely represents a sublabral sulcus or a foramen.[14]

MRI PATHOLOGIC ANATOMY ASSOCIATED WITH FEMOROACETABULAR IMPINGEMENT

Although the diagnosis of femoroacetabular impingement is primarily based on radiographs and clinical findings, MRI is important in confirming the diagnosis and assessing the labrum and cartilage.

Findings Associated with Cam Impingement

- The loss of normal femoral head-neck contour with asphericity of the femoral head (**Fig. 7**) and elevated α angle (**Fig. 8**).
- Chondrolabral separation (**Fig. 9**)
- Acetabular chondral loss (**Fig. 10**)

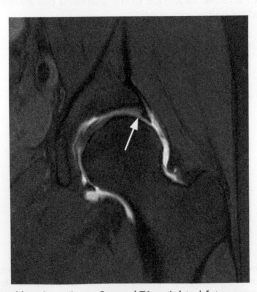

Fig. 5. Normal femoral head cartilage. Coronal T1-weighted fat-suppressed MR arthrogram image shows the normal superior chondrolabral junction (*arrow*).

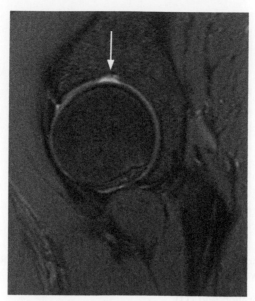

Fig. 6. Supra-acetabular fossa. Sagittal T1-weighted fat-suppressed MR arthrogram image shows supra-acetabular fossa at the superior acetabulum (*arrow*) that should not be mistaken for a focal chondral defect.

Findings Associated with Pincer Impingement

- Acetabular overcoverage
  - Focal overcoverage at the anterosuperior acetabular rim
  - Relative anterior overcoverage (acetabular retroversion)
  - Global overcoverage (coxa profunda, protrusio acetabuli)

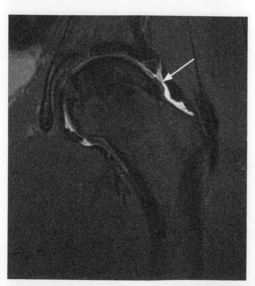

Fig. 7. Loss of normal femoral head-neck contour with asphericity of the femoral head. Oblique coronal T1-weighted fat-suppressed MR arthrogram image shows an ossoeus prominence with loss of the femoral head-neck contour (*arrow*).

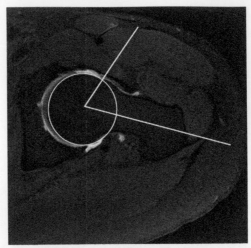

Fig. 8. Elevated α angle. Oblique axial T1-weighted fat-suppressed MR arthrogram image demonstrates an elevated α angle (66°).

- Labral degeneration (**Fig. 11**)
- Limited chondral injury
- Ossification of the rim (see **Fig. 2**)
- Contracoup injury to the posterior femoral head and acetabulum.

CASE EXAMPLES
Case 1. Pincer Impingement with Labral Tear and Synovial Proliferation

A 27-year-old woman presented with a 2-month history of left groin pain that began spontaneously after an extended walk. Physical examination was consistent with

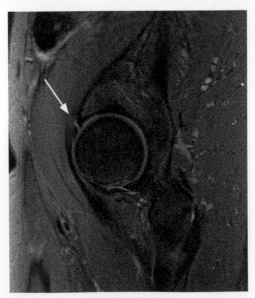

Fig. 9. Chondrolabral separation. Sagittal T1-weighted fat-suppressed MR arthrogram shows a linear signal at the base of the anterior superior labrum (*arrow*).

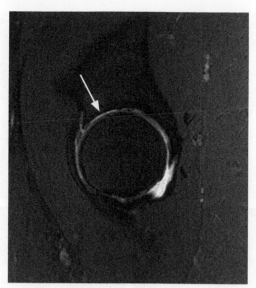

Fig. 10. Acetabular cartilage loss. Sagittal T1 weighted fat-suppressed MR arthrogram shows a large focus of full thickness cartilage loss of the anterior aspect of the superior acetabulum (*arrow*), and an anterior labral chondral separation.

the diagnosis of FAI. Roentgenography demonstrated radiographic features of pincer FAI. MRA revealed an anterosuperior labral tear and nonenhancing synovial mass inferior to the femoral head-neck junction. Intra-articular anesthetic injection provided immediate relief of her symptoms. Treatment consisted of arthroscopic acetabular rim reduction and labral refixation, followed by intra-articular excisional biopsy of hypertrophic synovial tissue (**Fig. 12**).

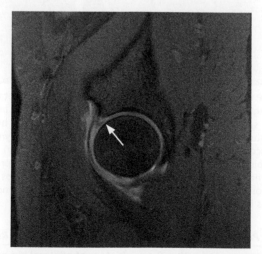

Fig. 11. Labral degeneration. Sagittal T1-weighted fat-suppressed MR arthrogram shows abnormal signal within the anterior aspect of the superior labrum compatible with degeneration (*arrow*).

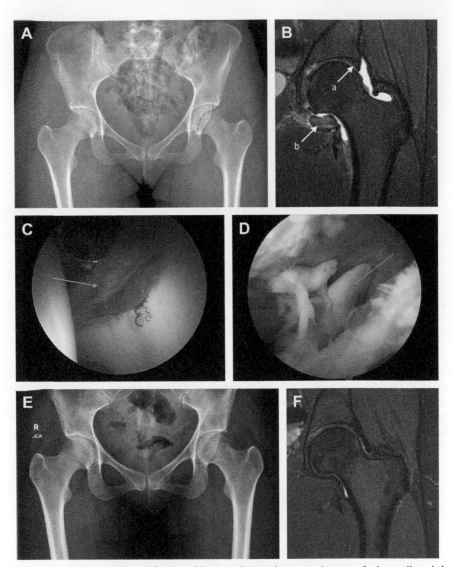

Fig. 12. (*A* and *E*) AP Pelvis with dotted line outlining the posterior acetabular wall and the dashed line outlining the anterior wall. (*B*) MRA of an anterosuperior labral tear (*arrow* a) and nonenhancing synovial mass (*arrow* b) inferior to the femoral head-neck junction. Intra-articular anesthetic injection provided immediate relief of her symptoms. Treatment consisted of arthroscopic acetabular rim reduction and labral refixation, followed by intra-articular excisional biopsy of hypertrophic synovial tissue. (*C*) Arrow represents the anterior labral tear with synovitis. (*D*) Arrow represents the soft tissue mass in the peripheral compartment/inferior medial femoral neck. (*F*) 1 year follow up MRI demonstrating repaired labrum and no mass in the inferior femoral neck region.

Case 2. Combined Pincer and Cam Impingement with Acetabular Rim Stress Fracture

A 22-year-old man presented with a 6-year history of bilateral hip pain, worsening on the left side over a 3-month period before his visit. A positive labral stress test and impingement test, as well as restricted range-of-motion with flexion and internal

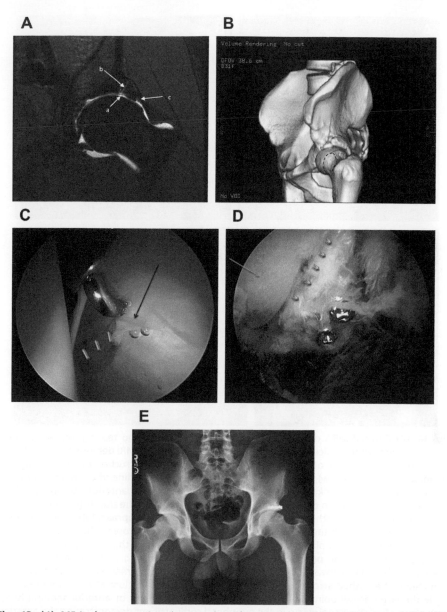

Fig. 13. (*A*) MRA demonstrating (*arrow* a) with articular cartilage thinning, (*arrow* b) demonstrating the fibrous line at the acetabular bony rim fracture and (*arrow* c), labral degeneration. (*B*) 3D CT scan reconstruction showing the bipartite acetabular rim fragments (*arrows*) and cam lesion (dashed line encircling the lesion). (*C*) Arthroscopic view from within the central compartment, demonstrating the acetabular rim injury (*short arrows*) and chondral lesion (*long arrow*). (*D*) Arthroscopic view from the peripheral compartment demonstrated the screws fixing the acetabular rim injury, with the long arrow pointing to the femoral head reduced in the joint, and the short arrowheads pointing to the labrum attached to the rim fragment, and sealing the joint over the femoral head. (*E*) Post op radiograph demonstrating the screws fixing the acetabular rim injury and restoration of femoral head-neck offset.

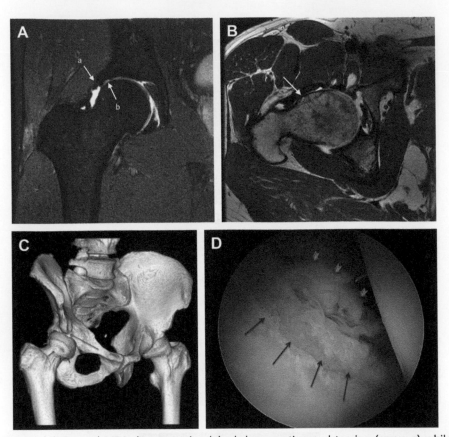

Fig. 14. (*A*) Coronal MRA demonstrating labral degeneration and tearing (*arrow* a) while (*arrow* b) points to the articular cartilage degeneration. (*B*) Axial MRI demonstrating anterior loss of femoral head neck offset (*arrow*). (*C*) A 3D CT Scan reconstruction demonstrating the elongated AIIS (*long arrow*), cam lesion (*short arrows*) and the outline of the normal location for the femoral head neck offset. (*D*) Arthroscopic view of the anterior acetabulum. The arrows point to the margin of damaged articular cartilage, while the stars highlight the badly damaged labrum. (*E*) Another arthroscopic view of the anterior supraacetabular region with the solid long arrow pointing to the femoral head, the dashed arrow to the anterior acetabular rim, after acetabuloplasty, and the arrowheads outlining the enlarged AIIS. (*F*) An arthroscopic view of the peripheral compartment demonstrating a crease in the femoral head, with the small arrows outlining the demarcation from normal femoral head and the cam lesion. The dashed arrow demonstrates the anterior acetabulum after acetabuloplasty, while the large arrow points to the cam lesion resulting in loss of anterior femoral head neck offset. (*G*) Arthroscopic view in the peripheral compartment demonstrating the anterior femoral head neck region after femoral osteoplasty (chielectomy) (*arrow*).

rotation, were demonstrated on physical examination. Radiographs revealed acetabular retroversion with a positive posterior wall and ischial spine signs, as well as an acetabular rim stress fracture and cam lesion of the proximal femur. CT scanning revealed a nondisplaced bipartite bony fragment located at the anterolateral acetabular rim. Anesthetic injection given at the time of MRA gave immediate relief of symptoms. MRA demonstrated elevated α angle, anterosuperior labral degeneration, and thinning of acetabular cartilage. Treatment consisted of debridement of delaminated

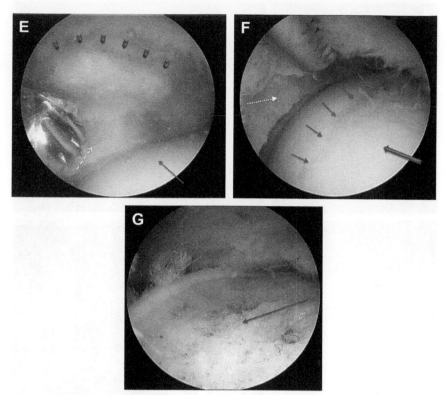

Fig. 14. (*continued*)

acetabular cartilage and microfracture to the corresponding area, acetabuloplasty, arthroscopic fixation of acetabular rim stress fracture, labral refixation, and femoral head osteoplasty (see **Fig. 2**; **Fig. 13**).

Case 3. Combined FAI with Anterior Inferior Iliac Spine Impingement

A 30-year-old man presented with a 13-year history of right-sided hip pain that started after a fall while snowboarding. Physical examination was consistent with femoroacetabular impingement and restricted range-of-motion. Radiographs revealed loss of anterolateral femoral head-neck contour, mild acetabular retroversion, and an enlarged anterior inferior iliac spine impingement (AIIS). Anesthetic intra-articular injection gave immediate partial pain relief. MRA was consistent with both cam and pincer pathologies and demonstrated anterosuperior labral tear and chondral thinning. CT scanning confirmed enlargement of the AIIS. Treatment consisted of arthroscopic partial labrectomy, removal of delaminated acetabular cartilage, acetabular rim resection, proximal femoral osteoplasty, and AIIS osteoplasty (**Fig. 14**).

Case 4. Combined Pincer and Cam Impingement

A 35-year-old man presented with a 4-month history of right groin and lateral-sided hip pain after falling down the stairs. On physical examination, the patient had pain with flexion and internal rotation of the hip. Radiographic analysis revealed anterolateral acetabular overcoverage and a cam lesion of the proximal femur. MRA demonstrated

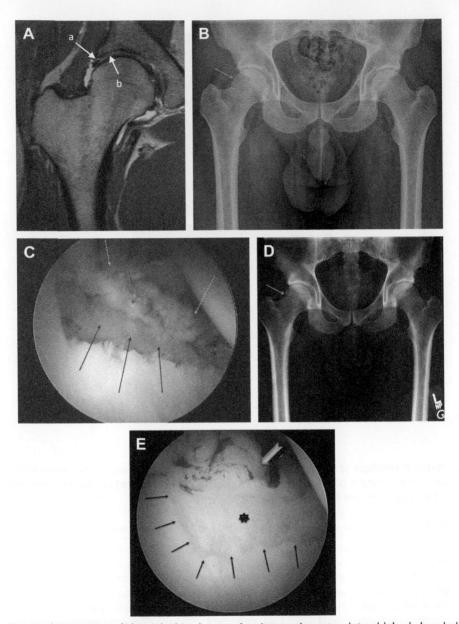

Fig. 15. (*A*) An MRA of the right hip. (*arrow* a) points to the anterolateral labral-chondral separation while (*arrow* b) points to an area of articular cartilage irregularity. (*B*) An AP pelvis radiograph demonstrating the loss of lateral femoral head-neck offset pre-operatively (*arrow*). (*C*) An arthroscopic view from the central compartment. The dashed arrows point the labrum which was refixed (blue sutures seen). The long solid arrows point to the area of chondral damage (exposed bone) which has undergone microfracture. (*D*) A post operative AP Pelvis radiograph demonstrating restoration of lateral femoral head neck offset (*arrow*). (*E*) Follow up arthroscopic image of this patient. The large, 3D arrow points to the healed labrum, with synovialization of the sutures (sutures not seen), while the star is in the center of the fibrocartilage at the anterior acetabulum as a result of the microfracture, and the multiple arrows outlining the demarcation between normal hyaline cartilage and the residual fibrocartilage resulting from the microfracture.

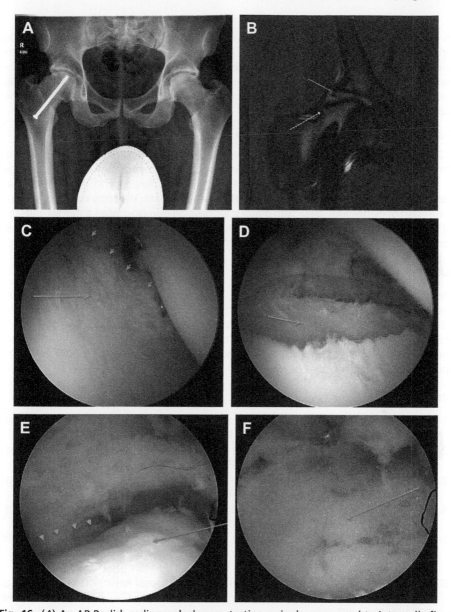

Fig. 16. (*A*) An AP Pevlish radiograph demonstrating a single screw used to internally fix a SCFE. The hip is in varus, with loss of femoral head neck offset. There is also acetabular retroversion as seen with the ischial spine and cross over signs, bilaterally. (*B*) Metal suppression MRI with the dashed arrow showing the loss of femoral head neck offset (cam lesion) and the solid arrow highlighting the anterolateral labral tear. (*C*) An arthroscopic view of the intra-articular acetabular chondral (*long arrow*) and labral tearing (*small arrows*). (*D*) Another arthroscopic view demonstrates the anterior acetabulum after partial labrectomy, acetabular rim reduction (shaded area) and chondroplasty wtih the arrow pointing to exposed acetabular bone. (*E*) An arthroscopic view of the peripheral compartment demonstrating the irregular anterior femoral neck with bumps, resulting in cam impingement, and the small arrows demarcating the acetabular rim after acetabuloplasty. (*F*) An arthroscopic view demonstrating the peripheral compartment after femoral osteoplasty, restoring the femoral head neck osteoplasty (*arrow*).

an anterolateral chondrolabral separation and an elevated α angle. CT reconstruction further delineated the cam deformity. The patient underwent arthroscopic labral takedown and chondroplasty of the delaminated acetabular cartilage, followed by acetabular microfracture and labral refixation. After addressing the pathologic condtion of the central compartment, a femoral head-neck osteoplasty was performed to debulk the existing cam deformity (**Fig. 15**).

Case 5. FAI from Residual SCFE Deformity

A 21–year-old collegiate football player with a history of right-sided slipped capital femoral epiphysis presented with hip pain since an in situ screw fixation at the age of 15. Physical examination demonstrated limited hip flexion and internal rotation and positive impingement testing. Intra-articular anesthetic injection resulted in complete relief of symptoms. MRA with metal suppression demonstrated anterolateral labral tearing and asphericity of the femoral head. Treatment consisted of arthroscopic partial labrectomy, acetabular rim reduction, and femoral osteoplasty (**Fig. 16**).

SUMMARY

FAI has been recognized with increasing frequency as a source of hip pain and dysfunction. MRI is useful for detecting both the morphologic features of and the pathologic changes associated with FAI. Understanding both normal and abnormal MRI anatomy of the hip is important for accurately diagnosing and treating FAI. An understanding of the technical considerations involved in MRI is essential for obtaining the appropriate imaging studies required for diagnosis.

REFERENCES

1. Ganz R, Bamert P, Hausner P, et al. Cervico-acetabular impingement after femoral neck fracture. Unfallchirurg 1991;94(4):172–5 [in German].
2. Myers SR, Eijer H, Ganz R. Anterior femoroacetabular impingement after periacetabular osteotomy. Clin Orthop Relat Res 1999;363:93–9.
3. Ganz R, Parvizi J, Beck M, et al. Femoroacetabular impingement: a cause for osteoarthritis of the hip. Clin Orthop Relat Res 2003;417:112–20.
4. Beck M, Kalhor M, Leunig M, et al. Hip morphology influences the pattern of damage to the acetabular cartilage. J Bone Joint Surg Br 2005;87(7):1012–8.
5. Hack K, Di Primio G, Rakhra K, et al. Prevalence of cam-type femoroacetabular impingement morphology in asymptomatic volunteers. J Bone Joint Surg Am 2010;92(14):2436–44.
6. Siebenrock KA, Wahab KH, Werlen S, et al. Abnormal extension of the femoral head epiphysis as a cause of cam impingement. Clin Orthop Relat Res 2004;(418):54–60.
7. Leunig M, Beck M, Kalhor M, et al. Fibrocystic changes at anterosuperior femoral neck: prevalence in hips with femoroacetabular impingement. Radiology 2005; 236(1):237–46.
8. Anderson LA. Acetabular cartilage delamination in femoroacetabular impingement risk factors and magnetic resonance imaging diagnosis. J Bone Joint Surg Am 2009;91(2):305–13.
9. Gosvig KK, Jacobsen S, Sonne-Holm S, et al. Prevalence of malformations of the hip joint and their relationship to sex, groin pain, and risk of osteoarthritis: a population-based survey. J Bone Joint Surg Am 2010;92(5):1162–9.
10. Ganz R, Leunig M, Leunig-Ganz K, et al. The etiology of osteoarthritis of the hip. Clin Orthop Relat Res 2008;466(2):264–72.

11. Ito K, Leunig M, Ganz R. Histopathologic features of the acetabular labrum in femoroacetabular impingement. Clin Orthop Relat Res 2004;429:262–71.

12. Rakhra KS, Sheikh AM, Allen D, et al. Comparison of MRI alpha angle measurement planes in femoroacetabular impingement. Clin Orthop Relat Res 2009; 467(3):660–5.

13. DuBois DF, Omar IM. MR imaging of the hip: normal anatomic variants and imaging pitfalls. Magn Reson Imaging Clin N Am 2010;18(4):663–74.

14. Chang CY, Huang AJ. MR imaging of normal hip anatomy. Magn Reson Imaging Clin N Am 2013;21(1):1–19.

15. Dietrich TJ, Suter A, Pfirrmann CW, et al. Supraacetabular fossa (pseudodefect of acetabular cartilage): frequency at MR arthrography and comparison of findings at MR arthrography and arthroscopy. Radiology 2012;263(2):484–91.

16. Saddik D, Troupis J, Tirman P, et al. Prevalence and location of acetabular sublabral sulci at hip arthroscopy with retrospective MRI review. Am J Roentgenol 2006;187(5):W507–11.

Imaging of Athletic Pubalgia and Core Muscle Injuries

Clinical and Therapeutic Correlations

Andrew Palisch, MD[a], Adam C. Zoga, MD[b],*,
William C. Meyers, MD[c,d,e,f]

KEYWORDS

- Core injury • Core muscle injury • Athletic pubalgia • Sports hernia
- Rectus abdominis/adductor aponeurosis • MRI

KEY POINTS

- MRI is the imaging modality of choice for diagnosis and delineation of core injuries or athletic pubalgia lesions.
- The rectus abdominis and thigh adductor muscle origins all attach to a fibrocartilaginous plate at the anterior pelvis, intimate to the pubic symphysis and pubic tubercles.
- Core injuries involving the rectus abdominis/adductor aponeurosis or the pubic plate can be unilateral, bilateral, or midline in location.
- Although hip injury is the most common confounding cause of groin pain in athletes, numerous other musculoskeletal and visceral injuries ranging from the iliac crest to the pubic symphysis should always be considered.

INTRODUCTION

Injuries to the groin are common in athletes. Clinical presentations of the various causes of groin pain in athletes overlap, and incomplete or incorrect diagnoses may lead to protracted pain syndromes and dysfunction. Such delays cause frustrations and consternation with respect to expected time frames for return to play, or even return to normal daily activities. The three broad categories of differential diagnoses for

[a] Department of Radiology, Thomas Jefferson University Hospital, 132 South 10th Street, Philadelphia, PA 19107, USA; [b] Department of Radiology, Thomas Jefferson University Hospital, 132 South 10th Street, Room 1083A, Philadelphia, PA 19107, USA; [c] Vincera Institute, 4623 South Broad Street, Philadelphia, PA 19112, USA; [d] Department of Surgery, Drexel University College of Medicine, 219 N Broad Street, Philadelphia, PA 19107, USA; [e] Department of Surgery, Thomas Jefferson University, 1015 Walnut Street, Curtis Building, Suite 620, Philadelphia, PA 19107, USA; [f] Department of Surgery, Duke University School of Medicine, 2301 Erwin Road Durham, Durham, NC 27710, USA
* Corresponding author.
E-mail address: Adam.zoga@jefferson.edu

Clin Sports Med 32 (2013) 427–447
http://dx.doi.org/10.1016/j.csm.2013.03.002
0278-5919/13/$ – see front matter © 2013 Elsevier Inc. All rights reserved.

activity-induced groin pain are (1) core muscle injury (athletic pubalgia); (2) ball-in-socket hip joint injury; and (3) other causes.[1] Clinicians managing these injuries need to be familiar with the three categories and broad array of causes, and perform histories and physical examinations comprehensively to come up with the correct diagnoses and appropriate treatment paths. Magnetic resonance imaging (MRI) plays a primary role in the diagnosis and grading of these lesions.[2]

Rapid acceleration, deceleration, twisting, lateral motion, or hyperextension/hyperabduction results in tension on the athlete's musculoskeletal core symmetrically arranged around the pubic bone. Some of the activities most frequently associated with core injury are soccer, American football, ice hockey, lacrosse, rugby, and baseball. Other activities, such as rodeo and basketball, may have a lower incidence of groin pain but are associated with more severe injuries. The pattern of groin injury may have a predilection for the sport type or position of the athlete. In American football, an injury to a right-sided defensive back or linebacker may involve the left groin as the player transitions from a "karaoke" style of running to backpedaling while in pass coverage. In baseball, a left-sided power hitter creates incredible torque across the left lower abdomen and groin. Very slight alteration in "opening the hips" during the swing may cause a left-sided core injury. Pitchers, however, may generate great force on the lower abdomen on either the throwing side or contralateral side. Depending on the specific mechanics and wear-and-tear foci, "transition" phases such as covering first base or fielding a bunt, may cause further alterations and lead to injury on one side versus the other. Hockey goalies may effectively separate their thighs from their abdomens to make a save and produce isolated adductor injuries or disrupt their entire rectus abdominis or adductors from the fibrocartilage plate surrounding the pubic bone. The authors have seen numerous severe cases in which this occurs; the injury extends to complete disruption of the pubic symphysis joint.

Core muscle injury and athletic pubalgia are current, roughly interchangeable descriptors of pelvic musculoskeletal injuries that do not originate from the ball-in-socket hip joint.[3] The authors favor the former term because it highlights the true pathophysiology. Despite its accuracy, athletic pubalgia does not exactly roll off the nonmedical tongue. Other terms including "sports hernia" and "sportsman's hernia" have fallen out of favor because of their misleading nature. These different lesions cannot be lumped into one injury type and they have nothing to do with true inguinal, femoral, obturator, or other types of hernias. True hernias do occasionally occur in athletes, but when they do, they are likely coincidental to the exertional pain that the core injuries produce. The authors emphasize the correct terminology because they continue to see many inappropriate traditional herniorrhaphies presumptively related to the use of this term and some studies in the literature without adequate definitions or compulsive long-term follow-up. They do recognize, however, that several procedures predicated on reinforcement or stabilization of the posterior wall of the rectus abdominis muscle have shown some short-term benefit for some lesions.[4]

The fulcrum of most core muscular injuries is the entire pubic bone with its investing fibrocartilage, which in the radiologic literature is often called the pubic plate (aponeurotic plate). The caudal rectus abdominis muscles, adductor longus, adductor brevis, and pectineus muscles of the adductor compartment blend into this plate over the anterior pubic bones and pubic symphysis joint. This large, plate-like attachment extends bilaterally from one pubic tubercle at the anteroinferior region of the superior pubic ramus just lateral to the pubic symphysis, confluently to the contralateral pubic tubercle. The interaction between the rectus abdominis and central adductor attachments provides much of the stability of the athlete's anterior core. Several other muscles pass in close proximity to this pubic plate including the rectus femoris, sartorius, iliopsoas, and obturators. Understanding this anatomy and associated biomechanics of this region is essential for accurate diagnosis and appropriate treatment.

MUSCULOSKELETAL CORE ANATOMY

The bony pelvis is made up of predominantly the two innominate bones, which are composed each of an ilium, ischium, and pubis and posteriorly by the sacrum and coccyx. The anterior aspect of the bony pelvis with its multiple muscle attachments and the midline pubic symphysis form the center of core injuries and athletic pubalgia. The bony pelvis is joined and stabilized anteriorly at the pubic symphysis, an amphiarthrodial joint, or one that permits limited range of motion and is connected by ligamentous structures.[5–7] Potential motion is limited in the craniocaudal direction, which distributes shear forces during ambulation.[8] A fibrocartilage articular disk is present between the pubic bones and is joined together by four ligaments and muscle attachments that stabilize the joint (**Fig. 1**).

The pubic bone is composed of the pubic body medially and the superior and inferior pubic rami. The pubic body is an ovoid structure with the pubic crest forming the superior and anterior margin. At the inferolateral aspect of the pubic crest lays the pubic tubercle, which is the site of rectus abdominis muscle attachment.[3,8,9] This attachment is important in unilateral rectus abdominis/adductor aponeurosis pattern of athletic pubalgia. The ligamentous attachments of the pubic symphysis include the arcuate, superior, anterior, and posterior pubic ligaments. The arcuate and superior pubic ligaments are the most functionally important for stability and resisting shear forces. The arcuate ligament lines the inferior aspect of the pubic symphysis superficial to the articular disk and deep to the rectus abdominis/adductor aponeurosis. The superior pubic ligament runs between the pubic tubercles. The anterior pubic ligament contains deep fibers that attach to the articular disk and superficial fibers that blend with the rectus abdominis/adductor aponeurosis. The posterior pubic ligament is thin and supplies the least support for stability.[8–10]

Musculoaponeurotic plate attachments at the pubic symphysis are important for core stability of the anterior pelvis. The abdominal musculature attachment includes the rectus abdominis, internal oblique, external oblique, and transversus abdominis. The medial thigh compartment attachments include the pectineus, adductor longus, adductor brevis, adductor magnus, and gracilius. The most important muscular

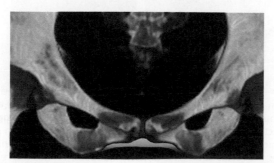

Fig. 1. Diagram of the pubic symphysis demonstrates the midline fibrocartilage pubic disk in *red* and the anteroinferior arcuate ligament in *green*. (*From* Khan W, Zoga AC, Meyers WC. Magnetic resonance imaging of athletic pubalgia and the sports hernia: current understanding and practice. Magn Reson Imaging Clin N Am 2013;21:98.)

attachments for anterior pelvic stabilization are where the rectus abdominis and three adductor muscles (longus, brevis, and pectineus) join to the fibrocartilage plate over the pubic symphysis.[5] This juncture spans the pubic tubercles superiorly at the caudal rectus abdominis attachments all the way to the anterior inferior pubic bodies. The rectus abdominis blends with the anterior pubic ligament medially in close proximity to the superficial inguinal ring laterally.[3] The central adductors also blend with the rectus abdominis laterally near the pubic tubercle at the caudal rectus attachment. The combination of the rectus abdominis, adductor longus, arcuate ligament, and anterior pubic periosteum forms the aponeurotic plate.[3,8,11]

BIOMECHANICS

The rectus abdominis and three adductors interplay tangentially and to some degree antagonistically, which turns out to be essential for anterior pelvic core stability. The rectus abdominis creates superoposterior tension, whereas the adductors create inferoanterior tension during core rotation and extension (**Fig. 2**). Disruption or injury to either the top or bottom component leads to abnormal biomechanical forces on the opposing component leading to instability of the muscle core and many of the lesions encountered in the setting of athletic pubalgia.[12] Detachment of the aponeurosis itself can lead to instability of the pubic symphysis joint, as can injury to the arcuate or anterior pubic ligaments. Such activities as running with an unstable pubic joint often lead to detachment of that fibrocartilage plate from the periosteum of the pubis, exacerbating the instability and shearing forces, ultimately allowing for fluid build-up within that potential space. Repetitive impaction at the symphyseal articular surfaces leads to fluid crossing the cortex, cystic formation, and even a painful pubic symphysis joint arthritis. This spectrum of bone and articular injury including fluid formation within subchondral bone (bone marrow edema), fluid around the symphyseal joint, bony cystic formation, and even classic arthritis is referred to as "osteitis pubis."[3,13]

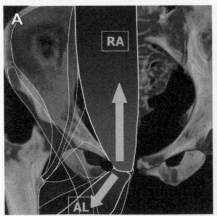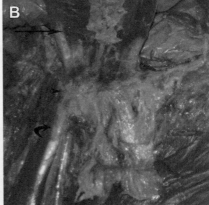

Fig. 2. (A) Diagram of the opposing forces of the rectus abdominis (RA) and adductor longus (AL) at the pubic tubercle. The rectus abdominis creates superoposterior tension, whereas the adductor longus creates inferoanterior tension. Disruption of either leads to altered biomechanics. The *black circle* represents the superficial inguinal ring. (B) Gross specimen demonstrates the rectus abdominis (*arrow*), adductor longus (*curved arrow*), and the pubic tubercle attachment of the rectus abdominis/adductor aponeurosis (*arrowhead*). ([A] *From* Khan W, Zoga AC, Meyers WC. Magnetic resonance imaging of athletic pubalgia and the sports hernia: current understanding and practice. Magn Reson Imaging Clin N Am 2013;21:98.)

Injury to the rectus abdominis or the three adductors can also lead to asymmetric forces across any number of biomechanical axes, often in a compensatory fashion. Strains of the hip flexors, hip rotators, and abdominal wall musculature are commonly encountered with core injuries. Altering biomechanics of the athlete's core may subsequently yield abnormal biomechanical forces and vectors throughout the upper or lower extremities, ultimately contributing to aggravation of hip impingement, hip labral tears, knee ligament injuries, and even ankle sprains. Core injuries in throwing athletes may alter the throwing mechanics and various upper torso and ultimately contribute to overuse syndromes at the shoulder, elbow, or flank musculature.

Accurate identification and treatment of core injuries should be considered essential for optimal timing of return to play and longevity of the athlete. Construction of an appropriate treatment plan and careful management prevent further injury.

HISTORY AND PHYSICAL EXAMINATION

Before modern MRI techniques for these injuries, the combination of history and physical examination provided the primary method of diagnosis. The combination revealed a wide variety of problems seen at surgery and remains the gold standard for diagnosis. As a result of that clinical correlation, two of the authors developed specific imaging techniques using fresh cadavers and then clinical, MRI, and pathologic correlation.

SPECIFIC PATTERNS OF CORE INJURY/ATHLETIC PUBALGIA LESIONS WITH MRI FINDINGS

History, physical examination, and MRI all play critical roles in the accurate diagnosis of core injuries at the rectus abdominis/adductor plate and elsewhere in the pelvic region. A routine large field-of-view bony pelvis MRI for groin pain may be capable of identifying the athlete's injury, but often falls short in accurate injury delineation and in identifying low-grade or chronic lesions. A dedicated athletic pubalgia MRI protocol including large field-of-view sequences of the bony pelvis along with smaller field-of-view sequences centered on the pubic symphysis has evolved as the imaging standard for characterization and delineation of the injury and treatment planning. When a core muscle injury (athletic pubalgia lesion, "sports hernia") is suspected clinically, and imaging is warranted, a dedicated protocol designed to detect such diagnoses should be requested. If an imager or imaging center is unfamiliar with such a protocol, guidance is available in numerous published reviews.[2,3,5]

Core muscle injury and athletic pubalgia manifest with variable patterns on MRI and correct identification of the pattern is essential for surgical planning and recovery. The injury description by the musculoskeletal radiologists at the authors' institution (Thomas Jefferson University) is used by the main referring surgeon to assist in treatment planning in core injuries. Core muscle injuries usually have overlap between the patterns of injury and the association of ball-and-socket hip joint problems. Rarely is just one pattern seen. For convenience, injury patterns are divided into five categories: (1) unilateral or bilateral rectus abdominis/adductor aponeurosis injury; (2) midline rectus abdominis/adductor aponeurosis plate injury (pubic plate injury); (3) osteitis pubis; (4) adductor tendon origin injury; and (5) other core muscle injury.

Unilateral or Bilateral Rectus Abdominis/Adductor Aponeurosis Injury

Injury to the rectus abdominis/adductor aponeurosis is the most common core injury pattern in athletic pubalgia at MRI. This lesion can either be unilateral or bilateral but does not typically extend across midline. The injury involves the caudal rectus abdominis attachment, the adductor longus origin, and the pubic tubercle periosteum off midline. Although an aponeurosis lesion most often originates in the region of the pubic tubercle 1 to 2 cm lateral to the symphysis, it often extends through the lateral edge of the rectus abdominis/adductor aponeurosis near the posteromedial margin of the superficial inguinal ring (**Fig. 3**).[3,12,14–17]

Large aponeurosis injuries are easily identified on MRI; however, small injuries can be subtle even with a dedicated athletic pubalgia protocol. Assessing for symmetry between the two sides of the caudal rectus abdominis and the aponeurosis is often essential for finding the lesion.

On coronal fluid-sensitive images, a secondary cleft almost always correlates with the site of symptoms.[18,19] Originally, the secondary cleft sign was an arthrographic finding, which was believed to represent a tear at the origin of the adductor longus and gracilis. The primary cleft is a normal developmental finding that has a vertical course at the pubic symphysis, whereas the secondary cleft appears as an inferolateral extension of the primary cleft coursing around the anteroinferior aspect of the pubic body.[5,19] At MRI, the secondary cleft is usually positioned between the rectus abdominis/adductor aponeurosis and pubic bone indicating a detachment of the aponeurotic insertion, but it may be subapophyseal in younger patients before pubic apophyseal maturation.[3]

Cross-sectional morphology on axial MR images is another imaging clue to a rectus abdominis/adductor aponeurosis lesion. The normal caudal rectus abdominis has curvilinear morphology laterally, whereas the injured side often shows an acutely angled or squared contour laterally leaving a more patulous superficial inguinal ring. This lateral rectus abdominis deficiency may be why some patients showed improvement with mesh inguinal hernia repairs.[4] Another common finding at MRI is focal subenthesial marrow edema on the pubic tubercle, likely reflecting avulsion of the aponeurosis. Osteitis pubis may or may not be a concomitant finding. The visible cleft often extends into the proximal adductor longus tendon with thickening and visible interstitial tearing, or simply peritendinous edema. More severe injuries can show complete detachment of the adductor longus from the pubic bone with retraction.

Clinically, a rectus abdominis/adductor aponeurosis lesion presents with focal tenderness at the pubic tubercle, anteroinferior on the pubic bone just lateral to midline. Pain occurs with various resistance tests designed to bring out pain with contraction of the associated muscles.

Although symptoms can improve with time off and physical therapy regimens, symptom recurrence is very common on resumption of activity. With rectus abdominis/adductor aponeurosis lesions, pelvic floor reconstruction is often considered the best option for a full recovery. After unilateral pelvic floor repair, an ipsilateral recurrence is very uncommon, but approximately 4% of patients develop a contralateral aponeurosis lesion at some point in the future.

An MRI report impression for a unilateral rectus abdominis/adductor aponeurosis injury may include (1) right rectus abdominis/adductor aponeurosis injury with detachment of the right caudal rectus abdominis extending laterally into the adductor origin, (2) tendinosis of the right adductor longus origin with interstitial tearing, (3) right pubic tubercle bone marrow edema, or (4) mild osteitis pubis.

Midline Rectus Abdominis/Adductor Aponeurotic Plate Injury

Midline pubic plate lesions are another common pattern of core muscle/athletic pubalgia injury encountered at MRI. With this lesion, bright signal on fluid-sensitive images (T2 hyperintense signal) extends bilaterally from the midline pubic symphysis forming the appearance of a bilateral secondary cleft. Fluid or granulation tissue extends from midline undercutting both rectus abdominis attachments medially and generally then

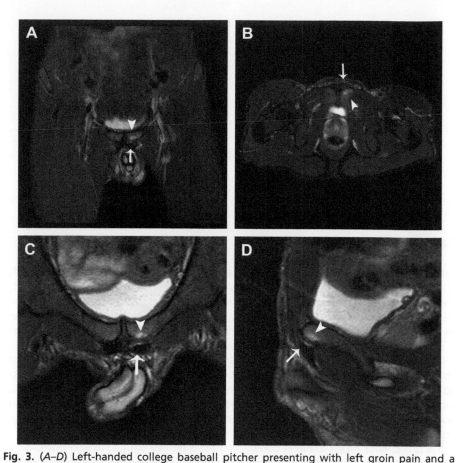

Fig. 3. (*A–D*) Left-handed college baseball pitcher presenting with left groin pain and a small unilateral detachment of the caudal rectus abdominis. (*A*) Large field-of-view coronal short TE inversion recovery (STIR) image of the bony pelvis shows a subtle transverse tear (*arrow*) in the left caudal rectus abdominis attachment at the pubic tubercle with focal edema localized to the pubic tubercle (*arrowhead*). (*B*) Large field-of-view axial T2 fat saturated fast spin echo (FSE) image of the bony pelvis shows a subtle transverse tear (*arrow*) in the left caudal rectus abdominis attachment at the pubic tubercle with focal edema localized to the pubic tubercle (*arrowhead*). (*C*) Small field-of-view coronal oblique T2 fat saturated FSE image using an athletic pubalgia protocol better demonstrates the detachment (*arrow*) of the left caudal rectus abdominis at the pubic tubercle with focal edema localized to the pubic tubercle (*arrowhead*) typical for a rectus abdominis/adductor aponeurosis lesion. The detachment may or may not extend into the adductor origin as a secondary cleft. (*D*) Small field-of-view sagittal T2 fat saturated FSE image using a pubalgia protocol demonstrates the detachment (*arrow*) of the left caudal rectus abdominis at the pubic tubercle with focal edema localized to the pubic tubercle (*arrowhead*). (*E, F*) Right-handed power hitting baseball player presenting with severe right groin pain and a large unilateral rectus abdominis/adductor aponeurosis defect. (*E*) Small field-of-view coronal oblique T2 fat saturated FSE image using an athletic pubalgia protocol demonstrates a large unilateral right aponeurotic tear with amputation of the right rectus abdominis (*arrow*) and avulsion of the right adductor longus (*arrowhead*). (*F*) Small field-of-view sagittal T2 fat saturated FSE image using a pubalgia protocol demonstrates a large unilateral right aponeurotic tear with detachment of the right rectus abdominis (*arrow*) and absence of the right adductor longus secondary to avulsion (*arrowhead*).

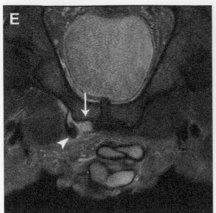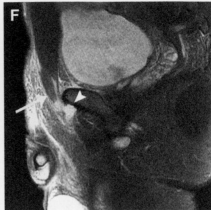

Fig. 3. (*continued*)

extending inferiorly involving both rectus abdominis/adductor aponeurosis (**Fig. 4**). The injury often extends asymmetrically to one side or the other and may extend to the lateral edge of the aponeurosis on one or both sides. With many midline pubic plate lesions, MRI shows visible extension of the injury into one adductor longus tendon where there is interstitial tearing, while sparing the other (**Fig. 5**). Osteitis pubis is common in the setting of pubic plate lesions.[15–17]

Clinically, midline pubic plate lesions can present in a similar fashion to unilateral aponeurosis lesions, and the symptomatic side often correlates with the side of adductor involvement at MRI. There is often, however, point tenderness at both pubic tubercles. For women with a core injury, midline pubic plate lesions are very common, possibly reflecting the strong anatomic raphe between the left and right rectus abdominis muscles.[3]

If a pelvic floor repair is being considered for a patient with a midline pubic plate lesion, even if symptomatology is predominately unilateral, a contralateral repair should at least be discussed because the midline defect could ultimately become symptomatic on the unrepaired side.

An MRI report impressions for pubic plate injury might include (1) midline pubic plate injury of the rectus abdominis/adductor aponeurosis, asymmetric to the right with extension to the right lateral edge into the adductor origin; (2) tendinosis of the right adductor origin with interstitial tearing; or (3) acute osteitis pubis, asymmetric to the right.

Osteitis Pubis

The pubic symphysis allows limited mobility in the cranial caudal direction and the shear forces transmitted from the axial to appendicular skeletal can lead stress across the pubic symphysis. Along with core muscle injury this can lead to altered biomechanics resulting in an inflammatory response leading to osteitis and periostitis.[5,13] The instability results in progressive core muscle injury and in turn progressive osteitis pubis.

Osteitis pubis has acute and chronic forms. Acute osteitis pubis on MRI shows bone marrow edema involving the subchondral bone at the pubic symphysis extending from anterior to posterior. The edema is usually bilateral but often asymmetric with more advanced edema involving the symptomatic side (**Fig. 6**). In chronic osteitis pubis, productive changes with osteophytes, sclerosis, and subchondral cysts are present

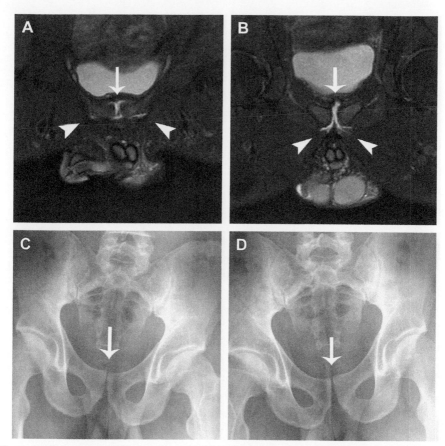

Fig. 4. Midline pubic plate detachment with unstable pubic symphysis. Professional hockey goalie with severe bilateral groin pain, unable to play. This is one of the most severe core muscle injuries seen at MRI. (*A*) Small field-of-view coronal oblique T2 fat saturated FSE image at the superior pubic plate using a pubalgia protocol demonstrates a severe midline detachment (*arrow*), which extends across the pubic symphysis suggestive of ligamentous instability. The midline detachment extends bilaterally to the lateral edge of the aponeurosis (*arrowheads*). (*B*) Inferiorly on the small field-of-view coronal oblique T2 fat saturated FSE sequence demonstrates the severe midline defect (*arrow*), which extends bilaterally into the adductor origins with interstitial tearing (*arrowheads*). (*C*) AP radiograph of the pelvis using a flamingo view (right leg straight and left knee flexed) demonstrates elevation (*arrow*) of the right pubic body relative to the left pubic body. This finding suggests instability across the pubic symphysis. (*D*) AP radiograph of the pelvis using a flamingo view (left leg straight and right knee flexed) demonstrates elevation (*arrow*) of the left pubic body relative to the right pubic body. This finding suggests instability across the pubic symphysis.

secondary to chronic instability. Often, patients present with acute on chronic osteitis pubis, which follows their clinical course. A variant pattern of severe osteitis pubis shows extensive subchondral bone marrow edema with articular erosion, similar to distal clavicular osteolysis at the acromioclavicular joint. The ability of the pubic symphysis to heal is unclear with these more advanced lesions.[20–22]

Clinically, osteitis pubis presents with pain and tenderness. However, it is often seen in conjunction with a rectus abdominis/adductor aponeurosis lesion or a pubic plate

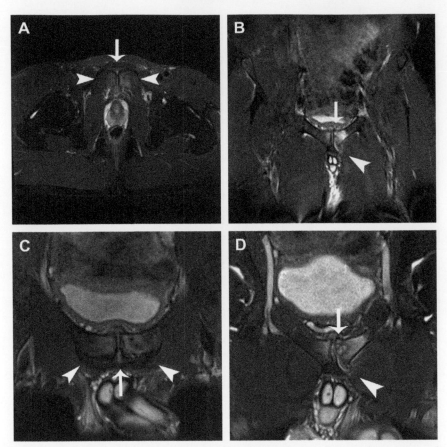

Fig. 5. Midline pubic plate detachment. Left-handed professional power hitter presenting with left groin pain. Typical core injury in hitters involves the rectus abdominis/adductor aponeurosis of the back leg. (*A*) Large field-of-view axial T2 fat saturated FSE image of the bony pelvis shows a midline pubic plate tear (*arrow*) with osteitis pubis (*arrowheads*). This is a severe core injury, which is poorly seen on the survey images of the bony pelvis. (*B*) Large field-of-view coronal STIR image of the bony pelvis shows a secondary cleft extending into the left adductor origin with interstitial tearing (*arrowhead*). Osteitis pubis is present (*arrow*). (*C*) Small field-of-view coronal oblique T2 fat saturated FSE image using a pubalgia protocol better demonstrates the midline pubic plate detachment (*arrow*), which extends bilaterally (*arrowheads*). (*D*) Inferiorly on the small field-of-view coronal oblique T2 fat saturated FSE sequences, the midline detachment extends inferiorly into the left adductor origin as a secondary cleft (*arrowhead*) with interstitial tearing of the left adductor origin. Asymmetric acute on chronic osteitis pubis (*arrow*) is present with severe edema with degenerative cystic and productive changes.

lesion. In these cases, treatment is generally directed at the soft tissue lesion and pain from the osteitis pubis itself is felt to dissipate with time away from activity and stabilization of the symphysis.

There are scenarios where osteitis pubis occurs without an aponeurosis or pubic plate lesion, including ligamentous instability syndromes related to pregnancy or axial loading traumas.[3,23] If the primary concern is alleviating pain from the bony inflammation of osteitis pubis, image-guided steroid injections are often effective.

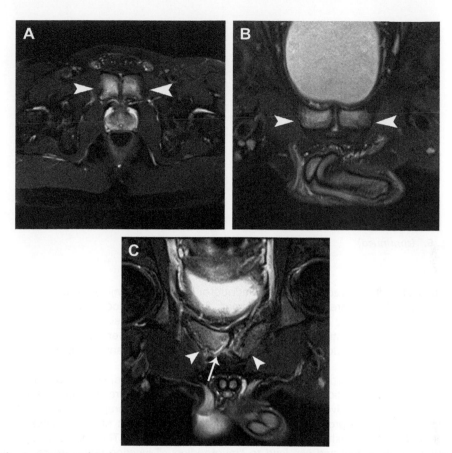

Fig. 6. Osteitis pubis. (*A, B*) College football player with typical appearance of severe acute osteitis pubis. (*A*) Large field-of-view axial T2 fat saturated FSE image of the bony pelvis shows severe acute osteitis pubis (*arrowheads*). Osteitis pubis extends in the anterior-posterior direction involving the pubic body rather than the focal edema localized to the pubic tubercle, which is often seen in unilateral caudal rectus abdominis detachments. (*B*) Small field-of-view coronal oblique T2 fat saturated FSE image using a pubalgia protocol demonstrates the severe acute osteitis pubis (*arrowheads*). No chronic changes are seen, such as degenerative cysts, sclerosis, or osteophytes in this case. (*C–E*) College soccer player with severe acute on chronic osteitis pubis. (*C*) Small field-of-view coronal oblique T2 fat saturated FSE image using a pubalgia protocol demonstrates severe acute on chronic osteitis pubis (*arrowheads*) with disorganization and resorption predominantly affecting the left pubis. A right secondary cleft is present (*arrow*). (*D*) Small field-of-view coronal oblique proton density image using a pubalgia protocol demonstrates severe acute on chronic osteitis pubis (*arrowheads*) with disorganization and resorption predominantly affecting the left pubis. (*E*) Large field-of-view axial T2 fat saturated FSE image of the bony pelvis demonstrates severe acute on chronic osteitis pubis (*arrowheads*) with disorganization and resorption predominantly affecting the left pubis.

Adductor Injury

The thigh adductor muscles and myotendinous units are frequently involved in athletic core injury syndromes. The three central adductor origins are intimately related to the caudal rectus abdominis and the osseous pubic periosteum. Even in the

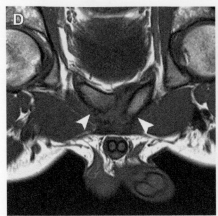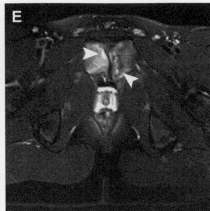

Fig. 6. (*continued*)

setting of a classic rectus abdominis/adductor aponeurosis injury, care should be taken at MRI interpretation to fully detail the degree of adductor involvement, including the specific muscles injured, asymmetric tendon size or peritendinous edema, and any interstitial tearing or complete avulsion. However, a subset of lesions is isolated to the adductor compartments without significant rectus abdominis involvement.

Chronic adductor origin pathologies are common in athletes. Low-grade isolated adductor lesions, particularly the ones away from the origins, are often treated effectively with conservative measures and focused physical therapy. An asymmetric enlargement of the proximal adductor longus is often seen at MRI in athletes who repeatedly extend against resistance, as in ice hockey skating. This can be a nagging source of groin pain and can lead to "myotendinous" junction strains more distal within the adductor compartment. The origins of the adductors are actually quite different from other muscles (eg, hamstring). They originate from the thick fibrocartilage plate and usually have very little true tendon. Some adductor injuries are centered at the proximal "myotendinous" junction, 8 to 15 cm distal to the origin. On MRI, strains present with increased T2 signal involving the muscle belly or "myotendinous" junction and are graded similarly to other muscle strains throughout the body (**Fig. 7**). A particularly difficult lesion in this location is a nonhealing strain with accompanying disruption of the regional epimysium, sometimes termed "baseball pitcher hockey goalie syndrome" (BPHGS). This particular injury appears at MRI as a relatively innocuous adductor myotendinous strain, most often involving the adductor longus, without significant fiber disruption but with a thickened and nodular central complex. The clinical presentation of BPHGS is that of a nagging medial thigh or groin strain, aggravated by specific activities with intermittent periods of improvement, and then subsequent reinjury. Usually these patients respond to time, physical therapy, and sometimes injection. Because healing tends to be slow in BPHGS, and activity may cause a new injury more proximal, near the aponeurosis, these patients sometimes go on to regional soft tissue debridement and compartment decompression similar to gastrocnemius compartmental releases in runners, and the patients generally do well.[24–26]

Although the common cause of adductor injury is most often chronic overuse, acute injuries also occur. Any of the adductor muscles may avulse from their pubic

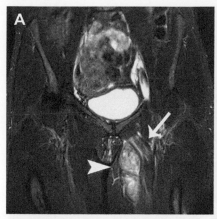 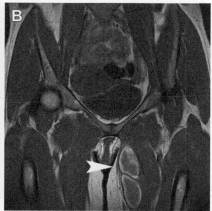

Fig. 7. Adductor longus strain and hematoma. Female patient presented with left groin pain after injury during yoga. (*A*) Large field-of-view coronal STIR image of the bony pelvis demonstrates a strain of the left adductor longus (*arrow*) and adjacent hematoma medially (*arrowhead*). (*B*) Large field-of-view coronal T1 image of the bony pelvis demonstrates the hematoma (*arrowhead*) medially to the adductor longus strain. Hematomas often show high T1 signal because of the degradation of blood products.

fibrocartilage plate origin. The adductor longus is most apt to avulse with up and down forceful jumping as in basketball rebounding, whereas the pectineus is more likely more sideways adductor action (eg, ice hockey, bull riding). With these avulsive proximal adductor injuries, care should be taken to exclude involvement of the rectus abdominis on physical examination and at MRI. Rarely, with extreme forced thigh abduction and extension, an osseous avulsion occurs with a fragment of the bony pubis detaching along with the adductor longus origin and retracting into the medial thigh, and ultimately requiring surgical fixation.[18,27–29]

Occasionally, and generally in the setting of a high-grade acute rectus abdominis/adductor aponeurosis lesion, a group of the adductor origins including at least the pectineus and the adductor longus avulse and retract together with a mushroom-like appearance of the avulsed common plate joining both muscles. This "anterior adductor avulsion" injury can often be reduced and stabilized at the time of pelvic floor repair to accelerate the return to play (**Fig. 8**).[3,5,18,30]

In the postoperative period after pelvic floor repair or tendon release, a common and almost expected MRI finding is edema about the distal adductor compartment myotendinous junctions. This is often located 15 to 20 cm from the muscle origin and may be bilateral. The cause is unclear, but may be secondary to an overall tightening of the postoperative core combined with prescribed physical therapy aimed at core strengthening and adductor flexibility.[3,31]

Rectus Abdominis Strain

Purely isolated strain or tear of the rectus abdominis muscle is an uncommon core injury pattern. Although the point of maximal tenderness may be well cephalad to the pubic symphysis, concomitant strains or degenerative lesions involving the more caudal rectus abdominis are common. Although a high rectus abdominis muscle injury, away from the insertion site, is generally treated nonoperatively, similar to other muscle belly injuries, more distal rectus abdominis lesions near the pubic symphysis are generally categorized as rectus abdominis/adductor aponeurosis lesions,

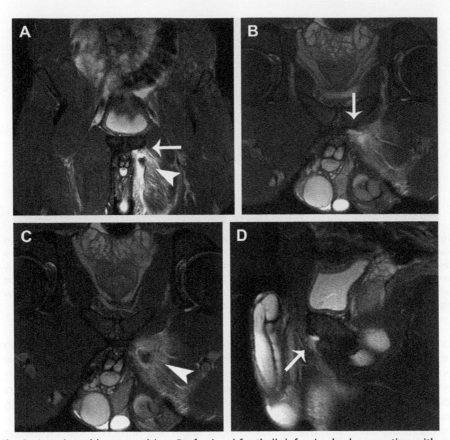

Fig. 8. Anterior adductor avulsion. Professional football defensive back presenting with severe left groin pain. Right-sided defensive backs often injury their left rectus abdominis/adductor aponeurosis when transitioning during pass coverage. (*A*) Large field-of-view coronal STIR image of the bony pelvis shows detachment of the left adductor origin from the aponeurosis (*arrow*) with the retracted tendon fibers distally (*arrowhead*). The distance of retraction is often best measured on the coronal STIR images. (*B*) Small field-of-view coronal oblique T2 fat saturated FSE image using a pubalgia protocol demonstrates the detachment of the left anterior adductor origin from the aponeurotic plate (*arrow*). Often the pectinius and adductor longus detach together and is referred to as an "anterior adductor avulsion" because these are the two most anterior muscles at the pubic attachment. (*C*) Inferiorly on the small field-of-view coronal oblique T2 fat saturated FSE sequence, the retracted tendon fibers are seen distally (*arrowhead*). (*D*) Small field-of-view sagittal T2 fat saturated FSE image using a pubalgia protocol demonstrates the detachment of the left adductors from the aponeurotic plate (*arrow*). The retracted fibers are not seen on this image.

and often warrant intervention depending on the clinical correlations. Sometimes at MRI, it is important to use markers to indicate the site of pain on the abdominal wall, because standard athletic pubalgia protocols may not cover this area. After the injured region is imaged with MRI, the salient finding is increased intramuscular signal on fluid-sensitive sequences and rectus abdominis surface area enlargement on short axis and sometimes visible fiber disruption with feathery edema on long axis (**Fig. 9**). The contralateral rectus abdominis can be used as an internal control, but it

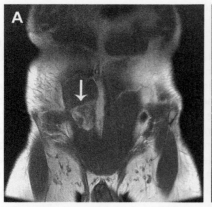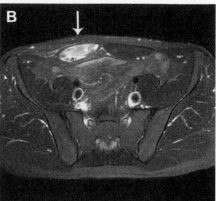

Fig. 9. Rectus abdominis muscle strain. Professional tennis player presenting with right abdominal wall pain after injuring during a serve. (*A*) Large field-of-view coronal T1 image of the bony pelvis shows a high-grade strain and hematoma (*arrow*) isolated to the right middle rectus abdominis muscle belly. The tendinous intersections and linea alba divide the rectus abdominis into the muscle bellies. (*B*) Large field-of-view axial T2 fat saturated FSE image of the bony pelvis shows a high-grade strain and hematoma (*arrow*) isolated to the right middle rectus abdominis muscle belly.

remains important to perform at least survey imaging of the pubic symphysis region.[17]

Inguinal Hernia

The close proximity of the inguinal canal to the caudal rectus abdominis attachment creates some of the confusion with true hernias. In the literature are papers that suggest that in athletes direct inguinal and femoral hernias are more common than indirect hernia.[31] Those types of studies help explain why the term "sports hernia" evolved. The term was banned from the medical literature in the 1970s because of poor results from hernia repair, in the absence of a palpable hernia. It remains nonetheless true that inguinal hernias do occur in this young population but rarely cause much discomfort in the absence of incarceration. Ironically, true inguinal hernias may be easily imaged on the coronal oblique non–fat-suppressed imaged from an athletic pubalgia MRI protocol sequence by evaluating asymmetry of the inguinal canal. Cord lipomas, however, create several false positives. Normal inguinal canal fat occurs in the spermatic cords or round ligaments.[32] Likewise, retroperitoneal fat extending into the inguinal canal occurs commonly common at MRI, but should not typically be considered a true hernia. Most often, at exploration, this fat is adherent to the spermatic cord, essentially functioning like a lipoma, and not sliding like a hernia. If a true hernia is suspected, alternative MRI or ultrasound techniques including prone imaging and dynamic sequences with and without Valsalva maneuver can be used, but definitive diagnosis of true hernia requires the presence of true intraperitoneal structures, such as the intestine, outside the peritoneal cavity or sliding within the inguinal canal or through the superficial ring.

A patulous superficial ring related to a rectus abdominis/adductor aponeurosis lesion can be addressed surgically at the time of pelvic floor repair. The concept of mesh should be preserved for true hernias. The presence of mesh on MRI may cause considerable distortion and is definitely associated with muscle atrophy.

DIFFERENTIAL CONSIDERATIONS REMOTE FROM THE PUBIC SYMPHYSIS
Hip Disorders

Hip pathology is often the most common differential diagnostic consideration in patients presenting with activity-related groin pain. Acetabular labral tears are exceedingly common in athletes with the most common locations along the anterosuperior and anterior aspects of the acetabulum.[33] Most athletic pubalgia MRI protocols offer a survey, such as limited assessment of the acetabular labra. Secondary signs of labral pathology, including paralabral cysts and joint effusions, and visible labral detachment should be identified, but chondral defects and nondetached labral tears are more difficult. Osseous morphologies predisposing the hip to femeroacetabular impingement and avascular necrosis and osteoarthritis can also be seen on the larger field-of-view sequences. If an acetabular labrum or cartilage lesion is suspected as the source of groin pain, dedicated imaging of the suspected hip with direct MR arthrography is the imaging standard (**Fig. 10**).

Concomitant hip and pubic symphysis lesions are a frequent occurrence in athletes. Even after a core injury is identified at physical examination, passive and active maneuvers dedicated to diagnosing hip lesions should be performed. Ultimately, if the clinical examination is unclear or suspicious for concomitant hip and groin injuries, a noncontrast athletic pubalgia MRI and a dedicated MR arthrogram of the hip with intra-articular contrast and anesthetic may be warranted. Ultimately, the response to intra-articular anesthetic may be the most useful diagnostic tool in effectively referring the patient to the most appropriate subspecialist hip surgeon or general surgeon.

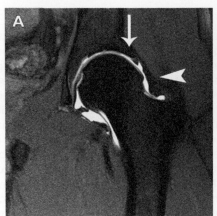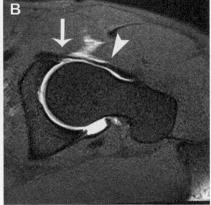

Fig. 10. Labral tear. Professional hockey player presented with groin pain for core muscle injury evaluation. An MRI with a pubalgia protocol was performed; however, no core injury was identified. On the large field-of-view images of the bony pelvis and small field-of-view sagittal images, there were findings of hip pathology including femeroacetabular impingement and a labral tear. Patient was evaluated in surgery clinic and dedicated MRI arthrography of the left hip was performed. (A) Coronal T1 fat saturated MR arthrogram image of the left hip demonstrates a nondetached tear of the superior labrum adjacent to a region of partial thickness cartilage loss of the superior acetabulum (*arrow*) and prominence of the left femoral head/neck junction (*arrowhead*) compatible with femeroacetabular impingement. (B) Axial oblique T1 fat saturated MR arthrogram image of the left hip demonstrates attenuation and tear (detached on other images) of the left anterior labrum (*arrow*) and prominence of the left femoral head/neck junction (*arrowhead*) compatible with femeroacetabular impingement.

Stress Fracture

Athletic patients perform activities that place atypical stresses on osseous structures during activity, particularly during initial training regimens or return to play. A soft tissue injury can cause altered biomechanics, exacerbating the atypical osseous stresses. The most common location for osseous stress response and stress fractures of the pelvis include the medial femoral neck, pubic rami, and parasymphaseal regions. With respect to many of these core muscle lesions, an intense osteitis may easily be overread as a stress fracture, even though the imaging may satisfy many of the characteristics that make that diagnosis. On MRI imaging there is initial focal T2 or STIR hyperintense signal, which progress to form a T1 hypointense fracture line perpendicular to the coursing trabeculae (**Fig. 11**).[34]

Skeletal immaturity introduces another spectrum of osseous stress injury with stress fracture at an immature growth plate. A stress fracture at the maturing triradiate fibrocartilage can mimic a unilateral rectus abdominis/adductor aponeurosis lesion clinically, but the most effective treatment is rest and limitation of weight bearing. Given the differences in therapy, distinguishing a primary soft tissue lesion from an osseous stress injury at MRI is imperative.

Accessory Flexor Lesions

Injuries to the accessory hip flexor tendons, including myotendinous strains, avulsions, and bursitis, are within the spectrum of core injury and are common sources of groin pain that can clinically mimic pubic symphysis lesions. The sartorius can be avulsed from the anterior superior iliac spine with an acute flexion injury or can be chronically enlarged and edematous at its muscle belly with overuse injury in such activities as yoga and cycling. The iliacus muscle and iliopsoas tendon are sometimes strained with repetitive flexion/rotation activities, such as gymnastics. External oblique avulsions are sometimes encountered in athletes who run while twisting at the waist as in football.

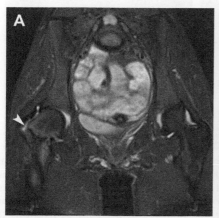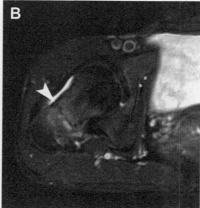

Fig. 11. Stress fracture. A long distance runner who persistently ran despite chronic right hip pain. The patient presented with right groin pain for core muscle injury. No prior radiographs were performed. (*A*) Large field-of-view coronal STIR image of the bony pelvis shows the stress fracture with a hypointense fracture line (*arrowhead*) with surrounding marrow edema. The fracture is dorsally angulated. (*B*) Large field-of-view axial T2 fat saturated FSE image of the bony pelvis shows the stress fracture with a hypointense fracture line (*arrowhead*) and surrounding marrow edema.

Any of these flexor strains may ultimately manifest as iliopsoas bursitis, and MRI can identify myotendinous edema, avulsive bony stress response, peritendinous edema or tendinous enlargement, and nodularity indicating an acute or chronic injury along the myo-teno-osseous unit. With iliopsoas bursitis, MRI shows T2 hyperintense fluid between the anterior hip capsule and distal iliopsoas tendon lateral to the femoral neurovascular bundle, with the position distinguishing it from a loculated joint effusion.[35,36]

Apophysitis

The biomechanical mechanisms discussed previously can cause apophysitis at several locations around the pelvis in a skeletally immature patient with athletic

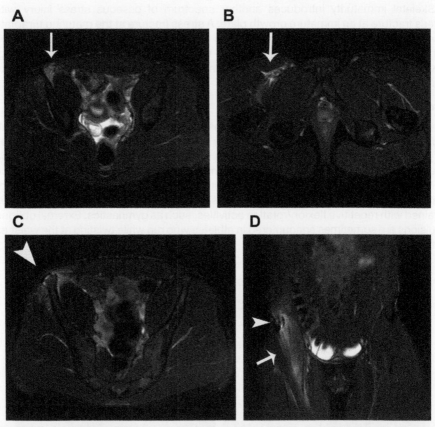

Fig. 12. Acute iliac muscle strain and chronic avulsion of the anterior superior iliac crest. Olympic-level female gymnast presented with right abdominal wall and right groin pain. (A) Large field-of-view axial T2 fat saturated FSE image of the bony pelvis demonstrated an acute strain of the right iliacus muscle (*arrow*) anterior to the psoas muscle. (B) Inferiorly on the large field-of-view axial T2 fat saturated FSE image of the bony pelvis shows the acute strain extending distally (*arrow*) in the region of the myotendinous junction. (C) Large field-of-view axial T2 fat saturated FSE image of the bony pelvis demonstrates a chronic avulsion of the anterior superior iliac crest (*arrowhead*) mildly displaced anterolaterally. Adjacent edema from the iliacus strain is seen medially. (D) Large field-of-view coronal STIR image of the bony pelvis demonstrates the chronic avulsion of the anterior superior iliac crest (*arrowhead*) and strain of the right iliacus muscle (*arrow*) involving the myotendinous junction.

pubalgia. Chronic, repetitive stress at an unfused apophyseal growth plate leads to delayed fusion or nonfusion, sometimes with fragmentation and even occasionally osteonecrosis.[3] This is generally a painful, nagging injury exacerbated by the specific activity and showing apophyseal and peritendinous edema at MRI. Ischial tuberosity apophysitis is common in the dominant lower extremity of teenaged soccer players. Anterior superior iliac spine apophysitis occurs with activities repetitively stressing the tensor fascia lata or the sartorius. Forceful thigh flexion activities can cause a painful apophysitis at the rectus femoris origin from the anterior inferior iliac spine. This lesion is common in hurdlers and kicking athletes, and can ultimately lead to frank apophyseal avulsion and displacement.

Apophysitis presents clinically with pain during active contraction of the involved myotendinous unit and point tenderness at the apophysis itself. Treatment may be operative or nonoperative depending on the specific situations. Interventional treatment should be directed toward stabilization of the apophysis until skeletal maturity (**Fig. 12**).

Surprises

Although common core injury lesions are observed at MRI, the imager must be leery of the unexpected MRI finding in patients with chronic groin pain. Osteoid osteoma and Langerhans cell histiocytosis (formerly eosinophilic granuloma) are benign but painful tumors of bone that tend to occur in children and young adults, often in the pelvis and proximal femur bones. Schwanomas may appear here. Soft tissue sarcomas, although rare, can also arise in pelvic region in this patient population. Inflammatory bowel disease, although a difficult diagnosis with MRI, can be a source of chronic lower abdominal and groin pain, as can endometriosis in women. When a patient presents with an athletic pubalgia history, and no injury is seen at the pubic symphysis or the hips, it is best to take a second and third look at the MRI to exclude uncommon lesions such as these.

SUMMARY

With an understanding of the anatomy, biomechanics, and common injury presentations at the musculoskeletal core or pelvic region, core muscle injuries (athletic pubalgia lesions) can be accurately diagnosed and treated. MRI plays an integral role in the process, not only in firming up the most common injuries, such as rectus abdominis/adductor aponeurosis lesions, but also in identifying the numerous other specific injuries that occur in this anatomic region. A dedicated noncontrast athletic pubalgia MRI protocol should be available at facilities where athletes are imaged.

REFERENCES

1. Meyers W, Zoga A, Joseph T, et al. Current understanding of core muscle injuries: athletic pubalgia, "sports hernia." In: Thomas Byrd JW, editor. Operative hip arthroscopy. New York: Springer; 2013. p. 67–77.
2. Khan W, Zoga A, Meyers W. Magnetic resonance imaging of athletic pubalgia and sports hernia: current understanding and practice. Magn Reson Imaging Clin N Am 2013;21(1):97–110.
3. Zoga A, Mullens F, Meyers W. The spectrum of MR imaging in athletic pubalgia. Radiol Clin North Am 2010;48:1179–97.
4. Srinivasan A, Schuricht A. Long-term follow-up of laparoscopic preperitoneal hernia repair in professional athletes. J Laparoendosc Adv Surg Tech A 2002;12(2):101–6.

5. Omar IM, Zoga AC, Kavanagh EC, et al. Athletic pubalgia and "sports hernia": optimal MR imaging technique and findings. Radiographics 2008;28:1415–38.
6. Walheim GG, Selvik G. Mobility of the pubic symphysis: in vivo measurements with an electromechanic method and a roentgen stereophotogrammetric method. Clin Orthop Relat Res 1984;191:129–35.
7. Walheim G, Olerud S, Ribbe T. Mobility of the pubic symphysis: measurements by an electromechanical method. Acta Orthop Scand 1984;55(2):203–8.
8. Gamble JG, Simmons SC, Freedman M. The symphysis pubis: anatomic and pathologic considerations. Clin Orthop Relat Res 1986;203:261–72.
9. Williams A. Thigh. In: Stranding S, editor. Gray's anatomy: the anatomical basis of clinical practice. 39th edition. Edinburgh (Scotland): Elsevier; 2008. p. 1349–87.
10. Putschar WG. The structure of the human symphysis pubis with special consideration of parturition and its sequelae. Am J Phys Anthropol 1976;45(3 pt 2):589–94.
11. Vix VA, Ryu CY. The adult symphysis pubis: normal and abnormal. Am J Roentgenol Radium Ther Nucl Med 1971;112:517–25.
12. Zoga AC, Kavanaugh EC, Omar IM, et al. Athletic pubalgia and the "sports hernia": MR imaging findings. Radiology 2008;247(3):797–807.
13. Harris NH, Murray RO. Lesions of the symphysis in athletes. Br Med J 1974; 4(5938):211–4.
14. Meyers WC, McKechnie A, Philippon MJ, et al. Experience with "sports hernia" spanning two decades. Ann Surg 2008;248(4):656–65.
15. Shortt CP, Zoga AC, Kavanagh EC, et al. Anatomy, pathology, and MRI findings in the sports hernia. Semin Musculoskelet Radiol 2008;12(1):54–61.
16. Kavanagh EC, Zoga AC, Omar I, et al. MR imaging of the rectus abdominis/adductor aponeurosis: findings in the "sports hernia." Proceedings of the American Roentgen Ray Society. AJR Am J Roentgenol 2007;188:A13–6.
17. Mullens FE, Zoga AC, Meyers WC. Review of MRI technique and imaging findings in athletic pubalgia and the "sports hernia". Eur J Radiol 2012;81(12):3780–92.
18. Robinson P, Barron DA, Parsons W, et al. Adductor-related groin pain in athletes: correlation of MR imaging with clinical findings. Skeletal Radiol 2004;33:451–7.
19. Brennan D, O'Connell MJ, Ryan M, et al. Secondary cleft sign as a marker of injury in athletes with groin pain. MR image appearance and interpretation. Radiology 2005;235:162–7.
20. Cunningham PM, Brennan D, O'Connell M, et al. Patterns of bone and soft-tissue injury at the symphysis pubis in soccer players: observations at MRI. AJR Am J Roentgenol 2007;188:W291–6.
21. Verrall GM, Slavotinek JP, Fon GT. Incidence of pubic bone marrow oedema in Australian rules football players: relation to groin pain. Br J Sports Med 2001; 35:28–33.
22. Kunduracioglu B, Yilmaz C, Yorubulut M, et al. Magnetic resonance findings of osteitis pubis. J Magn Reson Imaging 2007;25(3):535–9.
23. Gibbon WW, Hession PR. Diseases of the pubis and pubic symphysis: MR imaging appearances. AJR Am J Roentgenol 1997;169:849–53.
24. Meyers WC, Lanfranco A, Castellanos A. Surgical management of chronic lower abdominal and groin pain in high-performance athletes. Curr Sports Med Rep 2002;1:301–5.
25. Gokhale S. Three-dimensional sonography of muscle hernias. J Ultrasound Med 2007;26:239–42.
26. Zoga AC, Meyers WC. Magnetic resonance imaging for pain after surgical treatment for athletic pubalgia and the "sports hernia". Semin Musculoskelet Radiol 2011;15(4):372–82.

27. Akermark C, Johansson C. Tenotomy of the adductor longus tendon in the treatment of chronic groin pain in athletes. Am J Sports Med 1992;20:640–3.
28. Anderson K, Strickland SM, Warren R. Hip and groin injuries in athletes. Am J Sports Med 2001;29:521–33.
29. Garrett WE Jr. Muscle strain injuries. Am J Sports Med 1996;24(Suppl 6):S2–8.
30. Nicholas SJ, Tyler TF. Adductor muscle strains in sports. Sports Med 2002;32: 339–44.
31. Gullmo A. Herniography: the diagnosis of hernia in the groin and incompetence of the pouch of Douglas and pelvic floor. Acta Radiol Suppl 1980;361:1–76.
32. van den Berg JC, de Valois JC, Go PM, et al. Detection of groin hernia with physical examination, ultrasound, and MRI compared with laparoscopic findings. Invest Radiol 1999;34:739–43.
33. Overdeck KH, Palmer WE. Imaging of hip and groin injuries in athletes. Semin Musculoskelet Radiol 2004;8:41–55.
34. Hwang B, Fredericson M, Chung C, et al. MRI findings of femoral diaphyseal stress injuries in athletes. AJR Am J Roentgenol 2005;185(1):166–73.
35. Parziale JR, O'Donnell CJ, Sandman DN. Iliopsoas bursitis. Am J Phys Med Rehabil 2009;88(8):690–1.
36. Varma D, Richli W, Charnsangavej C. MR appearance of the distended iliopsoas bursa. AJR Am J Roentgenol 1991;156:1025–8.

Magnetic Resonance Imaging and Arthroscopic Appearance of the Menisci of the Knee

Kirkland W. Davis, MD*, Humberto G. Rosas, MD, Ben K. Graf, MD

KEYWORDS

- Knee • Meniscus • Magnetic resonance imaging • Arthroscopy • Tear

KEY POINTS

- On MRI, the criteria for diagnosing a meniscal tear include increased signal contacting the articular surface of the meniscus or abnormal morphology.
- Longitudinal-vertical tears are usually traumatic, parallel the circumference of the meniscus, and are often reparable.
- Bucket-handle tears are displaced longitudinal tears and may demonstrate a fragment in the notch, double PCL, double anterior horn, and truncated meniscal body on MRI.
- The central portion of a vertical flap tear resembles a radial tear but the more peripheral portion turns to run longitudinally.
- The displaced portions of horizontal flap tears may be easy to miss on MRI and should be specifically sought in the medial recesses, the posterior intercondylar notch, and the popliteal hiatus.

 Videos of arthroscopic treatment of meniscal tears accompany this article at http://www.sportsmed.theclinics.com/

The notion that the menisci of the human knee are vestigial structures with little practical function was abandoned decades ago. It is now known that the menisci are critical for healthy knee function and physiology. However, damaged menisci can be a source of acute and chronic pain and loss of mobility, which is sometimes disabling. Often, conservative measures are insufficient to return patients with meniscal tears to a satisfactory state of function and surgery is required. Since Fairbank's recognition that "Meniscectomy is not wholly innocuous..." in his 1948 landmark publication of

Disclosures: None (K.W. Davis, H.G. Rosas); Receives royalties from Smith and Nephew, unrelated to the current topic (B.K. Graf).
Department of Radiology, University of Wisconsin School of Medicine and Public Health, 600 Highland Avenue, Madison, WI 53792, USA
* Corresponding author.
E-mail address: kdavis@uwhealth.org

chronic maladaptive changes in patients after total meniscectomy,[1] surgical efforts have evolved to include meniscus preservation techniques. Long-term results are negatively associated with increasing degrees of meniscal resection,[2] thus encouraging less extensive degrees of partial meniscectomy and the development of meniscal repair techniques. Meniscal repair results in even better long-term results than partial meniscectomy.[3]

Since the introduction of magnetic resonance imaging (MRI) in the 1980s, MRI equipment and techniques have evolved substantially to the point where MRI provides an accurate depiction of anatomy and pathology of the human knee. MRI is now widely accepted as a critical tool for clinical decision making and surgical planning in many patients with signs and symptoms of internal derangement of the knee, sometimes obviating the decision to proceed with surgery,[4–6] and MRI often is a useful complement to skilled physical diagnosis to improve surgical planning and presurgical patient counseling.[7,8]

To be most helpful, MRI needs to not only help radiologists and sports medicine clinicians diagnose meniscal tears and other knee injuries accurately, but also describe the types and potential reparability of meniscal tears with precision. It is well known that successful repair of menisci depends on tear location and pattern: longitudinal and some oblique tears are reparable, whereas horizontal, radial, and complex tears generally are not; and repair of tears is most successful when they are located in the vascularized periphery of the meniscus, preferably with a peripheral rim that is less than 4 mm wide.[9,10] To date, published studies have reported mixed results with respect to accurate MRI diagnosis of tear type, extent, and location[11,12] but with precise description of meniscal tears, MRI should continue to improve in its ability to help with surgical planning. To that end, this article focuses on the correlation between the MRI depiction and arthroscopic appearance of the various types of meniscal tears.

NORMAL MENISCUS

The menisci are comprised of fibrocartilage and normally occur as incomplete oval structures that occupy the peripheral articular space between the femur and tibia but have a central gap. They are typically divided into thirds: the anterior horn, body, and posterior horn. In cross-section, menisci are triangular or wedge shaped, being thickest peripherally and tapering to a point at their central free edges. This triangular appearance is typical on cross-sectional sagittal and coronal MRIs through the menisci, although sagittal images through the body and coronal images through the anterior and posterior horns are not cross-sectional but instead cut along the longitudinal axis of the meniscus and demonstrate a variable slab or bow tie appearance (**Fig. 1**, Video 1).

The medial meniscus is larger, more C-shaped, and normally has a larger posterior horn than anterior horn in cross-section. The lateral meniscus is more circular and its anterior and posterior horns are nearly equivalent in size in cross-section (**Fig. 2**). The medial meniscus is more firmly attached to the tibia and capsule than is the lateral, presumably leading to the increased incidence of tears of the medial meniscus versus the lateral.[10,13,14]

The ends of the anterior and posterior horns are firmly attached to the tibia at their roots (root ligaments). The anterior root of the medial meniscus attaches to the anterior midline of the tibial plateau or less commonly the anterior surface of the tibia just below the plateau. The posterior root of the medial meniscus flattens at its attachment to the tibia, just anterior and medial to the posterior cruciate ligament (PCL). The anterior root of the lateral meniscus attaches to the tibia, just lateral to the midline and posterior to

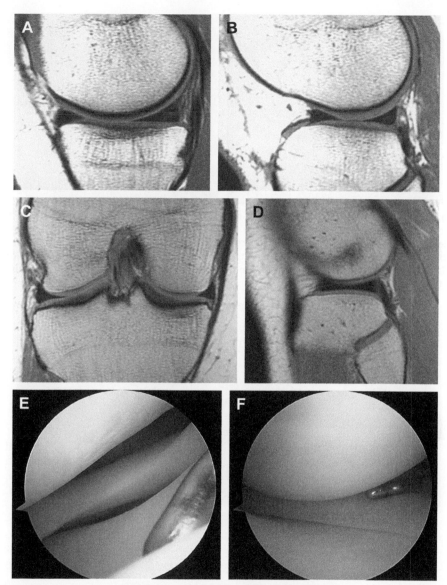

Fig. 1. Normal menisci. Sagittal proton density (PD) images through normal medial (*A*) and lateral (*B*) menisci in cross-section demonstrate the normal appearance of the anterior and posterior horns as black triangles. The posterior horn of the medial meniscus is normally larger than the anterior horn, whereas the anterior and posterior horns are more equivalent in the lateral meniscus. (*C*) Midcoronal PD image demonstrates the normal triangular appearance of the bodies of both menisci. (*D*) Far sagittal image of the lateral meniscus cuts through the edge, exhibiting the typical bow tie appearance. Arthroscopic images of the normal lateral (*E*) and medial (*F*) menisci demonstrate their smooth surfaces and tapered central free edges.

the anterior root of the medial meniscus attachment, and usually interdigitates with inserting fibers of the anterior cruciate ligament (ACL). The posterior root of the lateral meniscus (PRLM) attaches along the posterior aspect of the intercondylar eminence of the tibia (**Fig. 3**).[10,14–16]

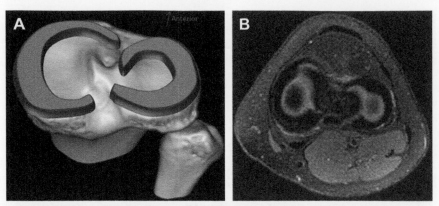

Fig. 2. Normal meniscal shape. (*A*) Three-dimensional rendition of the normal medial (*left*) and lateral (*right*) menisci superimposed on a three-dimensional computed tomography image of the tibial plateau. The medial meniscus is larger and more C-shaped and the lateral is more circular. The typical root attachments are depicted. (*B*) Fat suppressed thin-section axial PD image in the same orientation demonstrates the typical shape of the black menisci at the periphery of the joint.

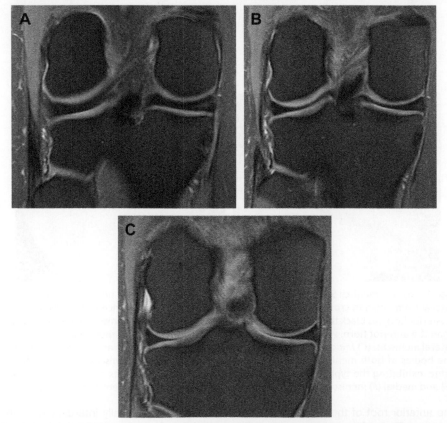

Fig. 3. Normal posterior meniscal roots. Sequential fat suppressed PD coronal images from posterior (*A*) to anterior (*C*) demonstrate the posterior horns of the menisci inserting into the tibia at the root ligament attachments alongside the posterior cruciate ligament.

There are several additional common attachments of the menisci. Most menisci have a transverse meniscal ligament (geniculate ligament) attaching the anterior horns of the two menisci to each other. Most knees also have one or two meniscofemoral ligaments (MFL), which attach the posterior horn of the lateral meniscus (PHLM) to the medial femoral condyle. The MFL of Humphry passes just anterior to the genu of the PCL, whereas the MFL of Wrisberg passes just posterior to the genu. Finally, there are several popliteomeniscal fascicles (PMF) that attach the periphery of the PHLM to the capsule.[14] On MRI of normal PHLMs, one almost always can see the anteroinferior and posterosuperior PMFs, which form the boundary of the popliteal hiatus (**Fig. 4**).[17] This hiatus is a posterior opening of the joint capsule through which the popliteus tendon passes on its way to its insertion along the peripheral lateral femoral condyle. Sagittal T2-weighted images are the best sequence to demonstrate the PMFs.[18]

The dominant structural scaffold of the meniscus is created by a series of circumferential type I collagen fibers oriented longitudinally in parallel (**Fig. 5**). A less extensive network of radially oriented collagen fibers helps protect against longitudinal splitting of the meniscus.[10,13] The primary functions of menisci include load transmission and shock absorption, helping protect articular cartilage from excessive peak weight-bearing stresses, and joint lubrication.[10,19] The ordered lattice of collagen fibers and the geometry of the knee and menisci allow the menisci to translate axial loads from weight bearing into radial loads on the circumferential collagen fibers known as "hoop strain."[13] However, if the circumferential fibers are torn, the ability of a meniscus to withstand hoop strain is diminished or lost altogether. Meniscal extrusion may result, dramatically increasing tibial-femoral peak loads. Radial tears and complex tears are especially likely to interfere with this normal physiology of the meniscus.

MRI OF MENISCAL TEARS: CRITERIA AND ACCURACY

Although the fine details of optimizing MRIs of the knee are beyond the scope of this article, a few brief points are in order. Diagnosis of meniscal tears on MRI should improve when these injunctions are followed to optimize signal-to-noise ratio: high-field-strength magnets are preferable (1.5 T and stronger); a high-resolution surface coil should be used; the field of view should only encompass the necessary structures and routinely be 16 cm or less; image slices should not be too thick (3–4 mm); and the matrix size should be at least 256 × 192 or higher.[20] Most tears are best seen on sequences with a low echo time, namely T1-weighted and proton density sequences[20]; some exceptions are noted subsequently.

The normal, intact meniscus is low signal on all sequences. In children, increased vascularity within the meniscus may cause increased signal within the meniscus, but usually the signal does not contact an articular surface. Mucinous degeneration of menisci also produces abnormal signal within a meniscus that does not contact an articular surface and which should not be mistaken for a tear.

The primary criteria for diagnosing meniscal tears on MRI include increased signal extending in a line or band to the superior articular surface, the inferior articular surface, or both surfaces; or abnormal morphology, size, or shape of the meniscus indicating missing portions or damaged surfaces.[14,21,22] Studies by Kaplan and colleagues[23] and De Smet and coworkers[24] showed that the abnormal signal must unequivocally contact the surface of the meniscus; menisci in which that was not true were no more likely to be torn than menisci with no abnormal signal approaching the surface at all.

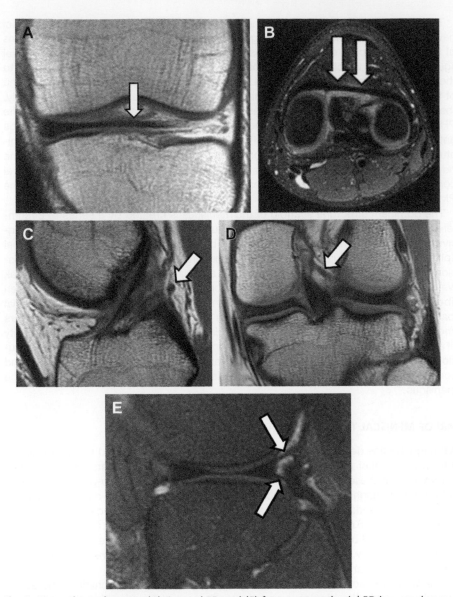

Fig. 4. Normal attachments. (*A*) Coronal PD and (*B*) fat suppressed axial PD images demonstrate the transverse meniscal ligament (*arrows*) attaching the anterior horns of the menisci to each other. (*C*) Sagittal and (*D*) coronal PD images demonstrate the meniscofemoral ligament of Wrisberg (*arrows*), attaching the PHLM to the medial femoral condyle, passing behind the PCL. (*E*) Sagittal fat suppressed T2 image depicts the popliteomeniscal fascicles (*arrows*) extending from the PHLM to the capsule, passing around the popliteus tendon.

To provide a greater degree of accuracy, De Smet advocated the "two-slice touch rule." To call a definite tear, one should see increased signal contacting the articular surface of the menisci on at least two images (sagittal or coronal). Increased signal to the surface on only one slice indicates a "possible tear." Cases of only one abnormal slice

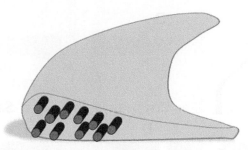

Fig. 5. Three-dimensional diagram of a meniscus cut in cross-section, simulating the dominant circumferential collagen bundles, which primarily resist hoop strain.

correlated to tears at arthroscopy 55% of the time for the medial meniscus and 30% for the lateral[24]; and only 43% and 18% in a follow-up study 13 years later.[25]

Using these criteria for diagnosing meniscal tears on MRIs, accuracy has been very good. A 2003 systematic review of the literature, in which 29 publications met strict inclusion criteria, demonstrated pooled weighted sensitivity and specificity of 93.3% and 88.4% for the medial meniscus and 79.3% and 95.7% for the lateral meniscus, respectively.[26] Subsequent studies continue to confirm and even improve on these numbers.[25,27] Noting that sensitivity for lateral meniscus tears continues to lag that for medial tears, one study revealed that all their missed lateral meniscus tears involved only one segment and were usually longitudinal tears of the posterior horn occurring in the setting of concomitant ACL tears.[28]

Most meniscal tears are visible and best seen on sagittal images. This is understandable because most tears occur in the posterior horns; as such, the sagittal images show longitudinal, horizontal, and complex tears of the posterior horns in cross-section.[14] However, experience with MRI interpretation quickly demonstrates that some tears are better seen or only seen on coronal images.[29] More recently, a few reports have surfaced advocating very thin axial images through the menisci to improve accuracy and tear description.[30] The current authors' practice has recently added a sequence of 1-mm thick proton density axial slices through the menisci and some surgeons find this sequence best depicts the tear configuration they should expect to see at arthroscopy.

PATTERNS OF MENISCAL TEARS

The primary features that determine whether a torn meniscus is reparable include the type or pattern of tear (longitudinal favorable); its location (peripheral favorable); and the quality of meniscal tissue. In this section, the major patterns of tears are described and depicted in MRIs, drawings, and arthroscopy images and videos. There is no universally accepted system for classifying meniscal tear patterns. A modification of the classification system developed by the International Society of Arthroscopy, Knee Surgery, and Orthopedic Sports Medicine[31] is used here and accompanying alternate names when they are in common use are provided. These patterns include longitudinal-vertical, bucket handle, horizontal, radial, vertical flap, horizontal flap, and complex.[31]

Longitudinal-vertical Tears

Longitudinal-vertical (longitudinal, peripheral-vertical) tears are vertically oriented and run parallel to the circumference of the meniscus along its longitudinal axis, separating the meniscus into central and peripheral portions (**Fig. 6**, Video 2). They may contact

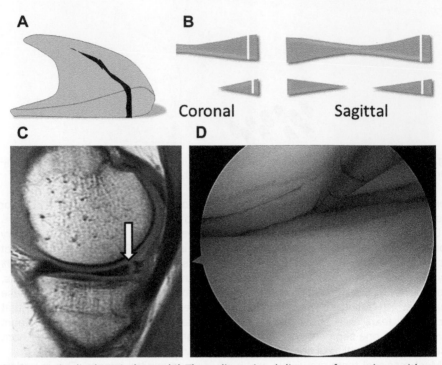

Fig. 6. Longitudinal-vertical tear. (*A*) Three-dimensional diagram of a meniscus with a peripheral longitudinal tear oriented in parallel to the circumference of the meniscus. This separates the meniscus into central and peripheral portions. (*B*) Two-dimensional depictions of portions of a meniscus in sagittal and coronal planes demonstrate that a longitudinal-vertical tear results in a vertical line of increased signal in the meniscus that maintains the same distance from the periphery. (*C*) Sagittal PD image shows a longitudinal tear (*arrow*) in the posterior horn of the medial meniscus (PHMM). (*D*) Arthroscopic image in the same patient demonstrates a probe buried in the undersurface of this longitudinal PHMM tear.

the superior surface, the inferior surface, or both articular surfaces of the meniscus. Longitudinal tears usually are the result of a specific injury, typically accompanying ACL tears, and usually start in the posterior horn.[13,14] Routinely occurring in the periphery of the meniscus, these lesions are usually amenable to repair if they are long enough to be unstable.

When seen in cross-section on MRI, longitudinal tears appear as a vertical line of abnormal signal contacting one or both surfaces. They maintain a constant distance from the periphery of the meniscus, parallel to the dominant collagen fibers.[22]

Bucket-handle Tears

If a longitudinal tear involves a long enough segment of the meniscus, the central fragment may displace from the peripheral portion of the meniscus.[22,32] Viewed from above, if the displaced fragment remains connected to the parent meniscus at both ends, it resembles the handle on a bucket (**Fig. 7**A). The fragment commonly displaces into the intercondylar notch, although it may predominantly displace anteriorly.[21] In the latter situation, a smaller portion of the displaced fragment should also be visible in the notch.

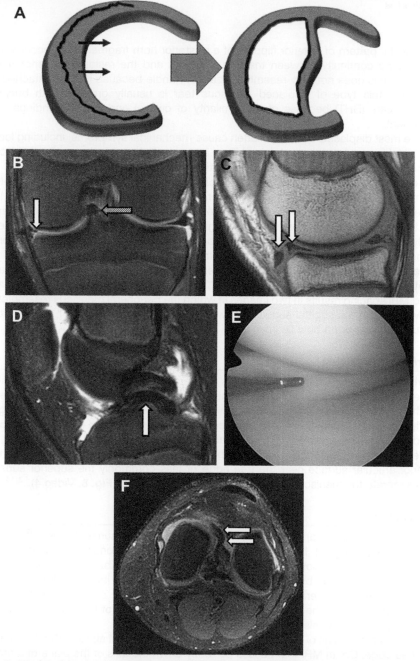

Fig. 7. Displaced bucket-handle tear. (*A*) Three-dimensional rendition of a longitudinal tear that is extensive enough to displace centrally as a bucket-handle tear. (*B*) Coronal fat suppressed PD image shows truncation of the body of the medial meniscus (*solid arrow*) with fragment displaced into the notch (*hashed arrow*). (*C*) Sagittal PD image through the medial meniscus demonstrates two "anterior horns" (*arrows*), one of which represents a displaced portion of the posterior horn. (*D*) Sagittal fat suppressed T2 image shows the double PCL sign, representing the displaced meniscal fragment (*arrow*) lying below the PCL. (*E*) Arthroscopic image demonstrates a pick reducing the bucket-handle meniscus fragment. (*F*) Axial fat suppressed PD image in another patient demonstrates the centrally displaced fragment from a bucket-handle tear (*arrows*).

A similar pattern of anterior flipping of a posterior horn fragment may occur when there is no continuity between the torn fragment and the residual posterior horn. Although this does not truly resemble a bucket handle because it is not attached at one end, this type of displaced meniscus tear is usually grouped with bucket-handle tears (BHT) because of the similarity of clinical and imaging findings and treatment.

Like most displaced tears, BHT often cause mechanical symptoms, including locking, catching, giving way, and pain.[21] They are more frequent in the medial meniscus than the lateral and often occur in conjunction with ACL tears.[32–34]

Several helpful MRI signs have been described. These include fragment in the notch sign; double anterior horn sign, in which there is an additional meniscal fragment in the anterior joint on top of or immediately posterior to the native anterior horn, representing the anteriorly flipped posterior horn fragment; double PCL sign, in which the centrally displaced fragment lies just anterior and parallel to the PCL; the coronal truncation sign, in which the free edge of the meniscal body appears clipped off on coronal images because of the displacement of the bucketed fragment; and the absent bow tie sign (see **Fig. 7**B–F, Video 3).[35–37] This final sign reflects the fact that standard MRI spacing results in two images in which the peripheral meniscus resembles a bow tie or slab on sagittal sequences; when there is a displaced BHT, this is often reduced to one or no bow tie images.

Horizontal Tears

Horizontal (cleavage, degenerative) tears run parallel to or at a slight angle to the surface of the meniscus, nearly parallel to the tibial plateau. Most horizontal tears extend to the inferior articular surface of the meniscus or the free edge. Typically occurring in patients older than 40, these tears are degenerative in nature and usually not associated with a discrete injury.[14,21] These tears may occur in the posterior horn, body, or anterior horn. On MRI, they exhibit abnormal horizontal linear signal contacting the inferior articular surface near the free edge or less commonly the superior surface and separate the meniscus into superior and inferior halves (**Fig. 8**, Video 4).[13,14]

Radial Tears

Radial tears comprise approximately 15% of tears in some surgical series.[38,39] They are vertically oriented but extend perpendicular to the longitudinal axis of the meniscus, akin to a spoke on a wheel. Radial tears always start at the central free edge of the meniscus but may extend through just part of its circumference or all the way to the peripheral margin.[22] These tears commonly occur at the center of the posterior horn of the medial meniscus or at the junction of the anterior horn and body of the lateral meniscus.[14]

The typical MRI sign of a radial tear is a linear, vertical cleft of abnormal high signal at the free edge. On an MRI that passes perfectly down the axis of the plane of a radial tear, there may be a "ghost" meniscus or a portion of the free edge may be truncated (**Fig. 9**, Video 5). For radial tears that are oriented obliquely to both sagittal and coronal images, one may observe the marching cleft sign, because the location of the vertical cleft of abnormal high signal shifts position from one image to the next.[14,38] Because radial tears are often filled with joint fluid, they usually stand out more on fluid-sensitive sequences, such as fat suppressed T2-weighted images.[39] Axial images can be especially helpful in identifying some radial tears and giving a realistic appreciation of their depth.[14] Because radial tears can lie between image slices in one plane, they may only be visible on one orthogonal image and are exceptions to the two-slice-touch rule.

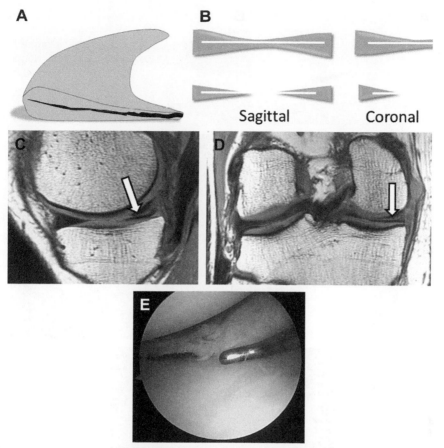

Fig. 8. Horizontal tear. (*A*) Three-dimensional diagram of a meniscus with a horizontal tear. This separates the meniscus into superior and inferior portions. (*B*) Two-dimensional depictions of portions of a meniscus in sagittal and coronal planes demonstrate the pattern of a horizontal tear. Sagittal (*C*) and coronal (*D*) PD images show a horizontal tear (*arrow*) contacting the superior surface of the PHMM. (*E*) Arthroscopic image in the same patient demonstrates this horizontal PHMM tear.

Vertical Flap Tears

Vertical flap (oblique, flap, parrot-beak) tears are unstable tears that occur in younger patients as the result of an acute injury.[21] At first glance, these tears may resemble radial tears: they are vertical tears that begin at the free edge of the meniscus and extend radially; however, they do not maintain their radial orientation perpendicular to the longitudinal axis of the meniscus but turn to run parallel to it.[21] The unstable portion of meniscus separated by this tear has been likened to a parrot's beak.

On MRI, these tears also resemble radial tears, with a linear cleft of abnormal signal seen at the free edge. However, close inspection reveals that the tear changes plane of orientation over its course. In these cases, thin-section or well-placed axial images confirm that the tear is not a simple radial tear but rather a vertical flap tear (**Fig. 10**, Video 6).

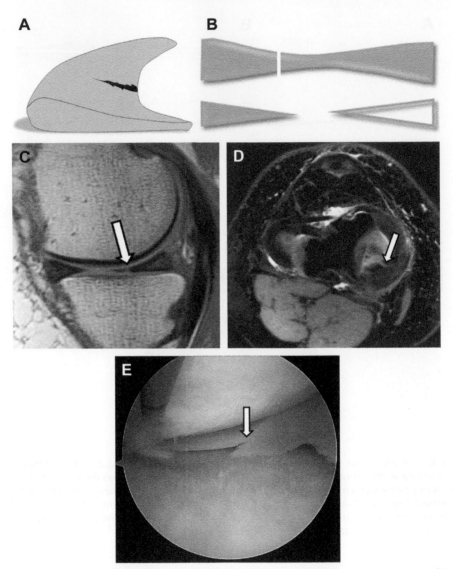

Fig. 9. Radial tear. (*A*) Three-dimensional diagram of a meniscus with a radial tear extending from the central free edge toward the periphery. (*B*) Two-dimensional depictions of portions of radial tears. In the upper image, the imaging plane is perpendicular to the tear, causing the tear to appear as a vertical line. In the lower image, the tear is in plane with the image slice, causing the "ghost meniscus" sign. Sagittal PD (*C*) and fat suppressed axial PD (*D*) images show a radial tear (*arrows*) at the junction of the body and PHMM. (*E*) Arthroscopic image in the same patient demonstrates this radial tear (*arrow*).

Horizontal Flap Tears

Horizontal flap tears are horizontal tears involving a short portion of the meniscus in which the subtended segment is unstable and displaced peripherally.[31,37,40] These tears often cause mechanical symptoms because they intermittently displace into the joint.[41]

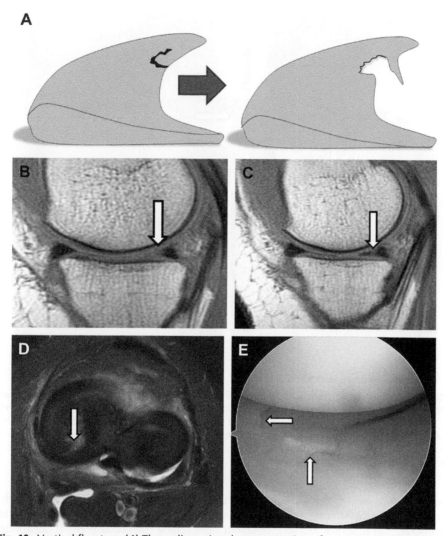

Fig. 10. Vertical flap tear. (*A*) Three-dimensional representation of a meniscus with a vertical flap tear. This has a radial component centrally and extends in a more longitudinal orientation more peripherally. These may displace, as indicated in the diagram. (*B*) Sagittal PD image shows truncation of the free edge from the radial component of a vertical flap tear (*arrow*) of the PHMM. (*C*) Adjacent sagittal PD image demonstrates the more peripheral, longitudinal component of the tear (*arrow*). (*D*) Axial fat suppressed T2 image more completely demonstrates the shape of the tear (*arrow*). (*E*) Arthroscopic image in the same patient demonstrates this vertical flap tear (*arrows*).

On MRI the nondisplaced portion of the tear demonstrates truncation or a horizontal tear[42]; however, the displaced flap of meniscus may not be obvious. As such, it is critical to search typical locations for the flaps because identifying these tears in advance of surgery is critical. When these tears occur in the body of the meniscus or nearby, the unstable fragment may displace into the superior recess underlying the medial collateral ligament or less commonly the inferior recess (**Fig. 11**, Video 7); similar displacement of tears of the lateral meniscal body are less common.[42] Fragments lying in the

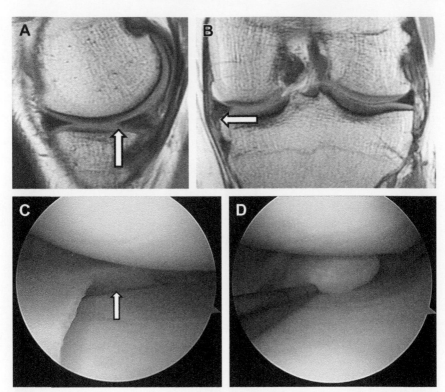

Fig. 11. Horizontal flap tear. (*A*) Sagittal PD image demonstrates a truncated, irregular appearance to the PHMM (*arrow*). Given the loss of meniscal tissue, one should be alert to displaced fragments. (*B*) Coronal PD image depicts the flap of meniscus displaced peripherally into the inferior gutter at the medial joint line (*arrow*). Arthroscopic images demonstrate the displaced flap extending inferiorly and peripherally (*arrow, C*) followed by reduction of the flap into the joint (*D*).

medial inferior recess are especially difficult to see at routine arthroscopy and only become evident when one slides a probe under the inferior surface of the peripheral meniscus.[40] In a similar fashion, posterior horn lateral meniscus (PHLM) horizontal flap tears may displace into the posterior notch or the popliteal hiatus and the surgeon should be alerted to their presence before arthroscopy for ease of discovery.[41,42]

Complex Tears

Complex meniscal tears are those in which there is more than one dominant plane of disruption. On MRI, there is considerable distortion of meniscal architecture and there are multiple lines of abnormal signal passing in different directions (**Fig. 12**, Video 8).[14,31] Because of the extent of these tears, they severely disrupt the ability of the meniscus to bear weight and to resist hoop strain.

Root Tears

Meniscal root tears are not part of the ISAKOS classification of tear type[31] presumably because they describe a location of tear rather than a pattern or appearance. However, root tears have received significant attention in the surgical and radiologic literature in the last decade. These tears are difficult to see at arthroscopy[13,43] and

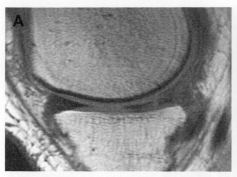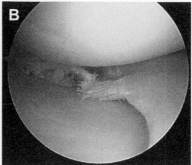

Fig. 12. (*A*) Sagittal PD image demonstrates horizontal and vertical components to this complex tear of the PHMM. (*B*) Arthroscopic image of this complex tear.

frequently are overlooked on MRI even when complete[44]; however, just as specific attention to the roots can aid arthroscopic diagnosis, direct attention to them on MRI improves radiologic diagnosis.[45]

Most root tears are radial tears with a much smaller number of complex tears.[45] Posterior root tears of the medial meniscus are more commonly degenerative and occur in patients older than 40, whereas posterior root tears of the lateral meniscus often are associated with ACL tears in younger patients.[43,46,47] Anterior meniscal root tears have not been reported.[15]

On MRI, one must inspect both the coronal and sagittal images, following the roots to their insertion points. Because artifactual signal may mimic tears, especially of the PRLM, and because fluid dissects into many radial root tears, fluid-sensitive sequences are often the most helpful.[13] Radial root tears demonstrate a fluid cleft on coronal images and often exhibit a ghost meniscus on consecutive sagittal images, in which the posterior root is the normal black signal on one image and essentially invisible on the next (**Fig. 13**).[14]

PRLM tears, however, may exhibit more irregular morphologic distortion and abnormal signal than the typical cleft and ghost meniscus.[47] Importantly, it should be noted that although increased signal in the PRLM indicates a tear in patients younger than 30 or who have suffered a concomitant ACL tear, it may indicate only synovitis and fraying in patients older than 40 with degenerative changes and no injury.[14]

In recent years, much has been made of the association of meniscal extrusion and root tears. Extrusion is defined as extension of the body of the meniscus more than 3 mm beyond the edge of the tibial plateau on a midcoronal MRI (see **Fig. 13**). Although it is true that many complete root tears, especially of the posterior root of the medial meniscus, exhibit extrusion,[44] extrusion is not a specific sign. Extrusion is also common in high-grade radial tears elsewhere in the meniscus, complex tears, and extensive chondrosis.[48–50]

SECONDARY MRI SIGNS OF MENISCAL TEARS

A discussion of several secondary MRI signs associated with meniscal tears is in order. In patients who have sustained acute injuries, the presence of a posterior tibial bone contusion underlying the meniscus strongly suggests an overlying meniscus tear.[14] In a 1999 study, Kaplan and coworkers[51] found MRI evidence of meniscocapsular separation or peripheral posterior horn meniscal tears overlying medial tibial

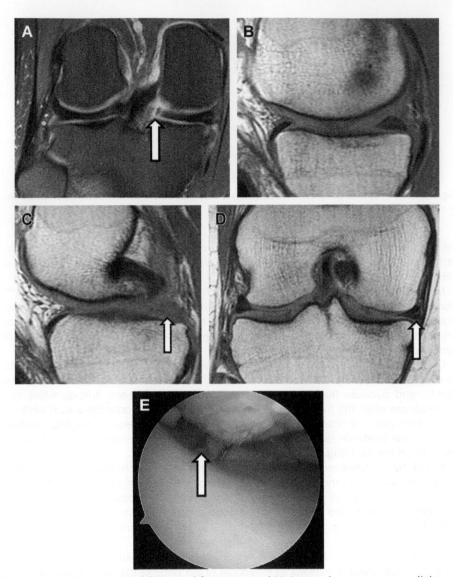

Fig. 13. Posterior root tear. (*A*) Coronal fat suppressed PD image demonstrates a radial tear of the root of the PHMM (*arrow*). Sequential sagittal images of the PHMM demonstrate a relatively normal appearance (*B*) followed by the ghost/absent meniscus sign (*arrow, C*) at the root tear. (*D*) Midcoronal PD imaging demonstrates 4-mm extrusion of the medial meniscus (*arrow*). (*E*) Arthroscopic image shows a probe adjacent to the root tear (*arrow*).

contusions in 24 of 25 patients with ACL tears. Several of the menisci with meniscocapsular separation had additional nonperipheral medial meniscus tears (**Fig. 14**).

A parameniscal cyst is a contained fluid collection immediately adjacent to the peripheral rim of a meniscus. These cysts have long been known to indicate underlying meniscus tears, with joint fluid seeping through the leaves of the tear to collect peripherally (**Fig. 15**). A recent study confirmed the high likelihood of a parameniscal cyst indicating an underlying tear of the medial meniscus (96% confirmed at arthroscopy)

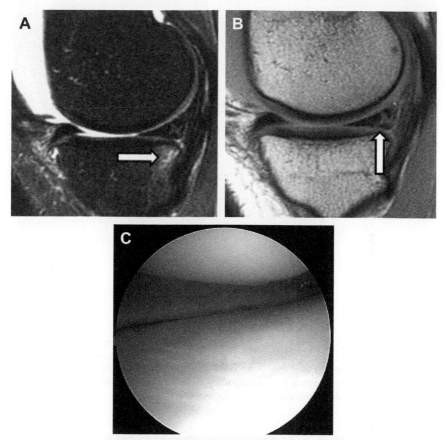

Fig. 14. Secondary sign: contusion. (*A*) Sagittal fat suppressed T2 image demonstrates high-signal contusion of the posterior medial tibial plateau (*arrow*) in a patient with an ACL tear (not shown). (*B*) Sagittal PD image at the same location shows the predominantly longitudinal-vertical tear of the PHMM (*arrow*), overlying the contusion. (*C*) Arthroscopic image demonstrates sutures in place after repair of this tear.

or the body or PHLM; however, parameniscal cysts at the anterior horn of the lateral meniscus were associated with a confirmed underlying tear only 64% of the time.[52]

Another helpful clue to the presence of subtle meniscal tears is abnormality of the PMF. The anteroinferior and posterosuperior PMFs should be visible on MRIs of normal knees. Abnormal morphology or frank disruption of the PMFs, especially the posterosuperior PMF, is strongly associated with PHLM tears at surgery (**Fig. 16**).[53,54]

PITFALLS AND NORMAL VARIANTS

There are several normal structures that may mimic or obscure meniscal tears. Similarly, there are normal variants that can confuse the uninitiated observer. These are discussed in brief in the following sections.

Transverse Meniscal Ligament

Where the transverse ligament attaches to the anterior horn lateral meniscus, there may be a line of increased signal that may be confused for a meniscus tear.

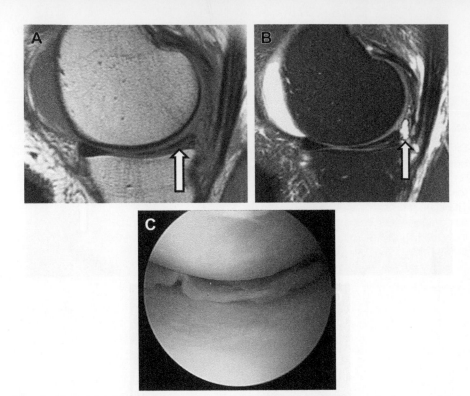

Fig. 15. Secondary sign: parameniscal cyst. (*A*) Sagittal PD image demonstrates a predominantly horizontal, mildly complex tear of the PHMM (*arrow*). (*B*) Sagittal fat suppressed T2 image shows a small, high signal fluid collection (*arrow*) adjacent to the periphery of the meniscus, consistent with a parameniscal cyst. These cysts can be clues to search for more subtle tears. (*C*) Arthroscopic image confirms the tear.

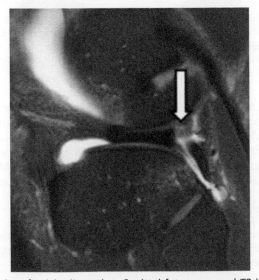

Fig. 16. Secondary sign: fascicle disruption. Sagittal fat suppressed T2 image demonstrates poor definition and presumed disruption of the posterosuperior popliteomeniscal fascicle (*arrow*). In this patient with an ACL tear, this indicates likely peripheral PHLM tear, confirmed at surgery.

Recognizing the location and following the transverse ligament away from this site on sequential sagittal images helps one not to mistake this normal attachment for a tear (**Fig. 17**A, B).[14]

Meniscofemoral Ligaments

Similar to the transverse ligament, the ligament of Humphry and the ligament of Wrisberg may demonstrate increased signal where they attach to the PHLM, simulating a tear (see **Fig. 17**C, D). Again, the astute observer, after noticing this concerning signal, follows the ligament away from its attachment to confirm that it is a normal structure.[14] The caveat to this point is that on occasion, subtle peripheral PHLM tears masquerade as particularly far lateral attachments of one of the MFLs to the posterior horn. Accordingly, one should not dismiss the attachment of the MFL to the PHLM if it extends more than 14 mm or four MR images lateral to the PCL but instead suspect a meniscal tear.[55]

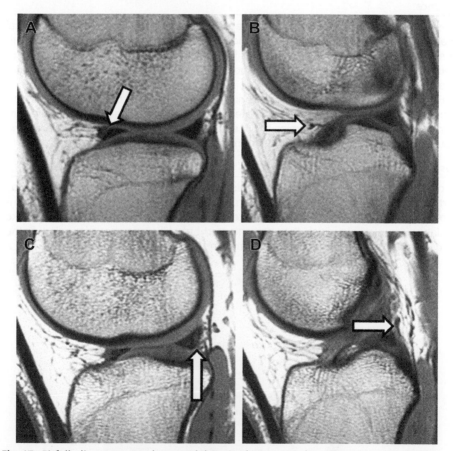

Fig. 17. Pitfalls: ligament attachments. (*A*) Sagittal PD image shows linear increased signal in the anterior horn lateral mensicus (AHLM, *arrow*), mimicking a tear; on following this finding medially, this proved to be the attachment of the transverse meniscal ligament, seen on an adjacent sagittal PD image (*arrow, B*). (*C*) Sagittal PD image demonstrate linear increased signal in the PHLM (*arrow*), possibly indicating a tear; on following this finding medially, this proved to be the attachment of the ligament of Wrisberg, seen on another sagittal PD image (*arrow, D*).

Striations of the Meniscal Roots

It is common to observe multiple lines of increased signal interspersed with the normal low signal of the anterior root of the lateral meniscus (**Fig. 18**). Similar findings have also been reported in the posterior root of the medial meniscus, although they are less common.[14] Both sites of "fissuring" have been shown to be normal at arthroscopy and should not be misinterpreted as tears.[56,57]

Chondrocalcinosis

One should also be aware that calcific deposits within the menisci from calcium pyrophosphate dihydrite deposition disease and other metabolic conditions may give spurious abnormal MRI signal within menisci, mimicking a tear. Chondrocalcinosis has been shown to reduce sensitivity and specificity for meniscal tears[58]; this is one of many good reasons that radiographs should be obtained to accompany knee MRIs.

Flounce

It is commonly recognized that one may see meniscal flounce in normal medial menisci routinely at arthroscopy.[59] Flounce is the appearance of rippling or smooth S-shaped undulation of the free edge of the meniscus. Arthroscopic visualization of flounce has been touted as having high positive predictive value and negative predictive value for an intact meniscus.[59]

Flounce also has been described as a normal variant at MRI, although quite uncommon (**Fig. 19**). Conversely, it has been noted that a destabilizing tear may cause redundancy of the meniscus that mimics flounce at MRI; as such, one should only presume flounce is a normal variant only if the meniscus appears normal otherwise.[60]

Discoid Menisci

A discoid meniscus is elongated and thicker than a typical meniscus and extends farther toward the center of the joint than expected. Discoid menisci are more common in Japanese and Korean than Western populations and may be complete, like a slab; incomplete, in which they are enlarged but still somewhat triangular; or the rare Wrisberg variant, in which the dominant attachment is the MFL in lieu of a

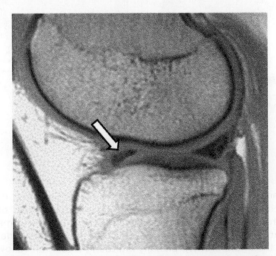

Fig. 18. Pitfall: striations. Sagittal PD image depicts striations in the root of the AHLM (*arrow*), a common normal finding. Also note longitudinal vertical tear in the posterior horn.

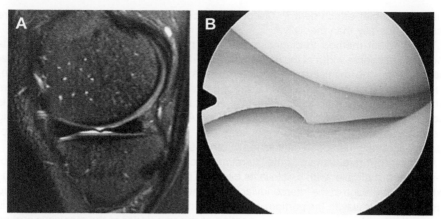

Fig. 19. Pitfall: flounce. (*A*) Sagittal fat suppressed T2 image demonstrates smooth S-shaped undulation of the free edge of the body of the medial meniscus. This uncommon finding is normal. (*B*) Arthroscopic image in a different patient demonstrates medial meniscal flounce, a common normal finding at arthroscopy.

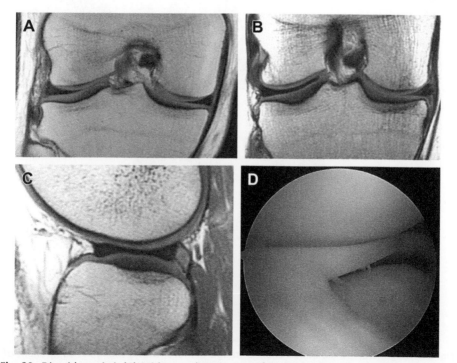

Fig. 20. Discoid menisci. (*A*) Midcoronal PD image of an incomplete discoid (type II) lateral meniscus demonstrates the body of the lateral meniscus to be larger than typical. This measured 18 mm wide. Midcoronal (*B*) and sagittal (*C*) PD images of a complete discoid (type I) lateral meniscus in a different patient show it to cover nearly the entire lateral tibial plateau. (*D*) Arthroscopic image in this latter patient shows the discoid meniscus protruding toward the intercondylar notch.

substantial tibial attachment.[61] Discoid menisci are approximately 10 times more common laterally than medially.[62,63]

The simplest method to diagnose a discoid meniscus on MRI is to measure the shortest transverse width of the meniscal body on coronal images; when this is greater than 14 mm, the meniscus is characterized as discoid (**Fig. 20**).[64] On sagittal sequences, three or more "bow ties" also suggests a discoid meniscus.[63] The literature remains inconclusive as to whether MRI accuracy for tears of discoid meniscus is reduced relative to that in nondiscoid menisci. Although abnormal signal contacting the surface and morphologic irregularity has been highly predictive of tear for some[65] accuracy has been diminished in other studies.[14,62]

A similar, but rare, variant of the lateral meniscus is the ring meniscus, which is not C-shaped but circular with a hole in its center. The central portion of a ring meniscus extends to the edge of the intercondylar notch and is typically mistaken for a displaced BHT on MRI. However, the portion at the notch does not appear irregular but instead is a smooth triangle, and there is no truncation of the remainder of the meniscus and no history of injury as would be expected with a BHT (**Fig. 21**).[14,61]

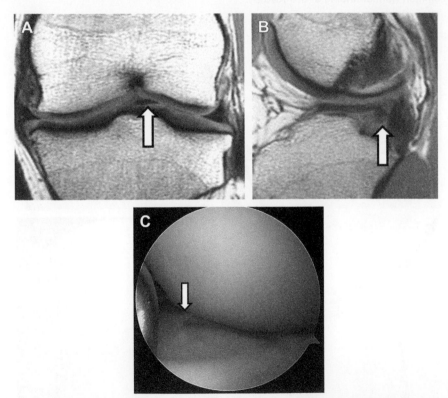

Fig. 21. Ring meniscus. (*A*) Midcoronal PD image demonstrates a triangular component of meniscus on the lateral edge of the intercondylar notch (*arrow*). Noting that the body of the lateral meniscus appears normal, this should not be a displaced bucket-handle tear. (*B*) Sagittal PD image of this portion of the meniscus, with irregularity and a displaced flap at the posterior margin (*arrow*), indicating the sole site concerning for tear. (*C*) Arthroscopic image depicts a ring lateral meniscus, with a focal tear at the posterior medial margin (*arrow*).

Oblique Meniscomeniscal Ligament

A total of 1% to 4% of knees exhibit an oblique meniscomeniscal ligament. These uncommon variants extend from the anterior horn of one meniscus to the posterior horn of the other and demonstrate homogeneously low signal, as does a normal meniscus. They pass obliquely through the intercondylar notch, between the ACL and PCL. An

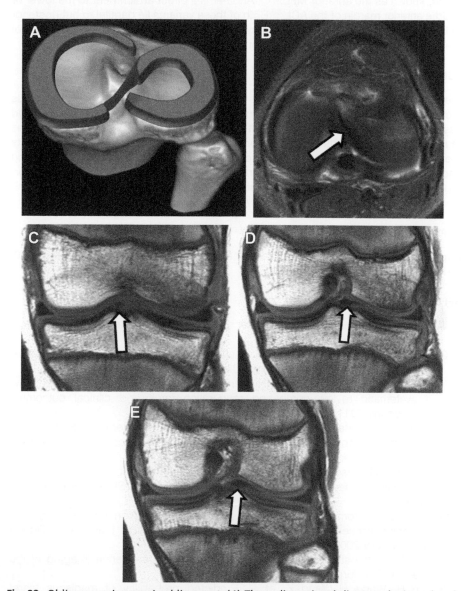

Fig. 22. Oblique meniscomeniscal ligament. (*A*) Three-dimensional diagram depicts a band of meniscal tissue connecting the AHLM to the PHMM. (*B*) Axial fat suppressed PD image shows a medial oblique meniscomeniscal ligament (*arrow*) attaching the anterior horn medial meniscus to the PHLM. (*C–E*) Sequential coronal PD images demonstrate the ligament passing through the notch (*arrows*).

oblique meniscomeniscal ligament is easily mistaken for a displaced meniscal fragment until one follows its course and recognizes the attachments to both menisci **(Fig. 22)**.[66]

Anterior Horn Medial Meniscal Variants

Finally, the anterior horn medial meniscus occasionally has an additional attachment extending into the midline. One variant is an attachment to the roof of the intercondylar notch, known as the anterior MFL.[67,68] Another is a direct attachment to the lower or middle anterior margin of the ACL.[69] Both of these variants lie parallel to but posterior to the ligamentum mucosum and are asymptomatic.[67] Awareness of the existence of these uncommon variants helps one not to mistake them for pathology.

SUMMARY

Treatment options and patient outcomes from torn knee menisci depend on numerous factors including tear pattern and extent, fragment stability and displacement, and associated injuries and joint damage. It is hoped that the descriptions and images of meniscal tears on MRIs and the accompanying arthroscopy images will aid sports medicine physicians and practitioners to better recognize meniscal tears at imaging and will help radiologists to better understand the important features to report regarding meniscal tears. Increasingly sophisticated MRI equipment only takes clinicians as far as their understanding allows them to go.

SUPPLEMENTARY DATA

Supplementary data related to this article can be found online at http://dx.doi.org/10.1016/j.csm.2013.03.005.

REFERENCES

1. Fairbank TJ. Knee joint changes after meniscectomy. J Bone Joint Surg Br 1948; 30B(4):664–70.
2. Higuchi H, Kimura M, Shirakura K, et al. Factors affecting long-term results after arthroscopic partial meniscectomy. Clin Orthop Relat Res 2000;(377):161–8.
3. Paxton ES, Stock MV, Brophy RH. Meniscal repair versus partial meniscectomy: a systematic review comparing reoperation rates and clinical outcomes. Arthroscopy 2011;27(9):1275–88.
4. Weinstabl R, Muellner T, Vecsei V, et al. Economic considerations for the diagnosis and therapy of meniscal lesions: can magnetic resonance imaging help reduce the expense? World J Surg 1997;21(4):363–8.
5. McNally EG, Nasser KN, Dawson S, et al. Role of magnetic resonance imaging in the clinical management of the acutely locked knee. Skeletal Radiol 2002; 31(10):570–3.
6. Elvenes J, Jerome CP, Reikeras O, et al. Magnetic resonance imaging as a screening procedure to avoid arthroscopy for meniscal tears. Arch Orthop Trauma Surg 2000;120(1–2):14–6.
7. Feller JA, Webster KE. Clinical value of magnetic resonance imaging of the knee. ANZ J Surg 2001;71(9):534–7.
8. Yan R, Wang H, Yang Z, et al. Predicted probability of meniscus tears: comparing history and physical examination with MRI. Swiss Med Wkly 2011; 141(w13314):1–7.
9. Tenuta JJ, Arciero RA. Arthroscopic evaluation of meniscal repairs. Factors that effect healing. Am J Sports Med 1994;22(6):797–802.

10. Rath E, Richmond JC. The menisci: basic science and advances in treatment. Br J Sports Med 2000;34(4):252–7.
11. Jee WH, McCauley TR, Kim JM, et al. Meniscal tear configurations: categorization with MR imaging. AJR Am J Roentgenol 2003;180(1):93–7.
12. Nourissat G, Beaufils P, Charrois O, et al. Magnetic resonance imaging as a tool to predict reparability of longitudinal full-thickness meniscus lesions. Knee Surg Sports Traumatol Arthrosc 2008;16(5):482–6.
13. Rosas HG, De Smet AA. Magnetic resonance imaging of the meniscus. Top Magn Reson Imaging 2009;20(3):151–73.
14. De Smet AA. How I diagnose meniscal tears on knee MRI. AJR Am J Roentgenol 2012;199(3):481–99.
15. Brody JM, Hulstyn MJ, Fleming BC, et al. The meniscal roots: gross anatomic correlation with 3-T MRI findings. AJR Am J Roentgenol 2007;188(5): W446–50.
16. Kohn D, Moreno B. Meniscus insertion anatomy as a basis for meniscus replacement: a morphological cadaveric study. Arthroscopy 1995;11(1):96–103.
17. Peduto AJ, Nguyen A, Trudell DJ, et al. Popliteomeniscal fascicles: anatomic considerations using MR arthrography in cadavers. AJR Am J Roentgenol 2008;190(2):442–8.
18. Johnson RL, De Smet AA. MR visualization of the popliteomeniscal fascicles. Skeletal Radiol 1999;28(10):561–6.
19. Jones AO, Houang MT, Low RS, et al. Medial meniscus posterior root attachment injury and degeneration: MRI findings. Australas Radiol 2006;50(4): 306–13.
20. Fox MG. MR imaging of the meniscus: review, current trends, and clinical implications. Magn Reson Imaging Clin N Am 2007;15(1):103–23.
21. Huysse WC, Verstraete KL, Verdonk PC, et al. Meniscus imaging. Semin Musculoskelet Radiol 2008;12(4):318–33.
22. Anderson MW. MR imaging of the meniscus. Radiol Clin North Am 2002;40(5): 1081–94.
23. Kaplan PA, Nelson NL, Garvin KL, et al. MR of the knee: the significance of high signal in the meniscus that does not clearly extend to the surface. AJR Am J Roentgenol 1991;156(2):333–6.
24. De Smet AA, Norris MA, Yandow DR, et al. MR diagnosis of meniscal tears of the knee: importance of high signal in the meniscus that extends to the surface. AJR Am J Roentgenol 1993;161(1):101–7.
25. De Smet AA, Tuite MJ. Use of the "two-slice-touch" rule for the MRI diagnosis of meniscal tears. AJR Am J Roentgenol 2006;187(4):911–4.
26. Oei EH, Nikken JJ, Verstijnen AC, et al. MR imaging of the menisci and cruciate ligaments: a systematic review. Radiology 2003;226(3):837–48.
27. Sampson MJ, Jackson MP, Moran CJ, et al. Three Tesla MRI for the diagnosis of meniscal and anterior cruciate ligament pathology: a comparison to arthroscopic findings. Clin Radiol 2008;63(10):1106–11.
28. De Smet AA, Mukherjee R. Clinical, MRI, and arthroscopic findings associated with failure to diagnose a lateral meniscal tear on knee MRI. AJR Am J Roentgenol 2008;190(1):22–6.
29. Magee T, Williams D. Detection of meniscal tears and marrow lesions using coronal MRI. AJR Am J Roentgenol 2004;183(5):1469–73.
30. Gokalp G, Nas OF, Demirag B, et al. Contribution of thin-slice (1 mm) axial proton density MR images for identification and classification of meniscal tears: correlative study with arthroscopy. Br J Radiol 2012;85:e871–8.

31. Anderson AF, Irrgang JJ, Dunn W, et al. Interobserver reliability of the International Society of Arthroscopy, Knee Surgery and Orthopaedic Sports Medicine (ISAKOS) classification of meniscal tears. Am J Sports Med 2011;39(5):926–32.

32. Rao N, Patel Y, Opsha O, et al. Use of the V-sign in the diagnosis of bucket-handle meniscal tear of the knee. Skeletal Radiol 2012;41(3):293–7.

33. Sparacia G, Barbiera F, Bartolotta TV, et al. Pitfalls and limitations of magnetic resonance imaging in bucket-handle tears of knee menisci. Radiol Med 2002; 104(3):150–6.

34. Magee TH, Hinson GW. MRI of meniscal bucket-handle tears. Skeletal Radiol 1998;27(9):495–9.

35. Dorsay TA, Helms CA. Bucket-handle meniscal tears of the knee: sensitivity and specificity of MRI signs. Skeletal Radiol 2003;32(5):266–72.

36. Ververidis AN, Verettas DA, Kazakos KJ, et al. Meniscal bucket handle tears: a retrospective study of arthroscopy and the relation to MRI. Knee Surg Sports Traumatol Arthrosc 2006;14(4):343–9.

37. Ruff C, Weingardt JP, Russ PD, et al. MR imaging patterns of displaced meniscus injuries of the knee. AJR Am J Roentgenol 1998;170(1):63–7.

38. Harper KW, Helms CA, Lambert HSIII, et al. Radial meniscal tears: significance, incidence, and MR appearance. AJR Am J Roentgenol 2005;185(6):1429–34.

39. Magee T, Shapiro M, Williams D. MR accuracy and arthroscopic incidence of meniscal radial tears. Skeletal Radiol 2002;31(12):686–9.

40. Lecas LK, Helms CA, Kosarek FJ, et al. Inferiorly displaced flap tears of the medial meniscus: MR appearance and clinical significance. AJR Am J Roentgenol 2000;174(1):161–4.

41. Vande Berg BC, Malghem J, Poilvache P, et al. Meniscal tears with fragments displaced in notch and recesses of knee: MR imaging with arthroscopic comparison. Radiology 2005;234(3):842–50.

42. McKnight A, Southgate J, Price A, et al. Meniscal tears with displaced fragments: common patterns on magnetic resonance imaging. Skeletal Radiol 2010;39(3):279–83.

43. Brody JM, Lin HM, Hulstyn MJ, et al. Lateral meniscus root tear and meniscus extrusion with anterior cruciate ligament tear. Radiology 2006;239(3):805–10.

44. Ozkoc G, Circi E, Gonc U, et al. Radial tears in the root of the posterior horn of the medial meniscus. Knee Surg Sports Traumatol Arthrosc 2008;16(9):849–54.

45. Lee YG, Shim JC, Choi YS, et al. Magnetic resonance imaging findings of surgically proven medial meniscus root tear: tear configuration and associated knee abnormalities. J Comput Assist Tomogr 2008;32(3):452–7.

46. Koenig JH, Ranawat AS, Umans HR, et al. Meniscal root tears: diagnosis and treatment. Arthroscopy 2009;25(9):1025–32.

47. De Smet AA, Blankenbaker DG, Kijowski R, et al. MR diagnosis of posterior root tears of the lateral meniscus using arthroscopy as the reference standard. AJR Am J Roentgenol 2009;192(2):480–6.

48. Choi CJ, Choi YJ, Lee JJ, et al. Magnetic resonance imaging evidence of meniscal extrusion in medial meniscus posterior root tear. Arthroscopy 2010; 26(12):1602–6.

49. Lerer DB, Umans HR, Hu MX, et al. The role of meniscal root pathology and radial meniscal tear in medial meniscal extrusion. Skeletal Radiol 2004;33(10): 569–74.

50. Costa CR, Morrison WB, Carrino JA. Medial meniscus extrusion on knee MRI: is extent associated with severity of degeneration or type of tear? AJR Am J Roentgenol 2004;183(1):17–23.

51. Kaplan PA, Gehl RH, Dussault RG, et al. Bone contusions of the posterior lip of the medial tibial plateau (contrecoup injury) and associated internal derangements of the knee at MR imaging. Radiology 1999;211(3):747–53.

52. De Smet AA, Graf BK, del Rio AM. Association of parameniscal cysts with underlying meniscal tears as identified on MRI and arthroscopy. AJR Am J Roentgenol 2011;196(2):W180–6.

53. De Smet AA, Asinger DA, Johnson RL. Abnormal superior popliteomeniscal fascicle and posterior pericapsular edema: indirect MR imaging signs of a lateral meniscal tear. AJR Am J Roentgenol 2001;176(1):63–6.

54. Laundre BJ, Collins MS, Bond JR, et al. MRI accuracy for tears of the posterior horn of the lateral meniscus in patients with acute anterior cruciate ligament injury and the clinical relevance of missed tears. AJR Am J Roentgenol 2009; 193(2):515–23.

55. Park LS, Jacobson JA, Jamadar DA, et al. Posterior horn lateral meniscal tears simulating meniscofemoral ligament attachment in the setting of ACL tear: MRI findings. Skeletal Radiol 2007;36(5):399–403.

56. Shankman S, Beltran J, Melamed E, et al. Anterior horn of the lateral meniscus: another potential pitfall in MR imaging of the knee. Radiology 1997;204(1): 181–4.

57. Shepard MF, Hunter DM, Davies MR, et al. The clinical significance of anterior horn meniscal tears diagnosed on magnetic resonance images. Am J Sports Med 2002;30(2):189–92.

58. Kaushik S, Erickson JK, Palmer WE, et al. Effect of chondrocalcinosis on the MR imaging of knee menisci. AJR Am J Roentgenol 2001;177(4):905–9.

59. Wright RW, Boyer DS. Significance of the arthroscopic meniscal flounce sign: a prospective study. Am J Sports Med 2007;35(2):242–4.

60. Yu JS, Cosgarea AJ, Kaeding CC, et al. Meniscal flounce MR imaging. Radiology 1997;203(2):513–5.

61. Kim YG, Ihn JC, Park SK, et al. An arthroscopic analysis of lateral meniscal variants and a comparison with MRI findings. Knee Surg Sports Traumatol Arthrosc 2006;14(1):20–6.

62. Ryu KN, Kim IS, Kim EJ, et al. MR imaging of tears of discoid lateral menisci. AJR Am J Roentgenol 1998;171(4):963–7.

63. Rohren EM, Kosarek FJ, Helms CA. Discoid lateral meniscus and the frequency of meniscal tears. Skeletal Radiol 2001;30(6):316–20.

64. Araki Y, Yamamoto H, Nakamura H, et al. MR diagnosis of discoid lateral menisci of the knee. Eur J Radiol 1994;18(2):92–5.

65. Yoo WJ, Lee K, Moon HJ, et al. Meniscal morphologic changes on magnetic resonance imaging are associated with symptomatic discoid lateral meniscal tear in children. Arthroscopy 2012;28(3):330–6.

66. Sanders TG, Linares RC, Lawhorn KW, et al. Oblique meniscomeniscal ligament: another potential pitfall for a meniscal tear–anatomic description and appearance at MR imaging in three cases. Radiology 1999;213(1):213–6.

67. Anderson AF, Awh MH, Anderson CN. The anterior meniscofemoral ligament of the medial meniscus: case series. Am J Sports Med 2004;32(4):1035–40.

68. Coulier B, Himmer O. Anteromedial meniscofemoral ligament of the knee: CT and MR features in 3 cases. JBR-BTR 2008;91(6):240–4.

69. Cha JG, Min KD, Han JK, et al. Anomalous insertion of the medial meniscus into the anterior cruciate ligament: the MR appearance. Br J Radiol 2008;81(961): 20–4.

Imaging of Cartilage and Osteochondral Injuries

A Case-Based Review

Robert A. Gallo, MD[a], Timothy J. Mosher, MD[a,b],*

KEYWORDS

- Cartilage • Osteochondral • MRI • Knee • Cartilage repair

KEY POINTS

- The evaluation of articular cartilage injury depends on magnetic resonance imaging (MRI) with high-contrast resolution, which requires the use of high-field magnets, state-of-the-art coil technology, and appropriate MRI acquisition sequences.
- The image signal intensity on turbo spin echo (TSE) or fast spin echo proton density and T2-weighted MR images is sensitive to structural properties of the extracellular cartilage collagen matrix.
- Acute injury of cartilage and the collagen matrix will increase the signal on TSE proton density or T2-weighted MR images, whereas more chronic injury results in heterogeneous areas of high and low signal.
- In addition to the articular surface, always evaluate the bone-cartilage interface for signs of chondral delamination.
- MRI is a sensitive tool for evaluating the degree of fill of cartilage repair tissue and monitoring for complications.

The continued development and advancement of magnetic resonance imaging (MRI) technology over the past 5 years has improved the visualization of articular cartilage and focal osteochondral injuries. Along with better noninvasive diagnosis of these injuries, there has been accumulating evidence that focal chondral lesions are a risk factor for the development of osteoarthritis[1–3] and a source of patient symptoms.[4] Development of new technologies for treating focal cartilage defects continues to be an active area of research, and MRI plays a prominent role in evaluating these techniques in clinical trials and monitoring patients for complications.

[a] Department of Orthopaedics, Penn State Milton S. Hershey Medical Center, 500 University Drive, Hershey, PA 17033, USA; [b] Department of Radiology, Penn State Milton S. Hershey Medical Center, MC H066, 500 University Drive, Hershey, PA 17033, USA
* Corresponding author. Department of Radiology, Penn State Milton S. Hershey Medical Center, MC H066, 500 University Drive, Hershey, PA 17033.
E-mail address: tmosher@hmc.psu.edu

Clin Sports Med 32 (2013) 477–505
http://dx.doi.org/10.1016/j.csm.2013.03.006
0278-5919/13/$ – see front matter © 2013 Elsevier Inc. All rights reserved.

In this article, the authors briefly review the technical factors for optimal MRI evaluation of articular cartilage. Although cartilage evaluation is critical for all joints, the authors' case focus remains the knee where MRI has been widely studied and applied. The authors review the important correlation of the MRI signal to the structure of the type II collagen matrix in normal cartilage and identify how alterations in this signal pattern can be an important sign of cartilage injury. Finally, the authors illustrate specific patterns of cartilage injury and application of MRI in evaluating cartilage repair through a series of selected cases.

TECHNICAL CONSIDERATIONS

The diagnosis of articular cartilage injuries requires images with high-contrast resolution. Optimal MRI techniques must enhance differences in signal intensity between (1) cartilage and synovial fluid and (2) cartilage and subchondral bone plate, while simultaneously achieving high spatial resolution. Historically, the clinical evaluation of articular cartilage has relied on 2 acquisition techniques: 3-dimensional (3D) fat-suppressed (FS) or water-excited (WE) T1-weighted spoiled gradient echo (SPGR) and 2D proton density (PD)–weighted turbo spin echo (TSE) or fast spin echo (FSE) techniques. Each technique has relative advantages and disadvantages with respect to contrast resolution and visualization of articular cartilage.

A comparison of 3 commonly used MRI sequences is illustrated in **Fig. 1**. When imaged with 3D WE T1-weighted SPGR sequence, articular cartilage has uniform high signal. Of the 3 sequences illustrated, this technique provides the highest spatial resolution, in this example, a voxel of 0.05 mm³. There is high contrast between cartilage and bone and moderate contrast between cartilage and the synovial fluid; however, there is little differentiation of signal within cartilage. As a result, it can be difficult to visualize the superficial flap tear within the lateral patellar facet. Despite having a spatial resolution and order of magnitude less than that of the SPGR technique, the PD-weighted TSE image better demonstrates the focal cartilage lesion. Because the TSE sequence is more sensitive to the effect of the type II collagen matrix on the cartilage water signal, it demonstrates regional variation in MRI signal within cartilage. Perturbation of this signal is a sensitive marker of early cartilage injury.

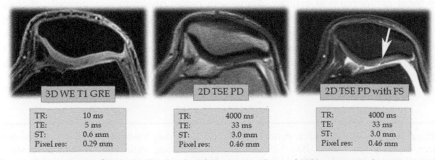

3D WE T1 GRE		2D TSE PD		2D TSE PD with FS	
TR:	10 ms	TR:	4000 ms	TR:	4000 ms
TE:	5 ms	TE:	33 ms	TE:	33 ms
ST:	0.6 mm	ST:	3.0 mm	ST:	3.0 mm
Pixel res:	0.29 mm	Pixel res:	0.46 mm	Pixel res:	0.46 mm

Fig. 1. *Comparison of images obtained with 3 commonly used MRI sequences* in a 52-year-old asymptomatic volunteer with an incidental flap tear of the lateral patellar facet (*arrow*). All images were obtained at 3.0 T with acquisition parameters as listed. The 2D TSE PD with FS image is an image with chemical shift FS. Note that the 3D WE T1 spoiled gradient echo SPGR image has substantially higher spatial resolution than the 2D TSE images. The 3D GRE voxel dimension of 0.05 mm³ is almost 13 times smaller than that of the 2D TSE images (0.64 mm³). ST, Section Thickness; TE, Time to Echo; TR, Time to Repetition.

Suppressing the signal from fat with chemical shift FS increases the dynamic range of the image and accentuates the internal contrast within cartilage, making the cartilage tear quite obvious (arrow). Fat suppression can be useful in identifying focal cartilage injuries occurring at the osteochondral junction (eg, delamination injuries). Furthermore, fat suppression makes the image sensitive to changes in bone marrow signal of the subchondral bone, which is a useful indirect indicator of acute osteochondral trauma or altered biomechanics related to an overlying chondral injury.

Given the small thickness of cartilage and the need for high image contrast, effective MRI requires a high signal-to-noise ratio (SNR), which is best accomplished using high-field MRI systems (1.5 T or 3.0 T). Although high SNR images can be obtained with low-field scanners, long image acquisition times are required to average the signal and, therefore, increase the probability of artifact from patient motion. Generally, as the thickness of the cartilage decreases, the more diagnostic accuracy depends on increased magnet-field strength. For example, diagnostic MRI of patellar cartilage can be obtained with low-field systems using appropriate acquisition techniques (**Fig. 2**). However, low-field images are limited in the evaluation of the thinner femorotibial cartilage (**Fig. 3**) and very limited in evaluating the thin cartilage of the hip or shoulder. A major advance in improving the specificity for the diagnosis of focal cartilage lesions has been the additional SNR provided by 3.0-T MRI and the continued improvement in phased-array coil technology.

For larger joints, such as the hip and knee, the PD-weighted TSE with or without fat suppression is generally preferred. Initial evaluation of this technique by Potter and colleagues[5] reported an accuracy of 92% for the diagnosis of focal cartilage lesions in the knee. Similar accuracy has been identified in subsequent studies[6,7] for full-thickness defects and partial-thickness defects involving greater than 50% cartilage thickness. Sensitivity is generally less than 50% for superficial fibrillation and surface erosion. The lack of sensitivity to surface lesions is partially a function of limited spatial resolution. However, spatial resolution of the image should not be increased at the expense of lowering the SNR. As illustrated in **Fig. 4**, the diagnosis

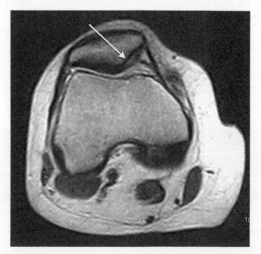

Fig. 2. Axial T2-weighted image obtained at 0.2 T of a 16-year-old girl with right knee pain following a twisting injury. There is focal increased signal at the osteochondral junction of the lateral patellar facet (*arrow*) indicating a cartilage delamination injury. The articular surface is intact. This pattern of cartilage injury can be seen with transient patellar dislocation.

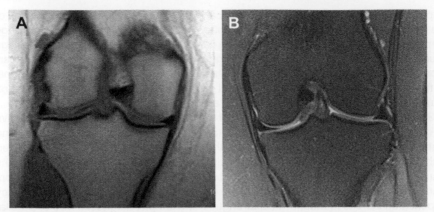

Fig. 3. Comparison of (*A*) coronal T2-weighted MRI obtained with a low-field (0.2 T) scanner and (*B*) coronal TSE PD-weighted FS image obtained with a high-field (3.0 T) scanner. The image obtained from the low-field scanner lacks sufficient contrast resolution to reliably delineate the articular surface. The poor contrast resolution decreases diagnostic accuracy for detection of partial-thickness defects. In contrast, the image obtained from the high-field scanner demonstrates sufficient contrast resolution to demonstrate regional differences in T2-weighted signal produced by the differences in the cartilage collagen matrix. The ability to resolve this intrinsic signal variation is a good indicator that the MRI technique is of sufficient quality to diagnosis focal cartilage injury.

depends on sufficient spatial resolution to resolve a clinically important defect. Pushing the spatial resolution too far will make the image noisy without improving the ability to visualize a clinically relevant cartilage defect. As a general rule, the authors recommend using an in-plane spatial resolution of approximately 7 pixels across the cartilage on a 3.0-T MRI scanner. For the knee, a pixel resolution in the range of 300 μm to 500 μm with a section thickness of 3 mm is suggested.

For imaging of small joints, such as the foot and hand, or small joints with curved surfaces, such as the elbow and ankle, obtaining sufficient spatial resolution using 2D sequences can be challenging. The 3D SPGR techniques can clearly delineate cartilage interfaces and minimize volume averaging in these instances.[8] Images with a 1.0- to 2.0-mm section thickness and in-plane resolution of 200 μm to 350 μm per pixel can be obtained using 3D SPGR techniques at 1.5 T. These sequences are also used in research applications of cartilage morphometry to quantitatively measure

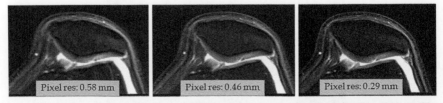

Fig. 4. *Effect of spatial resolution*: Axial PD-weighted images with FS (TR/TE: 4000 ms/33 ms and 3.0 mm section thickness) obtained at 3 different spatial resolutions (res). With the larger pixel dimension of 0.56 mm², it is difficult to resolve the superficial flap tear in the lateral patellar facet easily identified on images obtained at higher spatial resolution. Further decreasing the pixel dimension from 0.46 mm² to 0.29 mm² decreases the image SNR without improving conspicuity of the lesion. TE, Time to Echo; TR, Time to Repetition.

the volume, thickness, and surface area of cartilage in longitudinal clinical trials.[9] More recently, 3D TSE techniques have been used in joint evaluation. These techniques combine excellent tissue contrast of TSE imaging with the ability to retrospectively reconstruct images in any plane. In theory, this technique should be useful for curved articular surfaces such as the femoral trochlea whereby reconstructing image planes perpendicular to the subchondral bone would allow for more accurate estimates of lesion size and depth. Currently, routine use of these techniques is limited by the long image acquisition time and image blurring produced by the long echo train lengths.

STRUCTURE AND MRI APPEARANCE OF NORMAL CARTILAGE

The major components of articular cartilage are water, type II collagen, and the proteoglycan aggrecan. When PD- or T2-weighted MRI is obtained using TSE or FSE techniques, the signal intensity of cartilage is strongly influenced by the organization of the type II collagen matrix. This influence is caused by the efficient T2 relaxation and magnetization transfer by the highly anisotropic collagen matrix.[10–12]

Regional variation in the structural architecture of the collagen matrix, both with respect to depth from the articular surface and location in the joint, produces regional variation in signal intensity of cartilage on PD-weighted TSE images. Layers of signal intensity are most conspicuous in the patella and tibial plateau.[13] MR images of thin cartilage, such as the femoral condyle, ankle, and hip, generally lack sufficient spatial resolution to resolve zonal differences in cartilage T2. Recognizing the normal intensity variation in cartilage is necessary to (1) identify focal areas of cartilage injury associated with trauma and (2) to avoid erroneously interpreting nonuniform signal as disease.[14] As illustrated in **Fig. 5**, the T2 of articular cartilage on FS PD-weighted TSE images increases toward the articular surface. In cartilage subjected to repetitive compressive loading (**Fig. 6**), the organization of the type II collagen demonstrates a highly organized, zonal architecture.[15] With polarized light microscopy, the radial zone near bone is characterized by dense condensations of collagen fibrils oriented

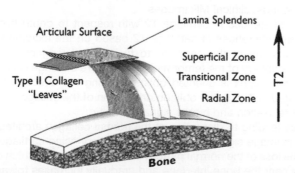

Fig. 5. *Type II collagen matrix of cartilage.* Collagen is organized into a leaflike architecture with a preferential orientation that varies with respect to depth from the articular cartilage. Near bone, the fibers are oriented perpendicular to the articular surface. This radial orientation is termed the *radial zone*. The high degree of collagen anisotropy in this layer produces efficient T2 relaxation. The short T2 results in low signal intensity on T2 or PD-weighted images. Toward the articular surface, fibers assume an oblique orientation (transitional zone) and finally are oriented parallel to the articular surface (superficial zone). The oblique orientation results in less efficient T2 relaxation and longer T2 times, which contributes to the higher signal intensity observed near the superficial layer of cartilage.

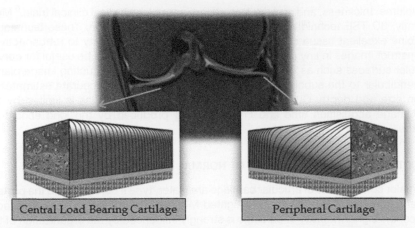

Fig. 6. *Regional variation in cartilage signal intensity.* In the central load-bearing region, cartilage has a thick radial zone and narrow transition zone. On MRI, this results in a thicker layer of low signal intensity cartilage near the bone with a relatively thin layer of superficial cartilage with higher signal intensity. In the periphery of the articular surface, the radial zone is relatively thin with a thicker transitional zone in which fibers are oriented along the lines of predominant shear strain. On MRI, this region has a relatively thin hypointense layer of cartilage near the bone corresponding to the radial zone, with a thicker layer of high-signal-intensity cartilage toward the surface related to the thicker transitional zone.

perpendicular to bone.[15] With very high-resolution images, the darker radial zone has a striated appearance with alternating fine bands of high- and low-signal intensity radiating from the bone-cartilage interface.[16–18] Closer to the articular surface, the higher water content, lower anisotropy, and oblique orientation of the collagen fibers increases the T2 relaxation time and causes a gradual increase in signal intensity. At the articular surface, collagen fibers are oriented parallel to the articular surface. This layer, termed the *lamina splendens*,[15] is approximately 200 μm thick and is too thin to resolve on most clinical MR images.

In addition to differences in cartilage T2 with respect to depth from the articular surface, there are differences in cartilage T2 based on the location within the joint and relative orientation of the cartilage to the applied magnetic field.[16,19–21] For example, in the periphery of the femorotibial joint where cartilage is exposed to shear strain, the collagen matrix is oriented obliquely along the direction of predominant strain. As illustrated in **Fig. 6**, the oblique orientation of the collagen matrix produces less efficient T2 relaxation and higher signal intensity.

Cartilage injury leading to disruption of the normal collagen architecture produces focal alteration in image signal intensity. A key to diagnosing cartilage injury on MRI is recognizing the loss of the normal pattern of signal intensity in which cartilage signal intensity is dark near the bone interface and gradually increases toward the articular surface.

PATTERNS OF CARTILAGE INJURY

The pattern of cartilage injury with acute trauma is a function of the rate of loading the tissue and the architecture of the collagen matrix. Cartilage demonstrates viscoelastic properties in response to compressive loading. With high rates of loading, such as with blunt injury in an automobile accident, the relatively stiff cartilage dissipates the energy within its superficial region of articular cartilage. This loading pattern can produce superficial fissures.[22] Conversely, lower rates of loading results in energy transferred to the deeper layers of the tissue.

With increasing age, the accumulation of advanced glycation end products and cross-linked collagen makes cartilage stiffer, brittle, and more susceptible to injury.[23] Age-related changes of the articular surface leads to greater friction and shear strain within the collagen matrix and further increases the potential for chondral injury. Excessive shear force applied to cartilage can produce oblique, surface-layer tears of cartilage along the obliquely oriented fibers in the transitional zone. Shear force at the osteochondral junction can debond the calcified layer of cartilage from the underlying bone plate. The sensitivity of the PD-weighted signal to disruption of the collagen matrix produces consistent patterns of MRI signal abnormalities used to diagnose focal cartilage injury. In the acute setting, fractures of the collagen matrix lead to a loss of the anisotropic organization of the collagen matrix and increases cartilage T2, making the signal brighter on T2- and PD-weighted images. In addition, the loss of the normal constraint of the collagen matrix on the hydrated aggrecan leads to a focal increase in water content and mobility of water within the extracellular matrix. All of these factors lead to an increase in the signal intensity of the injured tissue. With time, further degradation of the tissue and breakdown of the collagen matrix exposes more water-binding sites on collagen and produces T2 shortening and more efficient magnetization transfer. In the setting of subacute and chronic cartilage injury, areas of low signal intensity frequently develop adjacent to focal areas of high signal. This heterogeneous appearance of cartilage can be an important clue when estimating the chronicity of a cartilage lesion and its temporal correlation with patient symptoms.

In the following section, the authors use a case-based approach to illustrate characteristic patterns of cartilage injury and highlight diagnostic principles on MR images and surgical findings.

Case 1: Acute Cartilage Injury with Patellar Dislocation

History
A 41-year-old patient sustained a traumatic lateral patella dislocation during an all-terrain vehicle accident.

Radiographs
Immediate merchant view radiograph (**Fig. 7**) demonstrated an osteochondral impaction fracture of the medial patella and anterolateral cortex of the lateral femoral condyle consistent with transient patellar dislocation. Soft tissue edema in the medial

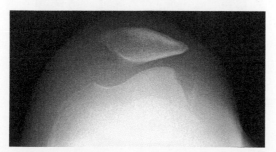

Fig. 7. An osteochondral impaction fracture of the medial patella and anterolateral cortex of the lateral femoral condyle consistent with transient patellar dislocation.

retinaculum and lateral patellar subluxation/tilt is suggestive of an injury to the medial patellofemoral ligament (MPFL).

MRI

The MRI obtained 1 week after injury better demonstrated the extent of cartilage and soft tissue injury. The axial TSE, PD with FS (**Fig. 8**) image demonstrated a large area of cartilage delamination from the lateral patellar facet. The margin of the cartilage defect was sharp with vertical shoulders. The lack of subchondral marrow edema beneath the cartilage defect was consistent with a delamination injury as opposed to the impaction fracture seen in the anterior femoral condyle, which characteristically demonstrates subchondral bone marrow edema (**Fig. 9**). The delaminated chondral fragment was displaced into the lateral gutter of the suprapatellar recess (**Fig. 10**). This image also demonstrated hemarthrosis related to the recent avulsion of the MPFL from the medial patella.

Surgery

Ten days after the injury, he underwent arthroscopy and open MPFL repair. He had a well-contained, full-thickness chondral defect (**Fig. 11**). The loose osteochondral fragments were too small for repair and were removed from the lateral gutter (**Fig. 12**).

Teaching points

- The case demonstrates several features of an acute cartilage injury: sharp margins of the cartilage defect, displaced chondral fragment, sites of diffuse, poorly defined bone marrow edema (indicating bone marrow contusion), and associated soft tissue injuries (MPFL tear, large joint hemarthrosis).
- In contrast to impaction injuries, areas of acute cartilage delamination often have scant marrow edema in the subchondral bone.

Case 2: Chronic Cartilage Impaction Injury

History

A 19-year-old woman involved in a motor vehicle collision struck the dashboard with her left knee and sustained a left acetabulum fracture, which was treated operatively.

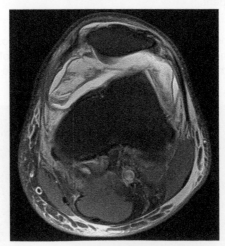

Fig. 8. (Same case as **Fig. 7**) A large area of cartilage delamination from the lateral patellar facet.

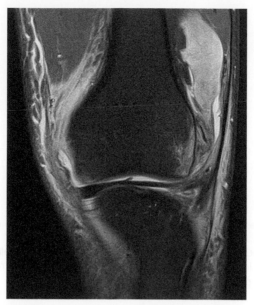

Fig. 9. (Same case as **Fig. 7**) A subchondral bone marrow edema.

Over the next 2 years, as her ambulation increased, she developed mechanical symptoms of the knee and sharp anterior knee pain that worsened with ascending and descending stairs.

MRI
The axial TSE, PD-weighted image with FS demonstrated linear fluid signal extending from the articular surface of the median ridge to subchondral bone (**Fig. 13**). This signal extended along the bone-cartilage interface of the lateral facet suggesting a

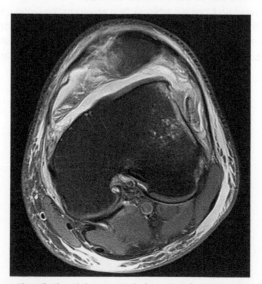

Fig. 10. (Same case as **Fig. 7**) The delaminated chondral fragment has been displaced into the lateral gutter of the suprapatellar recess.

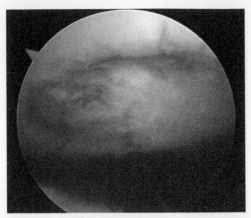

Fig. 11. (Same case as **Fig. 7**) A well-contained, full-thickness chondral defect.

larger area of chondral delamination and injury to the adjacent collagen matrix. Note the subtle areas of low T2 signal adjacent to the fissure. This heterogeneous appearance is suggestive of a chronic cartilage injury.

Surgery
Probing of the patellar cartilage demonstrated a flap tear of the lateral patellar facet (**Fig. 14**), which was debrided to stable lesions with margins measuring approximately 8 mm in diameter (**Fig. 15**).

Teaching points
- Cartilage fissures are characterized by a fluidlike signal (bright on T2 or PD images) typically oriented along the predominant direction of the type II collagen matrix. In this case, over the patellar ridge, the collagen matrix is oriented primarily perpendicular to the articular surface.
- High signal extending from a cartilage fissure along the bone cartilage interface is a useful sign that suggests a delamination-type tear and instability of the adjacent cartilage margin. This information can be helpful in preoperatively estimating the potential size of the cartilage defect following chondroplasty.

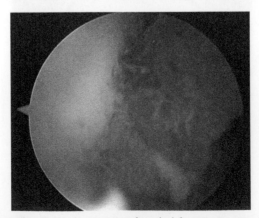

Fig. 12. (Same case as **Fig. 7**) The loose osteochondral fragments were too small for repair and were removed from the lateral gutter.

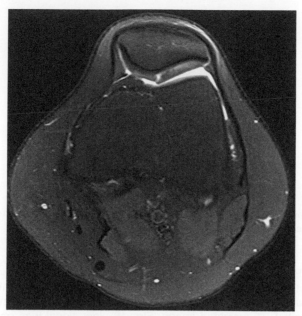

Fig. 13. MRI axial TSE PD-weighted image with FS demonstrates linear fluid signal extending from the articular surface of the median ridge to subchondral bone. This signal extends along the bone cartilage interface of the lateral facet suggesting a larger area of chondral delamination and injury to the adjacent collagen matrix. Note the subtle areas of low T2 signal adjacent to the fissure. This heterogeneous appearance is suggestive of a chronic cartilage injury.

- Heterogeneous low T2 signal in the cartilage adjacent to a site of a focal cartilage defect is an indicator of a more chronic cartilage injury.

Case 3: Chondral Delamination

History
A 39-year-old novice male runner began experiencing medial knee pain while training for a 5-km race. Although the pain limited him from running, he denied any locking or mechanical symptoms.

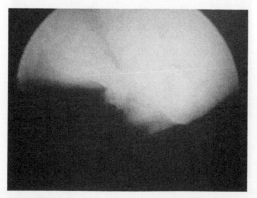

Fig. 14. (Same case as **Fig. 13**) Surgery: Probing of the patellar cartilage demonstrated a flap tear of the lateral patellar facet.

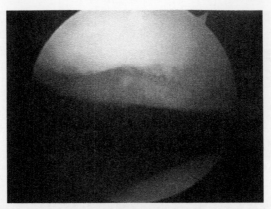

Fig. 15. (Same case as **Fig. 13**) Flap tear of the lateral patellar facet debrided to stable lesions with margins measuring approximately 8 mm in diameter.

MRI

Coronal, TSE, PD-weighted, FS image (**Fig. 16**) demonstrated a 1-cm, full-thickness cartilage defect with extensive chondral delamination of the adjacent anterior and posterior cartilage demonstrated on the sagittal TSE, PD-weighted image (**Fig. 17**). On the FS, sagittal, T2-weighted image (**Fig. 18**), low signal was observed in the superficial layer of the delaminated cartilage, which suggests a more chronic injury. The subchondral bone marrow signal is normal despite the presence of a full- thickness cartilage lesion. Other images from this case demonstrated a large joint effusion and synovitis, which likely contributed to the patient's report of significant pain.

Surgery

The patient was treated arthroscopically with the removal of the large flap and debridement of the surrounding diseased articular cartilage (**Fig. 19**). After the debridement, the cartilage defect measured approximately 1 cm wide by 2.4 cm long.

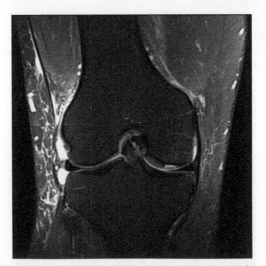

Fig. 16. A case of chondral delamination. MRI: Coronal TSE PD-weighted FS image demonstrates a 1-cm, full-thickness cartilage defect with extensive chondral delamination of the adjacent anterior.

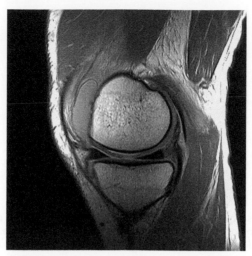

Fig. 17. (Same case as **Fig. 16**) Posterior cartilage demonstrated on the sagittal TSE PD-weighted image.

Companion case

A 54-year-old woman with a long history of knee pain and prior total knee arthroplasty of the contralateral knee demonstrated multifocal areas of cartilage delamination of the femur and patella (**Fig. 20**). This pattern of diffuse osteochondral injury is atypical for osteoarthritis and, in the absence of trauma, may indicate a genetic predisposition for cartilage debonding.[24]

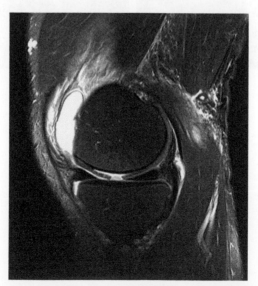

Fig. 18. (Same case as **Fig. 16**) FS, sagittal, T2-weighted image with low signal observed in the superficial layer of the delaminated cartilage, which suggests a more chronic injury. The subchondral bone marrow signal is normal despite the presence of a full-thickness cartilage lesion. Other images from this case demonstrated a large joint effusion and synovitis, which likely contributed to the patient's report of significant pain.

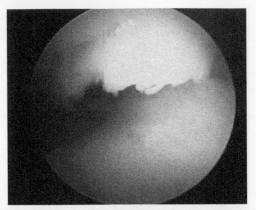

Fig. 19. (Same case as **Fig. 16**) Patient was treated arthroscopically with removal of the large flap and debridement of the surrounding diseased articular cartilage. After the debridement, the cartilage defect measured approximately 1 cm wide by 2.4 cm long.

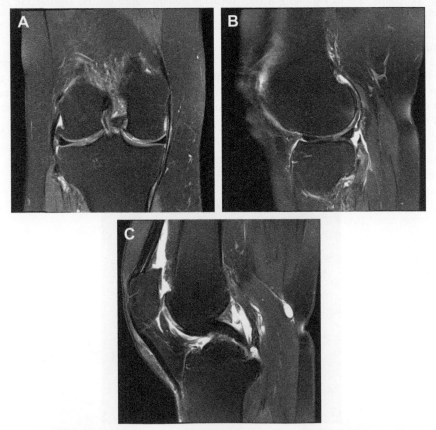

Fig. 20. (*A–C*) (A companion case to that presented in **Figs. 16–19**) A 54-year-old woman with a long history of knee pain and prior total knee arthroplasty of the contralateral knee demonstrates multifocal areas of cartilage delamination of the femur and patella. This pattern of diffuse osteochondral injury is atypical for osteoarthritis and, in the absence of trauma, may indicate a genetic predisposition for cartilage debonding.

Teaching points

- In addition to evaluating the articular surface for focal defects, cartilage evaluation should include careful evaluation of the osteochondral junction. Focal delamination injuries may be seen with loading or shear injuries to the articular surface and may not be associated with a focal defect at the articular surface. Arthroscopically, these delaminated lesions without a focal defect can be visualized and felt as soft spots using probing (see Case 5). Genetic studies indicate some individuals may have a genetic predisposition to cartilage delamination.
- The presence or absence of subchondral marrow edema should not be used to determine if a focal cartilage lesion is full thickness (outer bridge 4). Particularly, with chondral delamination injuries, marrow edema may be absent.
- The extent of high T2 fluid signal between the cartilage and bone can estimate the size of unstable cartilage.

Case 4: Pediatric Elbow Injury

History
A 12-year-old boy initially developed right elbow pain following a fall on an outstretched hand while playing football. Radiographs at that time were reportedly within normal limits. Intermittent pain ensued and was aggravated by baseball pitching the following spring.

Radiograph
The lateral radiograph of the right elbow approximately 6 months following the initial injury was normal (**Fig. 21**).

MRI
Sagittal T1 (**Fig. 22**A), TSE, T2-weighted with FS (see **Fig. 22**B) and 3D WE gradient Dual Echo in the Steady State (DESS) (see **Fig. 22**C) images demonstrated a focal 7-mm full-thickness chondral defect of the capitellum with a displaced chondral fragment within the anterolateral gutter. This fracture of the secondary physis of the capitellum is referred to as a *Kocher-Lorenz osteochondral fracture* and may be difficult to diagnose radiographically, especially when the displaced fragment lacks bone.

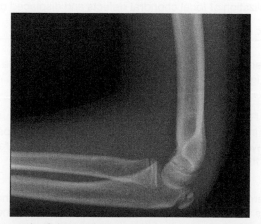

Fig. 21. Lateral radiograph of the right elbow approximately 6 months following the initial injury is normal.

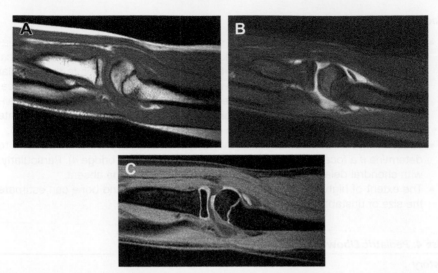

Fig. 22. (Same case as **Fig. 21**) MRI: Sagittal T1, TSE T2-weighted with FS and 3D WE Dual echo in the Steady State (DESS) images (*A–C*) demonstrate a focal 7-mm full-thickness chondral defect of the capitellum with a displaced chondral fragment within the anterolateral gutter. This fracture of the secondary physis of the capitellum is referred to as a *Kocher-Lorenz osteochondral fracture* and may be difficult to diagnose radiographically, especially when the displaced fragment lacks bone.

Surgery
Arthroscopic evaluation of the elbow demonstrated a 7-mm focal chondral defect of the defect with mild superficial chondrosis of the radial head. A hypertrophied, 1.5-cm cartilage body was located in the anterior gutter.

Teaching points
- MRI has high sensitivity for the diagnosis of occult fracture and epiphyseal fractures in the pediatric population when radiographic evaluation and clinical signs are equivocal.
- For small joints with curved articular surface, the 3D, FS, SPGR technique provides the best visualization of focal chondral defects and displaced chondral bodies.

Case 5: Basal Cystic Degeneration

History
A 31-year-old patient had progressive worsening of anterior knee pain 1 year after Anterior Cruciate Ligament (ACL) reconstruction.

MRI
Axial PD-weighted FS (**Fig. 23**) image demonstrated focal fluid signal in the deep layer of cartilage with an intact articular surface. The cystic lesion in the patella is confirmed on the sagittal T2-weighted FS (**Fig. 24**) images. There was a focal full-thickness cartilage defect of the femoral trochlea.

Surgery
At arthroscopy, there was a smooth focal contour abnormality of the articular surface (**Fig. 25**), which was soft when probed, consistent with cystic degeneration (**Fig. 26**). A focal full-thickness defect was present in the trochlea. Both lesions were treated with chondroplasty.

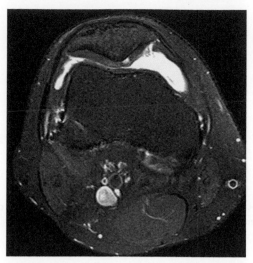

Fig. 23. A case of basal cystic degeneration. MRI axial PD-weighted FS demonstrate focal fluid signal in the deep layer of cartilage with an intact articular surface.

Teaching points

- Delamination injuries with disruption of the collagen matrix in the deep radial zone can lead to cystic degeneration of the deep radial zone[25] resulting in a focal cystlike area of fluid intensity beneath the articular surface.
- Delamination injuries may occur with an intact articular surface.

Case 6: Pediatric Knee Pain

History
A 9-year-old child with a history of juvenile idiopathic arthritis reported new onset of knee pain following a wrestling injury.

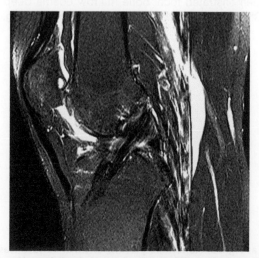

Fig. 24. (Same case as **Fig. 23**) Cystic lesion in the patella is confirmed on the sagittal T2-weighted FS images. There is a focal full-thickness cartilage defect of the femoral trochlea.

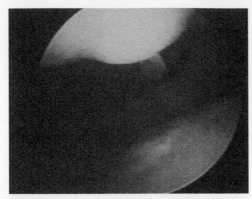

Fig. 25. (Same case as **Fig. 23**) At arthroscopy, there was a smooth focal contour abnormality of the articular surface.

Radiographs

Anteroposterior (AP) (**Fig. 27**A) and lateral (see **Fig. 27**B) radiographs of the right knee demonstrated a focal irregularity of the posterior lateral femoral condyle and raised concerns for a nondisplaced osteochondritis dissecans.

MRI

Coronal and sagittal PD-weighted, FS images (**Fig. 28**A, B) and sagittal TSE, T2-weighted, FS image (see **Fig. 28**C) demonstrated focal heterogeneous marrow signal of the posterior lateral femoral condyle with a normal appearance of the articular cartilage. The appearance was consistent with delayed ossification of the secondary physis, which is generally considered an asymptomatic developmental variant.

Companion case

Low-field (0.2 T) MR images of an 11-year-old boy with a several-month history of medial knee pain demonstrated focal bone marrow edema deep to the secondary physis on coronal Short Tau Inversion Recovery (STIR) images (**Fig. 29**). The overlying

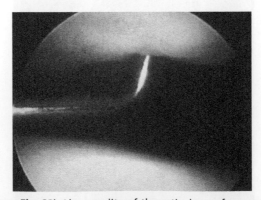

Fig. 26. (Same case as **Fig. 23**) Abnormality of the articular surface was soft when probed consistent with cystic degeneration. A focal full-thickness defect was present in the trochlea. Both lesions were treated with chondroplasty.

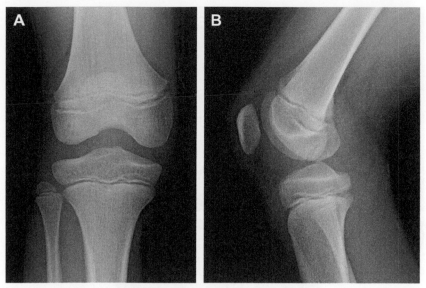

Fig. 27. AP (*A*) and lateral (*B*) radiographs of the right knee demonstrated a focal irregularity of the posterior lateral femoral condyle and raised concerns for a nondisplaced osteochondritis dissecans.

chondroepiphysis (nonossified epiphysis and articular cartilage) was intact on the sagittal T1- (**Fig. 30**A) and T2-weighted images (see **Fig. 30**B).

Teaching points

- Trauma or overuse injuries can lead to focal disruption of the secondary physis and delay in ossification of the epiphyseal cartilage resulting in juvenile osteochondritis dissecans.
- MRI is useful in evaluating the integrity of the overlying chondroepiphysis and may be useful in differentiating symptomatic lesions. Lesions located on the posterior femoral condyle with intact articular cartilage and lacking bone marrow edema likely represent an asymptomatic developmental variant.[26] Lesions with focal discontinuity of the secondary physis, widening of the overlying chondroepiphyseal cartilage, and subchondral bone marrow edema as in the companion case are more likely to be symptomatic.[27]

Case 7: Microfracture Repair

History
A 28-year-old woman had chronic intermittent medial right knee pain exacerbated with weight-bearing activities.

MRI
Coronal STIR 1.0-T MRI (**Fig. 31**) demonstrated a full-thickness chondral lesion of the medial femoral condyle with subchondral marrow edema. This lesion was subsequently treated with microfracture. Ten months after undergoing the microfracture procedure, the patient was reevaluated with MRI. Coronal (**Fig. 32**A) and sagittal (see **Fig. 32**B) PD-weighted FS images and sagittal PD-weighted (see **Fig. 32**C) images confirmed complete fill of the original chondral defect. Repair tissue

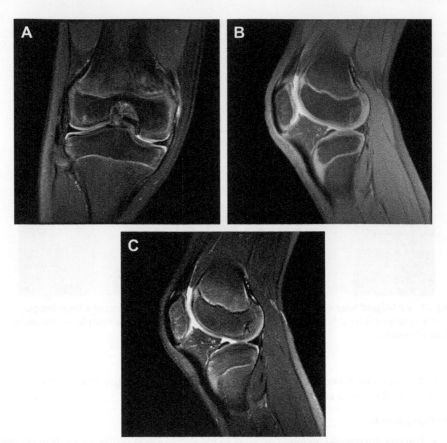

Fig. 28. (Same case as **Fig. 27**) Coronal (*A*) and sagittal (*B*) PD-weighted FS images and sagittal TSE T2-weighted FS image (*C*) demonstrate focal heterogeneous marrow signal of the posterior lateral femoral condyle with a normal appearance of the articular cartilage. The appearance is consistent with delayed ossification of the secondary physis, which is generally considered an asymptomatic developmental variant.

demonstrated heterogeneous bright signal on PD-weighted images with a loss of the normal zonal variation in signal intensity seen in normal native articular cartilage. Focal areas of marrow edema within the subchondral plate signaled bone remodeling at the sight of prior microfracture.

Surgery
Arthroscopic evaluation of the cartilage repair site confirmed a complete fibrocartilaginous fill of the defect (**Fig. 33**).

Teaching points
- MRI is a reliable noninvasive technique for evaluating cartilage repair. Semiquantitative scoring protocols, such as magnetic resonance observation of cartilage repair tissue (MOCART), are frequently used as outcome measures in longitudinal trials of cartilage repair.[28] This grading scale evaluates the degree of defect fill, integration of repair tissue to adjacent cartilage, integrity of the articular

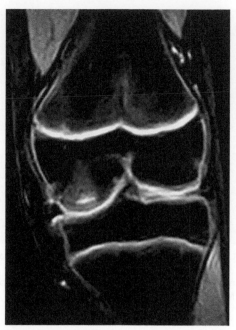

Fig. 29. (Same case as **Fig. 27**) Low-field (0.2 T) MRI of an 11-year-old boy with several-month history of medial knee pain demonstrate focal bone marrow edema deep to the secondary physis on coronal STIR images.

surface, signal intensity of the repair tissue, as well as features of subchondral bone, joint effusion, and adhesion. Since the introduction of the MOCART scoring system in 2006, the grading scale has undergone several revisions.[29,30]

- Cartilage repair tissue following marrow stimulation techniques, such as microfracture, lacks the normal zonal architecture of the cartilage type II collagen

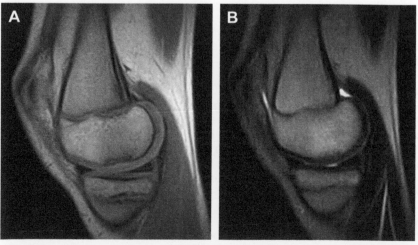

Fig. 30. (Same case as **Fig. 27**) The overlying chondroepiphysis (nonossified epiphysis and articular cartilage) is intact on the sagittal T1- (*A*) and T2-weighted images (*B*).

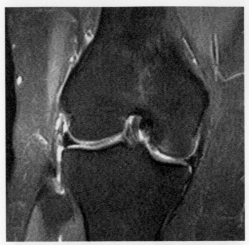

Fig. 31. Coronal STIR 1.0-T MRI demonstrates a full-thickness chondral lesion of the medial femoral condyle with subchondral marrow edema. This lesion was subsequently treated with microfracture. Ten months after undergoing the microfracture procedure, the patient was reevaluated with MRI.

matrix and generally demonstrates heterogeneous increased T2 signal. In comparison with histology, the heterogeneous MRI appearance correlates with a mixture of fibrocartilage and hyaline cartilage.

Case 8: Osteoarticular Transfer System Evaluation

History
An 18-year-old woman had continued pain in the posterior aspect of the knee 18 months following an osteoarticular transfer system (OATS) procedure.

Radiograph
AP (**Fig. 34**A) and lateral (see **Fig. 34**B) radiographs of the left knee demonstrated osseous integration of the transplant and suggested a loose body within the posterior recess.

MRI
Coronal (**Fig. 35**A) and sagittal (see **Fig. 35**B) PD-weighted FS MRI and sagittal PD-weighted MRI (see **Fig. 35**C) confirmed osseous integration of the allograft with subtle T2 hyperintensity compatible with bone remodeling of the graft margins. The cartilage defect was completely filled with minimal surface irregularity of the posterior margin. In contrast to the heterogeneous signal observed in the microfracture repair tissue, the cartilage overlying the transplant demonstrated the normal zonal variation in the T2-weighted signal.

Surgery
Arthroscopic surgery for the removal of a posterior loose body 20 months following the OATS procedure demonstrated congruity of the articular surface and integration of the autograft with the adjacent native tissue (**Fig. 36**).

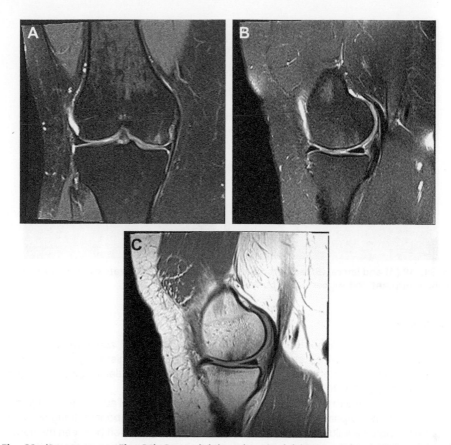

Fig. 32. (Same case as **Fig. 31**) Coronal (*A*) and sagittal (*B*) PD-weighted FS images and sagittal PD-weighted (*C*) images confirm complete fill of the original chondral defect. Repair tissue demonstrates heterogeneous bright signal on PD-weighted images with loss of the normal zonal variation in signal intensity seen in normal native articular cartilage. Focal areas of marrow edema within the subchondral plate signals bone remodeling at the sight of prior microfracture.

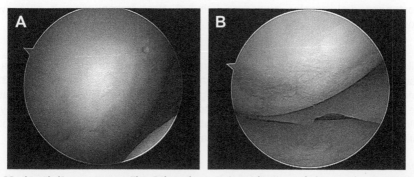

Fig. 33. (*A, B*) (Same case as **Fig. 31**) Arthroscopic evaluation of the cartilage repair site confirms complete fibrocartilaginous fill of the defect.

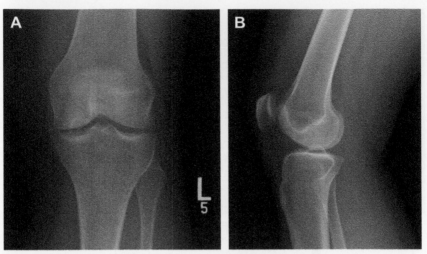

Fig. 34. AP (*A*) and lateral (*B*) radiographs of the left knee demonstrate osseous integration of the transplant and suggest loose body within posterior recess.

Teaching points

- Cartilage of osteochondral transplants retain the normal zonal variation in T2 signal intensity, which correlates with hyaline cartilage histology.[31] The repair tissue between the osteochondral grafts lacks this spatial variation in signal and correlates with fibrocartilage.
- MRI is sensitive to osseous incorporation of osteochondral autografts, allografts, and biphasic repair scaffolds that contain an osseous component. Imaging signs that indicate a failure to incorporate include a fluid signal cleft between the native bone and osseous graft, cyst formation, or change in position of the graft.

Case 9: Osteochondral Allograft Repair

History

A 39-year-old woman sustained cartilage injury 3 years before the initial presentation. She underwent chondroplasty and later microfracture for a focal chondral defect involving medial femoral condyle. After limited reparative tissue and continued pain, an osteochondral transfer procedure using 2 fresh-frozen allograft plugs was performed (**Fig. 37**).

MRI

A follow-up MRI obtained 7 months following allograft reconstruction of the articular surface demonstrated localized bright signal on PD-weighted FS imaging (**Fig. 38**A, B) and heterogeneous low signal on T1-weighted imaging (see **Fig. 38**C) in the native bone repair site, consistent with bone remodeling related to healing. The overlying cartilage demonstrated normal zonal variation in signal intensity indicating hyaline cartilage with congruity of the articular surface.

Surgery

Arthroscopic surgery 7 months following allograft transplantation confirmed the integrity of the articular margins and complete fill of the chondral defect (**Fig. 39**).

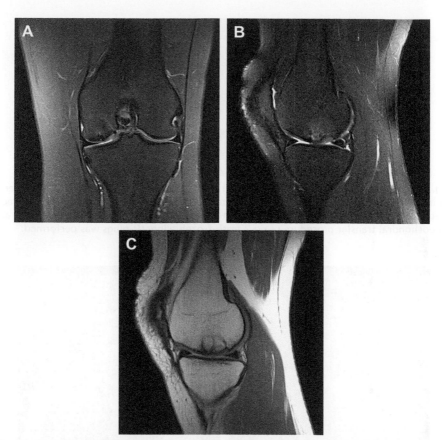

Fig. 35. (Same case as **Fig. 34**) Coronal (*A*) and sagittal (*B*) PD-weighted FS MRI and sagittal PD-weighted MRI (*C*) confirm osseous integration of the allograft with subtle T2 hyperintensity compatible with bone remodeling of the graft margins. The cartilage defect is completely filled with minimal surface irregularity of the posterior margin. In contrast to the heterogeneous signal observed in the microfracture repair tissue, the cartilage overlying the transplant demonstrates the normal zonal variation in T2-weighted signal.

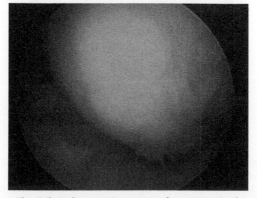

Fig. 36. (Same case as **Fig. 34**) Arthroscopic surgery for removal of a posterior loose body 20 months following OATS procedure demonstrates congruity of the articular surface and integration of the autograft with the adjacent native tissue.

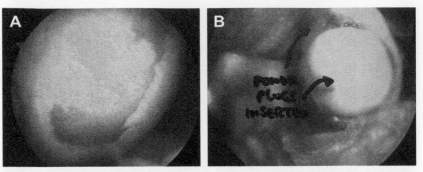

Fig. 37. (*A, B*) A 39-year-old woman sustained cartilage injury 3 years before initial presentation. She underwent chondroplasty and later microfracture for a focal chondral defect involving medial femoral condyle. After limited reparative tissue and continued pain, an osteochondral transfer procedure using 2 fresh-frozen allograft plugs was performed.

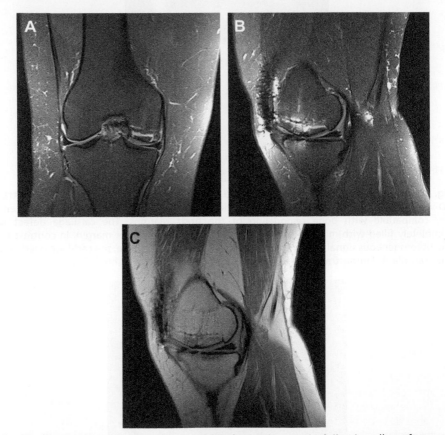

Fig. 38. (Same case as **Fig. 37**) Follow-up MRI obtained 7 months following allograft reconstruction of the articular surface demonstrates localized bright signal on PD-weighted FS imaging (*A, B*) and heterogeneous low signal on T1-weighted imaging (*C*) in the native bone repair site consistent with bone remodeling related to healing. The overlying cartilage demonstrates normal zonal variation in signal intensity indicating hyaline cartilage with congruity of the articular surface.

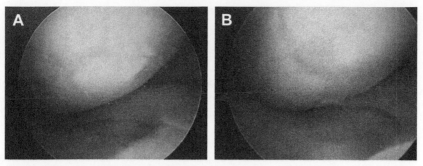

Fig. 39. (A, B) (Same case as **Fig. 37**) Arthroscopic surgery 7 months following allograft transplantation confirms the integrity of the articular margins and complete fill of the chondral defect.

Teaching points

- Localized fluid signal in the native bone adjacent to allograft reconstruction is associated with bone remodeling and healing, which may persist for several months following surgery.

SUMMARY

Continued advancement of MRI technology, leading to growth in 3-T magnet use and optimization of phased array coil technology, has improved visualization of articular cartilage. For large joints, TSE, PD-weighted imaging with or without FS provides the best contrast resolution and allows visualization not only of injury at the articular surface but also intrasubstance degeneration and injury of the osteochondral junction. This sensitivity is primarily driven by the strong influence of the type II collagen matrix on the water MRI signal in cartilage through T2 relaxation and magnetization transfer. Given the ability to directly visualize articular cartilage, MRI is playing an important role in research on the pathogenesis and natural history of focal cartilage injury and cartilage repair. Current active areas of research include the development of prognostic MRI biomarkers that may identify articular cartilage at risk for rapid deterioration, response markers that may be used to monitor cartilage repair, and the identification of MRI findings that are associated with specific patterns of joint pain. Translation of knowledge gained from these research studies will likely lead to further improvement in diagnosis and clinical management of focal osteochondral injuries in the near future.

REFERENCES

1. Schinhan M, Gruber M, Vavken P, et al. Critical-size defect induces unicompartmental osteoarthritis in a stable ovine knee. J Orthop Res 2012;30:214–20.
2. Widuchowski W, Widuchowski J, Faltus R, et al. Long-term clinical and radiological assessment of untreated severe cartilage damage in the knee: a natural history study. Scand J Med Sci Sports 2011;21:106–10.
3. Widuchowski W, Widuchowski J, Koczy B, et al. Untreated asymptomatic deep cartilage lesions associated with anterior cruciate ligament injury: results at 10- and 15-year follow-up. Am J Sports Med 2009;37:688–92.
4. Heir S, Nerhus TK, Rotterud JH, et al. Focal cartilage defects in the knee impair quality of life as much as severe osteoarthritis: a comparison of knee injury and

osteoarthritis outcome score in 4 patient categories scheduled for knee surgery. Am J Sports Med 2010;38:231–7.

5. Potter HG, Linklater JM, Allen AA, et al. Magnetic resonance imaging of articular cartilage in the knee. An evaluation with use of fast-spin-echo imaging. J Bone Joint Surg Am 1998;80:1276–84.

6. Bredella MA, Tirman PF, Peterfy CG, et al. Accuracy of T2-weighted fast spin-echo MR imaging with fat saturation in detecting cartilage defects in the knee: comparison with arthroscopy in 130 patients. AJR Am J Roentgenol 1999;172: 1073–80.

7. Yoshioka H, Stevens K, Hargreaves BA, et al. Magnetic resonance imaging of articular cartilage of the knee: comparison between fat-suppressed three-dimensional SPGR imaging, fat-suppressed FSE imaging, and fat-suppressed three-dimensional DEFT imaging, and correlation with arthroscopy. J Magn Reson Imaging 2004;20:857–64.

8. Link TM, Majumdar S, Peterfy C, et al. High resolution MRI of small joints: impact of spatial resolution on diagnostic performance and SNR. Magn Reson Imaging 1998;16:147–55.

9. Eckstein F, Wirth W. Quantitative cartilage imaging in knee osteoarthritis. Arthritis 2011;2011:475684.

10. Mosher TJ, Dardzinski BJ. Cartilage MRI T2 relaxation time mapping: overview and applications. Semin Musculoskelet Radiol 2004;8:355–68.

11. Dardzinski BJ, Mosher TJ, Li S, et al. Spatial variation of T2 in human articular cartilage. Radiology 1997;205:546–50.

12. Bruno MA, Mosher TJ, Gold GE. Arthritis in color: advanced imaging of arthritis. Philadelphia: Saunders/Elsevier; 2009.

13. Waldschmidt JG, Rilling RJ, Kajdacsy-Balla AA, et al. In vitro and in vivo MR imaging of hyaline cartilage: zonal anatomy, imaging pitfalls, and pathologic conditions. Radiographics 1997;17:1387–402.

14. Yoshioka H, Stevens K, Genovese M, et al. Articular cartilage of knee: normal patterns at MR imaging that mimic disease in healthy subjects and patients with osteoarthritis. Radiology 2004;231:31–8.

15. Jeffery AK, Blunn GW, Archer CW, et al. Three-dimensional collagen architecture in bovine articular cartilage. J Bone Joint Surg Br 1991;73:795–801.

16. Goodwin DW, Wadghiri YZ, Zhu H, et al. Macroscopic structure of articular cartilage of the tibial plateau: influence of a characteristic matrix architecture on MRI appearance. AJR Am J Roentgenol 2004;182:311–8.

17. Goodwin DW, Dunn JF. High-resolution magnetic resonance imaging of articular cartilage: correlation with histology and pathology. Top Magn Reson Imaging 1998;9:337–47.

18. Goodwin DW, Zhu H, Dunn JF. In vitro MR imaging of hyaline cartilage: correlation with scanning electron microscopy. AJR Am J Roentgenol 2000;174:405–9.

19. Goodwin DW, Wadghiri YZ, Dunn JF. Micro-imaging of articular cartilage: T2, proton density, and the magic angle effect. Acad Radiol 1998;5:790–8.

20. Xia Y. Magic-angle effect in magnetic resonance imaging of articular cartilage: a review. Invest Radiol 2000;35:602–21.

21. Mosher TJ, Smith H, Dardzinski BJ, et al. MR imaging and T2 mapping of femoral cartilage: in vivo determination of the magic angle effect. AJR Am J Roentgenol 2001;177:665–9.

22. Ewers BJ, Jayaraman VM, Banglmaier RF, et al. Rate of blunt impact loading affects changes in retropatellar cartilage and underlying bone in the rabbit patella. J Biomech 2002;35:747–55.

23. Verzijl N, DeGroot J, Ben ZC, et al. Crosslinking by advanced glycation end products increases the stiffness of the collagen network in human articular cartilage: a possible mechanism through which age is a risk factor for osteoarthritis. Arthritis Rheum 2002;46:114–23.

24. Holderbaum D, Malvitz T, Ciesielski CJ, et al. A newly described hereditary cartilage debonding syndrome. Arthritis Rheum 2005;52:3300–4.

25. Hwang WS, Li B, Jin LH, et al. Collagen fibril structure of normal, aging, and osteoarthritic cartilage. J Pathol 1992;167:425–33.

26. Gebarski K, Hernandez RJ. Stage-I osteochondritis dissecans versus normal variants of ossification in the knee in children. Pediatr Radiol 2005;35:880–6.

27. Laor T, Zbojniewicz AM, Eismann EA, et al. Juvenile osteochondritis dissecans: is it a growth disturbance of the secondary physis of the epiphysis? AJR Am J Roentgenol 2012;199:1121–8.

28. Marlovits S, Singer P, Zeller P, et al. Magnetic resonance observation of cartilage repair tissue (MOCART) for the evaluation of autologous chondrocyte transplantation: determination of interobserver variability and correlation to clinical outcome after 2 years. Eur J Radiol 2006;57:16–23.

29. Goebel L, Orth P, Muller A, et al. Experimental scoring systems for macroscopic articular cartilage repair correlate with the MOCART score assessed by a high-field MRI at 9.4 T–comparative evaluation of five macroscopic scoring systems in a large animal cartilage defect model. Osteoarthritis Cartilage 2012;20: 1046–55.

30. Welsch GH, Zak L, Mamisch TC, et al. Three-dimensional magnetic resonance observation of cartilage repair tissue (MOCART) score assessed with an isotropic three-dimensional true fast imaging with steady-state precession sequence at 3.0 Tesla. Invest Radiol 2009;44:603–12.

31. White LM, Sussman MS, Hurtig M, et al. Cartilage T2 assessment: differentiation of normal hyaline cartilage and reparative tissue after arthroscopic cartilage repair in equine subjects. Radiology 2006;241:407–14.

MRI of the Knee with Arthroscopic Correlation

Justin W. Griffin, MD, Mark D. Miller, MD*

KEYWORDS

- Ligament injuries • ACL • MRI • Multiligamentous

KEY POINTS

- In the acute setting, the appearance of the disrupted anterior cruciate ligament (ACL) has been described as an edematous mass with increased T2-signal and abnormal morphology; ACL reconstruction can be accomplished using a variety of both autografts and allografts.
- Posterior cruciate ligament (PCL) injuries are often subtle with indirect signs, such as posterior displacement of the tibia in relation to the medial femoral condyle, pseudo-laxity of the ACL, and late affects of the PCL deficiency.
- T2-weighted magnetic resonance imaging is key in examining which structures have been damaged in the posterolateral corner on T2 imaging and arthroscopically manifests as a drive-through sign.
- The double anterior horn sign and double PCL sign represent what will be a bucket handle meniscus tear arthroscopically, which ideally undergoes repair.
- The presence of contrast completely surrounding an osteochondritis dissecans fragment indicates an unstable fragment when using magnetic resonance arthrography.

INTRODUCTION

The growth of arthroscopic knee surgery has been explosive with the knee being the first joint to be examined arthroscopically. Although knee arthroscopy had its roots in Japan and Europe, it became popular in the United States in the 1960s and significant progress has been made over the past 5 decades.[1]

Any candidate for knee arthroscopy should first have a complete history and physical examination. After a review of the appropriate imaging and a discussion with the patient, a thorough and systematic approach to knee arthroscopy should be performed and all compartments and structures should be probed carefully and evaluated before performing therapeutic maneuvers. Knee arthroscopy can be performed

---

Department of Orthopaedic Surgery, University of Virginia, 400 Ray C. Hunt Drive, Suite 300, P.O. Box 800159, Charlottesville, VA 22908, USA
* Corresponding author.
E-mail address: mdm3p@virginia.edu

Clin Sports Med 32 (2013) 507–523
http://dx.doi.org/10.1016/j.csm.2013.03.004
0278-5919/13/$ – see front matter © 2013 Elsevier Inc. All rights reserved.

sportsmed.theclinics.com

with a standard leg holder or a simple post for countertraction. Standard portals include the inferolateral and inferomedial portal. The inferolateral portal is the primary viewing portal for arthroscopy; however, additional portals can be used for viewing and instrumentation. Remarkable correlations can been drawn between what one sees on magnetic resonance imaging (MRI) and what the surgeon sees at the time of knee arthroscopy.

ACL INJURY

The classic mechanism of injury for an ACL tear is a noncontact pivoting injury resulting in immediate swelling after hearing a "pop." The patient is typically unable to return to play because of difficulty with pivoting and cutting. The key physical examination is the Lachman, performed in 20° to 30° of knee flexion. The pivot shift is also helpful, but the maneuver is sometimes difficult to perform in the clinic because of guarding by the patient.

Findings on MRI

The normal ACL is best evaluated in the sagittal imaging plane using a T2-weighted pulse sequence (**Fig. 1**); however, the axial and coronal imaging planes are also useful in the evaluation of the proximal and distal attachment sites, respectively. The ACL arises proximally along the medial aspect of the lateral femoral condyle and inserts distally onto the tibia adjacent to the anterior tibial spine and is composed of an anteromedial and posterolateral bundle. The knee is often imaged in full extension so the ACL should parallel the roof of the intercondylar notch but should touch the roof of the notch.

There are several direct MRI signs, which indicate a complete disruption of the ACL.[2] Discontinuity of the ACL fibers seen in any of the 3 imaging planes is evidence of a complete tear. In the acute setting, the appearance of the disrupted ACL has been described as an edematous mass with increased T2-signal and abnormal morphology

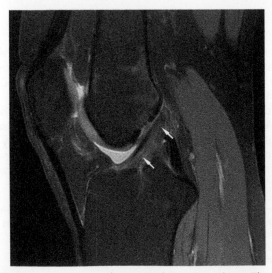

Fig. 1. Normal ACL, best depicted in the sagittal imaging plane. The fibers of the ACL (*arrows*) appear taut parallel the roof of the intercondylar notch, but should not touch the roof of the notch.

(**Fig. 2**). In the subacute setting, the discontinuous ACL fibers demonstrate a more linear fragmented appearance. The "empty notch" sign refers to an MR finding in which fluid signal rather than normal ACL fibers are seen at the proximal attachment site, usually best depicted on axial T2-weighted images. Finally, an avulsion fracture of the anterior tibial spine may be seen with a distal ACL injury, often in young patients (**Fig. 3**).

Indirect imaging signs may be seen with disruption of the ACL, including a large hemarthrosis.[3] A characteristic bone contusion pattern on the lateral femoral condyle and posterolateral tibial plateau occurs during pivot shift, resulting from a noncontact injury, and is often seen after an ACL disruption.[4] Other indirect signs of ACL disruption include the deep sulcus sign (irregular-appearing lateral femoral sulcus >2 mm in depth) and Segond fracture, which is a capsular avulsion injury fracture of the lateral tibial plateau (**Fig. 4**). The tibia may also translate in relation to the femur tipping off injury to the ACL.

Arthroscopic Findings

As a part of routine diagnostic arthrosocopy, the intact ACL is viewed and often appears with 2 distinct bundles (**Fig. 5**). When examined arthroscopically, the normal ACL has a diameter of approximately 11 mm and has broad insertions. Injury to the ACL will often result in an obvious "stump" of residual tissue, especially on the tibial side, which may need to be debrided to prevent impingement. ACL reconstruction can be accomplished using a variety of grafts, both autografts and allografts. Recently, an emphasis has been made on placing the graft in a more "anatomic" position, using either a single-bundle or a double-bundle technique. This involves placing

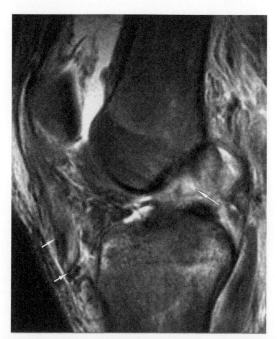

Fig. 2. Acute ACL disruption sagittal T2-weighted image shows an edematous mass appearance of the ACL with a complete disruption of the mid substance (*long arrow*). Also noted is a high-grade tear of the patellar tendon (*short arrows*).

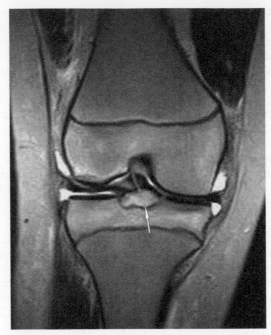

Fig. 3. Anterior tibial spine avulsion injury coronal T2-weighted image demonstrates an avulsion fracture (*long arrow*) of the anterior tibial spine at the distal attachment site of the ACL.

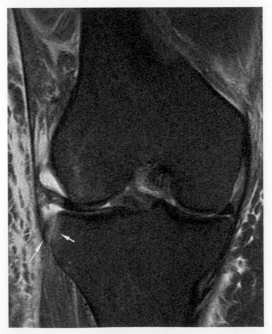

Fig. 4. Segond fracture (*long arrow*), which is an indirect signs of ACL injury, indicating an avulsion injury of the capsule along the peripheral aspect of the lateral tibial plateau with adjacent marrow edema (*short arrow*).

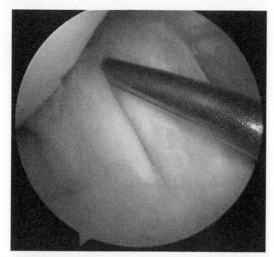

Fig. 5. Arthroscopic appearance of the normal ACL demonstrating the two bundles.

the graft in the center of the ACL footprint on both the tibia and the femur in a more horizontal and slightly more anterior position.[5] This can be accomplished with the use of an accessory medial portal for placement of the femoral tunnel.

PCL INJURY

After PCL injury, the history and examination findings are often more subtle. For PCL tears with associated multiple ligament injuries, the findings are not so subtle and usually involve a motor vehicle accident with posterior directed force on the tibia and potentially even frank dislocation. Certain tests can be performed in the office to allow for identification and characterization of PCL injuries. The posterior drawer test (done in 70°–90° of flexion) is the classic examination performed for a PCL deficient knee. Recent studies by Sekiya and colleagues[6] suggest a posterior drawer in excess of 12 mm is associated with combined posterolateral corner injuries in most cases. Stress radiographs are routinely used in the authors' office to quantify side-to-side differences in PCL injuries.

MRI Features

The posterior cruciate ligament (PCL) is typically about twice the thickness of the ACL and is best evaluated on MRI using the T2-weighted sagittal images. The PCL originates along the intercondylar portion of the medial femoral condyle and inserts distally on the slanted portion of the posterior tibia.[7] With the knee imaged in full extension, the PCL has an arcuate-shaped bandlike appearance of homogeneous low-signal intensity (**Fig. 6**).

The PCL is often injured as a result of a "dashboard" mechanism of injury (direct trauma to the anterior aspect of the tibia with the knee in flexion) and this injury may result in a bone contusion of the anterior aspect of the proximal tibia (**Fig. 7**).[4] The dashboard mechanism of injury places posteriorly directed forces on the proximal tibial, resulting in PCL injury. The PCL is more often partially torn when compared with the ACL and, while injury can occur anywhere along the course of the ligament, most injuries occur within the mid substance of the PCL. A partial thickness tear will appear as thickening and edema of the ligament, possibly with fluid signal extending

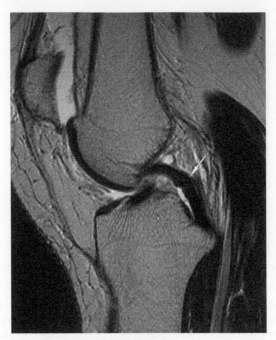

Fig. 6. Normal PCL on sagittal T2-weighted image.

partially through the substance of the ligament, but with visualized intact fibers.[8–10] A full-thickness tear will demonstrate a complete disruption with discontinuity of the fibers (**Fig. 8**). A "peel-off" injury refers to an avulsion injury at the femoral attachment of the PCL.

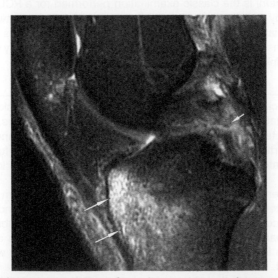

Fig. 7. "Dashboard" contusion pattern from direct trauma to the anterior aspect of the proximal tibia with the knee in flexion with bone contusion (*long arrows*).

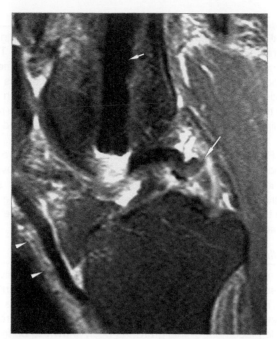

Fig. 8. Complete tear mid substance PCL (*long arrow*) with a lax-appearing PCL. An intrame-dullary rod (*short arrow*) has been placed within the femur with soft tissue contusion (*arrowheads*) along the anterior aspect of the lower leg.

Arthroscopic Findings

From an arthroscopic standpoint, Fanelli and colleagues[11] have described both direct and indirect signs for PCL disruption with direct signs, including a torn graft. However, more often than not, the findings are most subtle and usually involve indirect signs, such as posterior displacement of the tibia in relation to the medial femoral condyle, pseudo-laxity of the ACL, and late affects of the PCL deficiency, including chondrosis of the medial femoral condyle and patellofemoral joint. A high index of suspicion is needed to diagnose PCL rupture arthroscopically. Arthroscopic-aided reconstruction can be performed several different ways and remains controversial.

POSTEROLATERAL CORNER INJURY

Posterolateral corner (PLC) injuries are most often associated with combined ligament injuries (especially the PCL), but have been reported in isolated cases. Disruption of one or all of the PLC structures can result in rotational instability. These injuries clas-sically involve some rotational force. The essential structures in the posterolateral corner include the biceps tendon, the iliotibial band, the lateral collateral ligament, the popliteus and the popliteofibular ligament, and the posterolateral capsule. The dial test is the classic examination finding for posterolateral corner laxity demon-strating external rotation asymmetry. This test is performed at both 30° and 90° of knee flexion with a positive test being greater than 15° asymmetry or more and 30° and not 90° of knee flexion. In the authors' experience, this often represents a com-bined posterolateral corner and anterior cruciate ligament injury. Asymmetry at more than 15° at both 30° and 90° of knee flexion suggests a combined posterolateral corner and posterior cruciate ligament injury.

MRI Features

The posterolateral corner is anatomically complex with several distinct and separate anatomic structures, which are responsible for providing stability. These structures include the posterior capsule, arcuate ligament, popliteofibular ligament, popliteomeniscal fascicles, popliteus tendon, fibular collateral ligament, biceps femoris tendon, and the conjoined tendon (**Fig. 9**).[12] MRI is key in examining which structures have been damaged in the PLC. Injury to one or more of the structures can result in posterolateral pain, buckling into hyperextension during weight-bearing, and instability of the knee.

Following an MRI, the posterolateral corner structures are best evaluated using T2-weighted sequences and all 3 imaging planes are required to provide an accurate assessment of each of these individual structures. Each anatomic structure should be described individually when injury is present. A 3-point grading system is used to describe injury to each individual structure: grade I—strain; grade II—partial thickness tear; and grade III—complete disruption (**Fig. 10**).[13]

Arthroscopic Findings

Arthroscopic findings of a posterolateral corner injury include excessive opening of the lateral compartment. This has been described by LaPrade as the "arthroscopic drive-through sign."[13] Treatment of posterolateral corner injuries requires open treatment. This is best performed with primary repair supplemented by free graft augmentation (**Fig. 11**). Anatomic placement of this graft has been shown to be important in long-term results.[14] Multiple techniques have been described.

TRANSIENT PATELLA DISLOCATION/SUBLUXATION

Instability of the patella largely occurs in the lateral direction. The shearing force generated by this event sometimes results in an osteochondral injury to either the medial

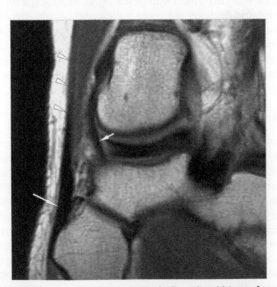

Fig. 9. Normal posterolateral corner structures including distal biceps femoris musculotendinous junction (*arrowheads*), conjoined tendon (*long arrow*), and popliteus tendon (*short arrow*).

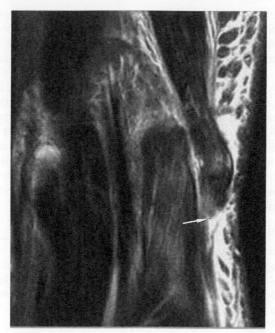

Fig. 10. Grade III complete tear of the MCL demonstrating a complete disruption of the MCL at the distal attachment site (*arrow*).

facet of the patella or the lateral femoral condyle, or both. It also often results in an injury to the medial patellofemoral ligament (MPFL). This important structure is the primary restraint to lateral translation of the patella.[15] There may be tenderness over its insertion. The key examination findings for an acute patella dislocation include an effusion and apprehension with lateral translation of the patella.

MRI Features

MRI evidence of a recent dislocation of the patella usually includes bone contusions of the anterior peripheral aspect of the lateral femoral condyle and of the inferior aspect

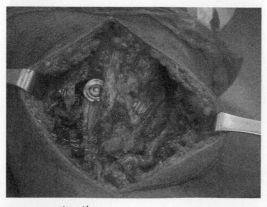

Fig. 11. MCL after open reconstruction.

of the medial patellar facet.[16,17] Osteochondral shearing or impaction-type injuries can occur along the mid to lower pole of the medial patellar facet of along the peripheral margin of the lateral femoral condyle (**Fig. 12**).[16] A large joint effusion usually presents and the MRI should be thoroughly evaluated for the presence of a loose intra-articular body.

The MPFL is the most important of the medial patellar stabilizers. Disruption of the MPFL most often occurs at the femoral attachment site near the adductor tubercle, but can also occur in the mid substance or at the patellar attachment site. Injuries are graded on a 3-point scale. Grade I is a sprain, seen as adjacent edema but with intact MPFL fibers. Grade II is a partial-thickness tear, seen on MRI as partial disruption of the MPFL fibers with adjacent soft tissue edema. Grade III is a full-thickness tear, seen as a complete disruption of the MPFL with retraction and laxity of the fibers, often associated with an adjacent hematoma, uplifting and displacement of the overlying vastus medialis obliquus muscle (**Fig. 13**).[17]

Arthroscopic Findings

Treatment of acute patellar dislocations is controversial. If there is an associated osteochondral fragment, many surgeons would recommend excision or repair of these fragments. Acute repair of the medial patellofemoral ligament is also controversial; however, success has been reported with treatment of these lesions, especially avulsions off the femoral side including loose body removal when indicated (**Fig. 14**). Current trends include reconstruction of the MPFL opening using hamstring autograft or other allograft.

MEDIAL COLLATERAL LIGAMENT INJURY

Medial collateral ligament injuries are common and are usually caused by a valgus force during activities such as soccer and football. The key examination finding is

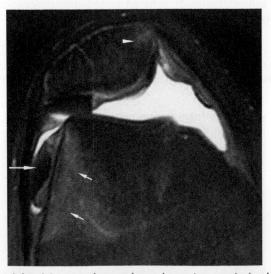

Fig. 12. Axial T2-weighted images show a large loose intra-articular body (*long arrow*) within the suprapatellar pouch. Bone contusions indicate prior transient dislocation of the patella with contusions of the lateral femoral condyle (*short arrows*) and medial patellar facet (*arrowhead*).

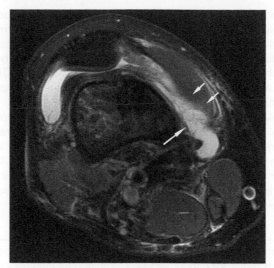

Fig. 13. Medial patellofemoral ligament (MPFL) disruption with axial image showing a complete disruption of the MPFL near the medial femoral condyle attachment site with a large adjacent hematoma (*long arrow*) and VMO displacement (*short arrows*).

opening with valgus stress in both 30° of flexion and full extension. Opening in 30° of flexion only suggests an isolated tear of the medial collateral ligament; however, opening in full extension connotes a combined injury to the medial collateral ligament and at least one of the cruciate ligaments.

MRI Features

The medial collateral ligament (MCL) is composed of a superficial and deep component. The superficial component originates on the adductor tubercle of the medial

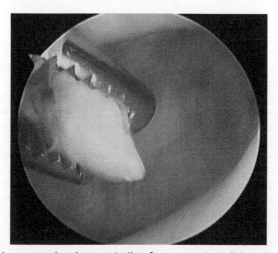

Fig. 14. Loose body removed arthroscopically after a transient dislocation of the patella.

femoral condyle and inserts distally on the tibia approximately 5 cm below the joint line just deep to the insertion of the pes anserine tendons. The ligament measures approximately 1.5 cm in anteroposterior diameter. The deep fibers attach to the medial capsule and medial meniscus. There is a tibial collateral ligament bursa, a potential space between the superficial and deep components of the MCL.[18] The normal MCL appears as a continuous low signal intensity bandlike structure located along the medial joint line.

Medial collateral ligament injuries occur as a result of valgus stress to the knee. Grade I injury is a sprain of the MCL and grade II injury represents a partial-thickness tear. Grade III represents a full-thickness disruption. MRI will show a complete discontinuity of the fibers with laxity and retraction of the torn ligament ends. A full-thickness tear may occur near the proximal or distal attachment site.[19] The term Pelligrini-Stieda refers to calcification or ossification within the substance of the MCL associated with an old injury.

Surgical Findings

Typically, treatment of medial collateral ligament injuries is nonoperative and involves the use of a hinged brace for 8 to 12 weeks. Combined injuries may require operative intervention to include multiple ligament reconstruction. Injuries of the tibial side are more ominous and may require surgery. This is because synovial fluid from the knee can escape and prevent healing of the tibial-sided lesions. A modified Bosworth reconstruction can supplement the repair. This involves the use of a semitendinosus, which is harvested with an open-ended tendon stripper, preserving the distal insertion. The free end of the tendon is looped over a screw on the medial epicondyle and fixed distally on the tibia.

BUCKET HANDLE TEAR OF THE MENISCUS

Some of the earliest arthroscopic surgeries were to address meniscal tears. This remains one of the most common diagnoses requiring arthroscopic surgery. Unfortunately, most of the tears are irreparable. The bucket handle tear is a notable exception. Meniscal tears are often caused by a twisting injury and can be associated with ACL tears. Physical examination may note loss of full extension, signifying a "locked" knee.

MRI Features

Given the common occurrence of meniscal injuries and corresponding knee arthroscopy, MRI has evolved into an accurate means of noninvasively detecting meniscal abnormalities before arthroscopy. With regard to detecting meniscal tear, MRI accuracy ranges between 90% and 95%. It is critical to assess the meniscus in both the sagittal and the coronal imaging planes. Low-sequence imaging T1-weighted imaging is most accurate for detecting meniscal tears, while abnormalities seen on T2-weighted images are very specific.[20]

The menisci are composed of fibrocartilage and therefore appear dark on all MR pulse sequences. On the sagittal images, the peripheral portion of the menisci has been described as demonstrating a "bow-tie" configuration, whereas more centrally, the meniscus demonstrates a triangular appearance tapering toward the free edge. The anterior and posterior horns of the lateral meniscus are nearly equivalent in size, whereas the posterior horn of the medial meniscus is nearly twice the size of the anterior horn.[21]

Direct signs of meniscal tear include unequivocal surfacing signal, missing meniscal tissue, and displaced meniscal fragment. There are several MRI signs that have been described with regard to the identification of a bucket handle tear of the menisci. The double PCL sign indicates a buckle handle tear of the medial meniscus displaced into the intercondylar notch (**Fig. 15**). The double anterior horn sign indicates a lateral meniscus bucket handle tear that has flipped into the anterior aspect of the lateral compartment of the knee. The absent "bow-tie" sign indicates that a meniscal fragment has been displaced and no longer sits in its normal anatomic position.[22–24]

Arthroscopic Findings

The classic arthroscopic appearance of a bucket handle meniscal tear includes displacement of the meniscal tear into the notch that blocks full extension and can give a false end point to Lachman examination. Treatment involves reduction of the meniscus preparation of the periphery by rasping and meniscal repair. Although new devices allow arthroscopic all-inside treatment, the classic repair technique is inside-out vertical mattress sutures.

MENISCUS TEAR WITH DISPLACED FRAGMENT
MRI Findings

Meniscal tears can have multiple other configurations with displaced fragments involving either the medial or the lateral meniscus. All meniscus tears should be probed to unveil any trapped unstable fragments (**Fig. 16**). Evaluating the gutters and sometimes the posterior capsular area can identify unstable meniscal flap fragments.[21,25] In the medial compartment, meniscal fragments are most commonly seen along the medial joint line with the fragments displaced into either the superior or the inferior recesses. The pattern is more variable in the lateral compartment of the knee.

Arthroscopic Findings

Arthroscopic partial meniscectomy is the most common procedure performed by orthopedic surgeons. Unfortunately, most of these tears are irreparable because

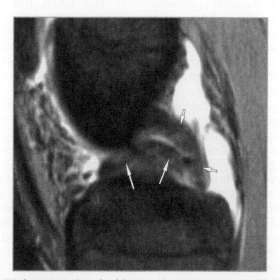

Fig. 15. Sagittal MRI demonstrating double PCL sign representing a bucket handle tear of the medial meniscus with the displaced fragment (*long arrows*) sitting just behind the native anterior horn (*short arrows*).

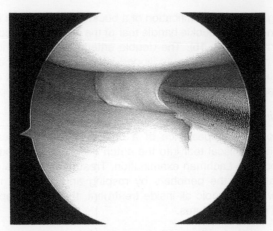

Fig. 16. Arthroscopic appearance of a displaced meniscal flap fragment.

they involve complex cleavage planes and avascular fragments in areas with poor blood supply of the meniscus. It is important to retain as much normal meniscus because the amount of meniscus removed is directly proportional to the arthrosis that can develop subsequently. Accessory posterior portals are often helpful to ensure a complete meniscectomy is accomplished with no residual fragments.

OSTEOCHONDRAL DEFECT
MRI Features

Osteochondritis dissecans (OCD) refers to a lesion of the articular cartilage and underlying bone typically occurring in adolescents or young adults. This lesion commonly occurs in the knee, although it also can occur in other locations including the capitellum. Lesions are described as juvenile OCD if the growth plates are still open or adult if the growth plates are closed. Open growth plates are the best prognostic sign in OCD. In the knee, OCD most often occurs in the lateral aspect of the medial femoral condyle. Management of OCD has evolved significantly and the treatment is largely based on MRI and arthroscopic appearance.

T2-weighted image with fat-saturation or proton density images with fat saturation are the best images for evaluating OCD lesions. The primary role of imaging is to detect the presence of an OCD lesion and to determine the stability of the fragment that will guide management regarding the need for surgical versus nonsurgical intervention. The MRI grading system uses a 4-point scale. Grade I lesions present with subchondral marrow edema with intact overlying cortex and articular cartilage. Grade II lesions present with partially detached osteochondral lesion and grade III lesions present with completely detached fragment in situ (**Fig. 17**). Grade IV lesions are completely detached and displaced. MRI signs indicating an unstable fragment include linear high T2 signal at the interface of the fragment and the underlying bone measuring more than 5 mm in length, the presence of a subchondral cystic change, and a focal chondral defect measuring greater than 5 mm in diameter. MR arthrography may improve specificity for detecting an unstable fragment. The presence of contrast completely surrounding the fragment indicates an unstable fragment when using MR arthrography.[26,27]

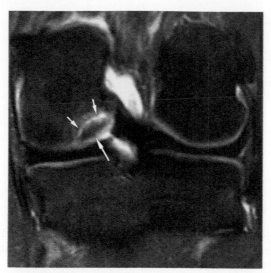

Fig. 17. OCD of the medial femoral condyle on coronal MRI. The fragment (*long arrow*) demonstrates undermining bright T2-signal (*short arrow*), representing fluid completely undermining the fragment and indicating an unstable fragment.

Arthroscopic Findings

After reviewing the MRI, arthroscopy can help characterize an OCD lesion more specifically. This review may help identify whether a cartilage lesion is a focal osteochondral defect caused by a shearing injury or an osteochondritis dissecans lesion, which typically occurs in the juvenile population and cause is unclear. Focal osteochondral lesions can be treated with a variety of techniques including microfracture (**Fig. 18**), osteoarticular transfer, and autologous chondral site implantation to name a few (**Fig. 19**). Osteochondritis dissecans is best treated with drilling or in situ repair and bone grafting if possible. For all cartilage lesions, it is appropriate to make sure the

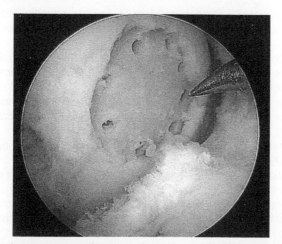

Fig. 18. Arthroscopic appearance after microfracture of a focal chondral defect within the medial femoral condyle.

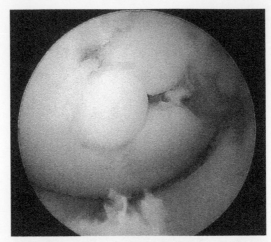

Fig. 19. Arthroscopic appearance after osteochondral plug transfer within a focal chondral defect of the medial femoral condyle.

mechanical axis is restored so that excessive force is not transmitted across the affected compartment.

REFERENCES

1. Ishibashi Y, Yamamoto Y. The history of arthroscopy. In: Miller MD, Cole BJ, editors. Textbook of arthroscopy. Philadelphia: Elsevier; 2004. p. 3–7.
2. Robertson PL, Schweitzer ME, Bartolozzi AR, et al. Anterior cruciate ligament tears: evaluation of multiple signs with MR imaging. Radiology 1994;193:829–34.
3. Tung GA, Davis LM, Wiggins ME, et al. Tears of the anterior cruciate ligament: primary and secondary signs at MR imaging. Radiology 1993;188:661–7.
4. Sanders TG, Medynski MA, Feller JF, et al. Bone contusion pattern of the knee at MR imaging: footprint of the mechanism of injury. Radiographics 2000;20: S135–51.
5. van Eck C, Lesniak BP, Schrieber VM, et al. Anatomic single- and double-bundle anterior cruciate ligament reconsturction flowchart. Arthroscopy 2010;26(2): 258–68.
6. Sekiya JK, Whiddon DR, Zehms CT, et al. A clinically relevant assessment of posterior cruciate ligament and posterolateral corner injuries. J Bone Joint Surg Am 2008;90(8):1621–7.
7. Gross ML, Grover JS, Bassett LW, et al. Magnetic resonance imaging of the posterior cruciate ligament: clinical use to improve diagnostic accuracy. Am J Sports Med 1992;20:732–7.
8. Grover JS, Bassett LW, Gross ML, et al. Posterior cruciate ligament: MR imaging. Radiology 1990;174:527–30.
9. Rodriquez W Jr, Vinson EN, Helms CA, et al. MR appearance of posterior cruciate ligament tears. AJR Am J Roentgenol 2008;191:1031.
10. Sonin AH, Fitzgerald SW, Hoff FL, et al. MR imaging of the posterior cruciate ligament: normal, abnormal and associated injury patterns. Radiographics 1995;15: 552–61.
11. Fanelli GC, Giannotti BF, Edson CJ. The posterior cruciate ligament: arthroscopic evaluation and treatment. Arthroscopy 1994;10:673–88.

12. Yu JS, Solomen DC, Hodler J, et al. Posterolateral aspect of the knee: improved MR imaging with a coronal oblique technique. Radiology 1996;198:199–204.
13. Vinson EN, Major NM, Helms CA. The posterolateral corner of the knee. AJR Am J Roentgenol 2008;190:449–58.
14. LaPrade RF. Arthroscopic evaluation of the lateral compartment of knees with grade 3 posterolateral knee complex injuries. Am J Sports Med 1997;25:596–602.
15. Sallay PI, Poggi J, Speer KP, et al. Acute dislocation of the patella: a correlative pathoanatomic study. Am J Sports Med 1996;24:52–60.
16. Sanders TG, Paruchuri NB, Zlatkin MB. MRI of osteochondral defects of the lateral femoral condyle: incidence and pattern of injury after transient lateral dislocation of the patella. AJR Am J Roentgenol 2006;187:1332–7.
17. Sanders TG, Morrison WB, Singleton BA, et al. Medial patellofemoral ligament injury following acute transient dislocation of the patella: MR findings with surgical correlation in 14 patients. J Comput Assist Tomogr 2001;25:957–62.
18. De Maeseneer M, Van Roy F, Lenchik L, et al. Three layers of the medial capsule and supporting structures of the knee: MR imaging-anatomic correlation. Radiographics 2000;20:S83–9.
19. Scheweitzer MS, Tran D, Deely DM, et al. Medial collateral ligament injuries: evaluation of multiple signs, prevalence and location of associated bone bruises, and assessment with MR imaging. Radiology 1995;194:825–9.
20. De Smet AA, Norris MA, Yandow DR, et al. MR diagnosis of meniscal tears of the knee: importance of high signal in the meniscus that extends to the surface. AJR Am J Roentgenol 1993;161:101–7.
21. Ruff C, Weingardt JP, Russ PD, et al. MR imaging patterns of displaced meniscus injuries of the knee. AJR Am J Roentgenol 1998;170:63–7.
22. Rangger C, Klestil T, Kathrein A, et al. Influence of magnetic resonance imaging on indications for arthroscopy of the knee. Clin Orthop 1996;330:133–42.
23. Wright DH, De Smet AA, Norris M. Bucket-handle tears of the medial and lateral menisci of the knee: value of MR imaging in detecting displaced fragments. AJR Am J Roentgenol 1995;165:621–5.
24. Magee TH, Hinso GW. MRI of meniscal bucket-handle tears. Skeletal Radiol 1998;27:495–9.
25. McKnight A, Southgate J, Price A, et al. Meniscal tears with displaced meniscal fragments: common patterns on magnetic resonance imaging. Skeletal Radiol 2009;39(3):279–83.
26. Mosher TJ. MRI of osteochondral injuries of the knee and ankle in the athlete. Clin Sports Med 2006;25:843–66.
27. De Smet AA, Ilahi OA, Graf BK. Reassessment of the MR criteria for stability of osteochondritis dissecans in the knee and ankle. Skeletal Radiol 1996;25:159–63.

Foot and Ankle Injuries in Sport
Imaging Correlation with Arthroscopic and Surgical Findings

Kenneth J. Hunt, MD[a],*, Michael Githens, MD[a],
Geoffrey M. Riley, MD[b], Michael Kim, MD[b], Garry E. Gold, MD[a,c,d]

KEYWORDS

- Ankle • Arthroscopy • Sports injuries • Magnetic resonance imaging • Impingement

KEY POINTS

- When using advanced imaging studies to evaluate an athlete with a foot or ankle injury, direct communication between the treating physician and radiologist regarding the clinical question can optimize information from the study.
- Correlation of radiographic findings with physical examination is crucial for appropriate clinical diagnosis and treatment decisions.
- Magnetic resonance imaging (MRI) is a highly sensitive and specific tool for the diagnosis of sports-related injuries, and can aid in decision making regarding treatment. For some injuries, MRI can facilitate minimally invasive surgical approaches.
- Arthroscopy is a safe and effective technique for the treatment of many sports-related injuries in the foot and ankle. Its use continues to expand, particularly in smaller joints and tendon injuries.
- A thorough knowledge of normal ankle and subtalar anatomy is critical in identifying and addressing pathologic structures and injuries.

INTRODUCTION

Injuries to the foot and ankle are common among both competitive and recreational athletes. In recent decades, surveillance programs have quantified the frequency and breadth of foot and ankle injuries in many sports and at various levels of

Funding Sources: None.
Conflict of Interest: None.
[a] Department of Orthopaedics, Stanford University, 450 Broadway Street, MC 6342, Redwood City, CA 94063, USA; [b] Department of Radiology, Stanford University, 300 Pasteur Drive, S0-56, Stanford, CA 94305, USA; [c] Department of Radiology, Stanford University, 1201 Welch Road, P271, Stanford, CA 94305, USA; [d] Department of Bioengineering, Stanford University, 1201 Welch Road, P271, Stanford, CA 94305, USA
* Corresponding author.
E-mail address: kjhunt@stanford.edu

competition.[1,2] Although many of these injuries can be managed conservatively, surgical intervention is often necessary to allow safe return to play and/or prevent long-term dysfunction. Fundamental to successful, efficient, and effective treatment of sports-related injuries is a thorough understanding and appropriate implementation of radiographic imaging. This article reviews current magnetic resonance imaging (MRI) techniques for the foot and ankle, the appearance of normal structures on MRI and arthroscopy, and several common injuries and chronic conditions that occur in athletes.

MRI TECHNIQUES FOR THE FOOT AND ANKLE

- MRI of the foot and ankle requires careful attention to detail for optimal results.
- Imaging at high field strength (1.5 T or 3 T) results in the best resolution and imaging quality.
- A dedicated foot and ankle radiofrequency coil is needed for an ideal signal.
- The foot and ankle should be positioned at the isocenter of the magnetic field to maximize the amount of signal obtained.
- Imaging of the foot and ankle typically consists of 3 planes using a variety of MR sequences:
  - Standard planes include transverse (axial), coronal, and sagittal.
  - Oblique variations of these can also be used to answer specific questions, such as imaging the calcaneofibular ligament.
  - Inclusion of water-sensitive sequences is critical, usually consisting of T2-weighted or proton density–weighted sequences with the application of fat suppression.
- A typical protocol may include the 3 standard planes of imaging with T1-weighted and T2-weighted images with fat suppression, and last between 30 and 45 minutes.

Fat Suppression

- Suppressing the signal from fat is necessary to highlight edema in the fatty marrow.
- Fat suppression also allows easy identification of soft-tissue edema, which in turn can indicate underlying tendon or ligament injury.
- Chemical fat suppression is usually added to a T2 or proton density weighting sequence to highlight fluid.
- However, in areas of significant magnetic-field inhomogeneity (eg, metal or at the distal end of the foot where conventional fat suppression may fail), it is often helpful to use short-tau inversion recovery (STIR) or fat-water separation (IDEAL) to reduce the fat signal.

Clinical Area of Interest

It is particularly important when ordering a foot and/or ankle MRI to indicate the specific clinical question, which is crucial in helping the radiologist develop the ideal protocol to address the anatomic area of interest.

- Specific sequences, planes, field of view, and the use of contrast are all variables that can be adjusted based on the clinical concern.
- If there is need to cover a large area (eg, to evaluate the entire Achilles tendon), a large field of view is used at the expense of anatomic detail.

- If there is need to cover a small anatomic area (ie, a plantar plate injury), a smaller field of view is preferred. While excluding other structures, it provides superior anatomic detail for the anatomic area of interest.
- The decision to use intravenous or intra-articular contrast may also be determined based on the clinical question.
  - If the concern is for a mass or complicated osteomyelitis, intravenous contrast may be beneficial.
  - Intra-articular contrast (MR arthrography) can be considered when conventional MRI has not sufficiently answered the clinical question, particularly with intra-articular abnormality (ie, subtle cartilage injury or loose-body formation).

MRI CORRELATIONS WITH ANATOMY: NORMAL ARTHROSCOPIC APPEARANCE
Anatomy of the Ankle Joint

Many structures in the ankle joint can be readily accessed via arthroscopic techniques. Ankle arthroscopy is routinely performed through the standard anterolateral and anteromedial portals,[3] which serve as both viewing and utility portals. Accessory anterolateral and anteromedial portals can be helpful in accessing gutters,[4] and posterior portals may help in visualizing and accessing posterior structures and abnormalities.[5]

- During any ankle arthroscopic procedure, is important to inspect the entire joint to ensure no injuries or abnormalities are missed.
  - Ferkel's 21-point examination[6] can be a useful, thorough checklist.
  - From the anterior viewing portals, the normal smooth rounded talar dome and concave tibial plafond can be visualized (**Fig. 1**).
  - All articular surfaces should have the uniform appearance of smooth and healthy hyaline cartilage. Articular surfaces should be thoroughly evaluated for chondromalacia, chondral injuries, and other disorders.[7]

Ligamentous Structures

- Viewed from the anteromedial portal, the intra-articular portion of the anterior inferior tibiofibular ligament (AITFL) should appear as a shiny white band running in a steep oblique fashion from the tibia inferiorly to the fibula (**Fig. 2**).

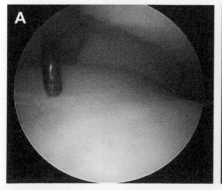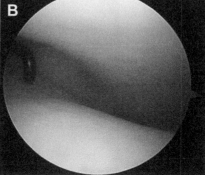

Fig. 1. Arthroscopic images illustrating normal talar dome viewed from the anteromedial (*A*) and anterolateral (*B*) portals.

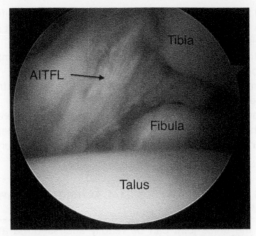

Fig. 2. Arthroscopic image showing that the anterior inferior tibiofibular ligament (AITFL) is visualized easily from the anteromedial portal (*arrow*).

- o The AITFL can be easily identified on T1-weighted axial MRI of the ankle (**Fig. 3**).
- o A more pronounced thickening of the distal fascicles of this ligament, as described by Bassett and colleagues,[8] can be a normal anatomic variant but may be the source of symptomatic impingement in some patients (**Fig. 4**).
- The intra-articular portion of the anterior talofibular ligament (ATFL) may be seen anterolaterally as well.

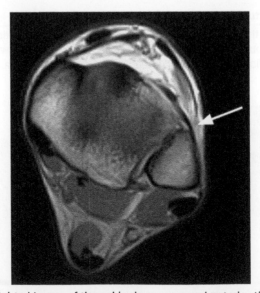

Fig. 3. Axial T1-weighted image of the ankle shows a normal anterior tibiofibular ligament (*arrow*).

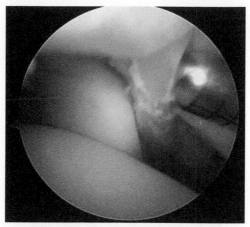

Fig. 4. Arthroscopic image illustrating the Bassett ligament as a thickened variant of the distal fascicles of the AITFL.

Medial and lateral gutters

- The medial and lateral gutters should both appear smooth with no loose bodies, and be free of excessive synovium (**Fig. 5**).
- Coronal MRI allows excellent visualization of the deep and superficial layers of the deltoid, and evaluation of the content of the gutters (**Fig. 6**).

Posterior Structures

The gutters can be followed posteriorly to visualize posterior structures.

- The posterior talofibular ligament (PTFL) can be visualized spanning between the posterior aspect of the fibula in a shallow oblique fashion to the posterolateral tubercle of the talus (**Fig. 7**A).
- The transverse tibiofibular ligament can also be evaluated here (see **Fig. 7**B).[7]
- Axial and coronal plane MRI afford the best views for assessing posterior ligamentous structures (**Figs. 8** and **9**).

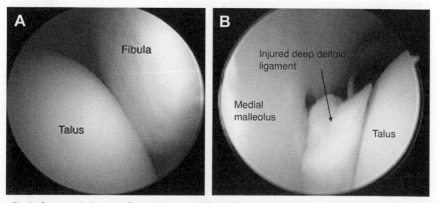

Fig. 5. Arthroscopic image showing normal lateral gutter (*A*), and medial gutter with abnormally thickened deep deltoid reflection consistent with deltoid ligament injury (*B*) (*arrow*).

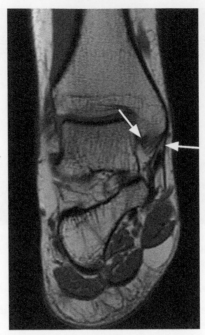

Fig. 6. Coronal proton density image of the ankle demonstrates the normal deep and superficial components of the deltoid ligament complex (between *arrows*). The lateral gutter can also be evaluated.

Syndesmosis

- The syndesmosis should be visualized and examined during arthroscopy (**Figs. 10** and **11**).
- The syndesmosis can have a normal gap no greater than 1 to 2 mm. Any widening greater than 2 mm is abnormal.

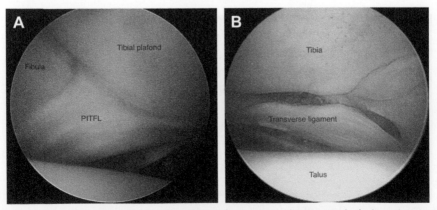

Fig. 7. (*A, B*) Arthroscopic images illustrating the posterior ligaments, including the posterior inferior tibiofibular ligament (PITFL) and transverse ligament.

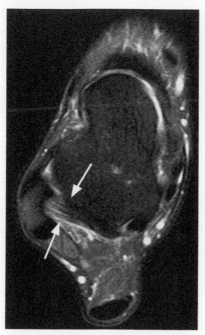

Fig. 8. Axial T2-weighted fat-suppressed image of the ankle showing a normal posterior talo-fibular ligament (between the *arrows*). This ligament often appears striated in its normal state.

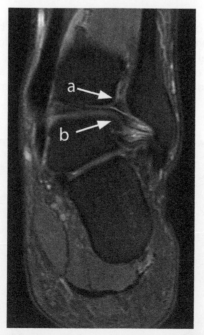

Fig. 9. Coronal T2-weighted image with fat suppression at the level of the posterior ankle shows the components of the posterior syndesmotic ligament complex, including the inferior aspect of the posterior inferior tibiofibular ligament (*arrow* a) and the inferior transverse ligament (*arrow* b).

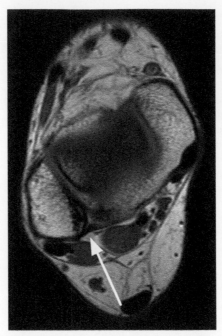

Fig. 10. Axial T1-weighted image of the ankle shows a normal posterior tibiofibular ligament (PTFL) (*arrow*).

- Dynamic instability can be evaluated during arthroscopy by manual manipulation or by advancing a probe or shaver into the syndesmosis to attempt to distract the fibula from the tibial incisura.[6]
- The talar neck and corresponding anterior tibia and the anterior capsular space can be evaluated for osteophytes, synovitis, or scar tissue, which can produce impingement.

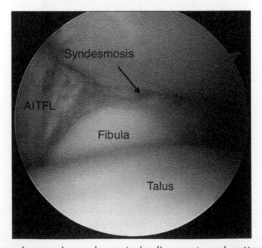

Fig. 11. Normal-appearing syndesmosis; posterior ligaments and gutter are apparent.

Anatomy of the Subtalar Joint

Arthroscopy of the subtalar joint is useful for the management of intra-articular abnormalities, and is an adjunct to assessing the quality of reduction in fracture treatment.

- The subtalar joint is made up of 3 articulations or facets: anterior, middle, and posterior.
- The posterior facet is separated from the others by the tarsal canal and the interosseous talocalcaneal ligament (**Fig. 12**).
- The posterior facet is easily visualized during standard subtalar arthroscopy, whereas the anterior and middle facets are more difficult to access and treat.[9]
- The primary viewing and working portals are all laterally based: anterior, middle, and posterolateral:
  - The anterior portal is the first established portal and is the primary viewing portal.
    - Anterior structures visualized include ligaments of the sinus tarsi, the anterior process of the calcaneus, and occasionally the anterior joint.
    - Viewing posteriorly, one can examine the articular surfaces of the posterior facet, the posterior pouch, and an os trigonum if present (**Fig. 13**).
    - Lateral structures to be evaluated include the lateral talocalcaneal and calcaneofibular ligaments.[9,10]
    - Viewing from the posterior portal allows better visualization of anterior structures, posteromedial and posterolateral gutters, the posterior pouch, and the flexor hallucis longus (FHL) tendon.
- The primary indications for subtalar arthroscopy include symptomatic os trigonum, posterior impingement, chondromalacia, subtalar impingement lesions, osteophytes, posttraumatic arthrofibrosis, synovectomy, and removal of loose bodies.

Anatomy of the First Metatarsophalangeal Joint

As is the case with many small joints in the body, arthroscopy of the first metatarsophalangeal (MTP) joint has increased in recent years.

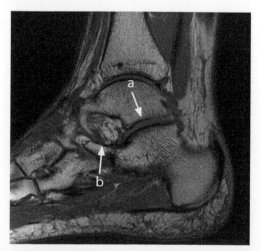

Fig. 12. Sagittal T1-weighted image of the ankle shows the posterior subtalar facet (*arrow* a) and the sinus tarsi anteriorly (b *arrow*).

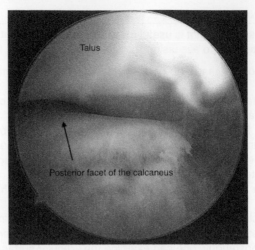

Fig. 13. Arthroscopic image of a normal subtalar joint posterior facet viewed from the anterolateral portal; the posterior facet of the calcaneus is well visualized (*arrow*).

- Commonly accepted indications include low-grade hallux rigidus, focal chondral defects, loose bodies, synovitis, and sesamoid abnormalities.[11,12]
- First MTP joint arthroscopy is performed through the standard dorsolateral and dorsomedial portal, with manual longitudinal distraction applied to enhance visualization and working space.[11]
- Readily visible structures include:
  - First metatarsal head and intracapsular portion of the metatarsal neck
  - Proximal phalangeal base
  - Tibial and fibular sesamoids and plantar plate (**Fig. 14**)
- The integrity of the plantar plate and articular surfaces can be assessed with a probe.

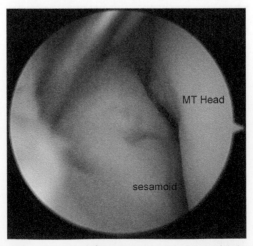

Fig. 14. Arthroscopic view of normal first metatarsophalangeal joint anatomy as viewed from the dorsomedial portal. MT, metatarsal.

- Osteochondral lesions of the metatarsal (MT) head, degenerative changes of MT and sesamoid cartilage, impinging synovium, and plantar plate injuries can be accessed arthroscopically.
- Dorsal osteophytes (hallux rigidus) and inflamed synovium can be removed.[13,14]

SPORTS INJURIES IN THE FOOT AND ANKLE
Injuries to the Ankle Joint

Osteochondral lesions of the talus

Osteochondral lesions of the talus (OLT) are most often located on the posteromedial aspect (typically deep, cup shaped) or anterolateral shoulder (more superficial, thin wafer-like) of the talar dome. A history of ankle trauma is noted in 61% of patients with medial lesions and 93% in those with lesions of the lateral talus.[15] Although not all OLTs are symptomatic,[16] painful OLTs commonly require surgical treatment because of a high failure rate with nonoperative management.[17] Given the current lack of well-controlled studies on the treatment of OLTs, bone marrow stimulation (BMS) via arthroscopic debridement, curettage, and microfracture is generally considered the best initial treatment.[17] There are many considerations during the treatment of OLTs:

- OLTs can be highly variable in appearance depending in part on etiology and acuity.[18]
- In nontraumatic or chronic OLTs, etiology may include morphologic, genetic, metabolic, vascular, endocrine, and degenerative factors.[19]
- OLTs can have subtle appearance and may present with:
  - Chondral flap, which may be stable or unstable
  - Discoloration of cartilage, indicating delamination
  - Delamination, which may only be noted after probing an area of soft ballotable cartilage (**Fig. 15**)[18]
- Underlying bone may have cystic changes (**Fig. 16**).
- Corresponding kissing lesions involving the tibial plafond are often noted in traumatic OLTs.
- Chronic lesions typically have partial or full thickness cartilage loss with associated loose chondral fragments in the joint and sclerotic subchondral bone (**Fig. 17**).[18,20]

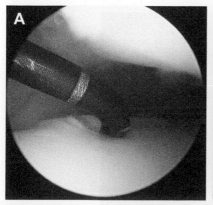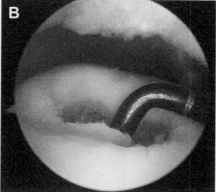

Fig. 15. Arthroscopic images illustrating soft ballotable articular cartilage indicating an osteochondral lesion of the talus (OLT), before (A) and after (B) curettage in preparation for microfracture.

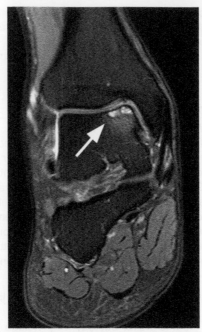

Fig. 16. Coronal proton density–weighted fat-suppressed image of the ankle demonstrates subchondral cystic change with adjacent bone marrow edema compatible with a talar dome osteochondral defect (*arrow*).

- Outcomes are superior for lesions smaller than 10 mm in diameter,[21] which corresponds with the threshold size for deviation in joint stresses.[22]
- OLTs treated with BMS techniques typically heal with smooth fibrocartilage, which improves pain and mechanical symptoms and is able to withstand physiologic loading and fluid ingress (**Figs. 18** and **19**).

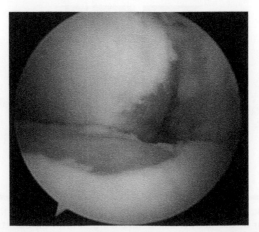

Fig. 17. Arthroscopic image demonstrating exposed sclerotic subchondral bone of an OLT.

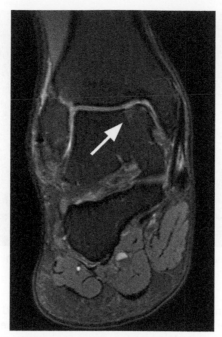

Fig. 18. Coronal proton density–weighted fat-suppressed image obtained 1 year after microfracture, demonstrating resolution of the subchondral cystic change with minimal residual bone marrow edema (*arrow*).

Synovitis

- Inflammation of the synovial lining of the ankle joint has many causes.
- Synovitis appears red and injected, and large fronds develop as it hypertrophies (**Fig. 20**).
  - These fronds may then become entrapped in the joint (**Fig. 21**), and joint motion, which compresses the irritated tissue, becomes very painful.[7]

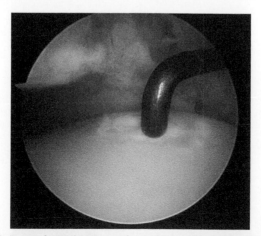

Fig. 19. Arthroscopic image from that anterolateral portal illustrating the presence of stable fibrocartilage, indicating healing of a talar osteochondral defect 1 year after microfracture.

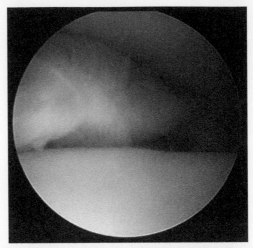

Fig. 20. Arthroscopic image demonstrating inflamed synovium in the anterior tibiotalar articulation.

- Findings on MRI may be subtle, but in cases of advanced inflammation heterogeneous, irregular increased signal intensity may be present (**Fig. 22**).
- Synovitis is very commonly seen alone or in conjunction with ankle instability,[23] OLTs, or other intra-articular abnormalities.

Loose bodies

Loose bodies in the ankle joint are a frequent cause of pain and mechanical symptoms. Because these lesions can result in damage to the articular surface and, ultimately, posttraumatic arthritis, it is generally accepted that symptomatic or loose bodies or fragments be removed arthroscopically. Loose bodies are often the result of a traumatic injury or ankle instability, although they can also result from synovial chondromatosis, osteochondromatosis, and degenerative arthritis. For patients undergoing removal of a loose body from the ankle, there are several important considerations:

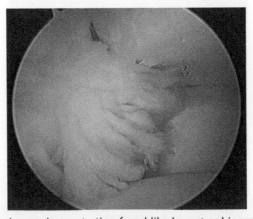

Fig. 21. Arthroscopic image demonstrating frond-like hypertrophic synovium.

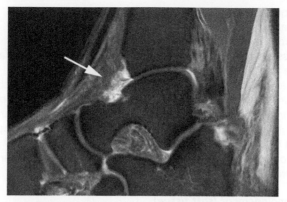

Fig. 22. Sagittal proton density–weighted fat-suppressed image of the ankle demonstrates a small tibiotalar joint effusion anteriorly with heterogeneous irregular signal intensity, compatible with synovitis (*arrow*).

- MRI and computed tomography can help assess the location and nature of loose bodies (**Fig. 23**).
- During arthroscopy, thorough assessment of all gutters and recesses, including the posterior gutter and syndesmosis, is important in ensuring no loose bodies are missed.

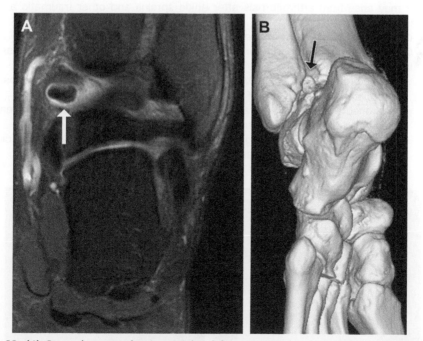

Fig. 23. (*A*) Coronal proton density–weighted fat-suppressed image of the ankle demonstrates a 10-mm ovoid hypointense lesion in the posteromedial tibiotalar joint (*arrow*). (*B*) Three-dimensional reformatted computed tomography image of the ankle demonstrates a loose body in the distal tibiofibular joint (*arrow*).

○ Use the posterolateral portal for access.
○ Inspect synovial lining, as some fragments may be adherent.
○ Use fluoroscopy as needed to locate loose bodies.
- Dynamic assessment of the ankle by passive dorsiflexion and plantarflexion can help to free loose bodies from gutters and recesses.
- Inspect for a donor site, which may or may not be readily identifiable. If needed, a microfracture of the donor site can be performed in the same setting.
  ○ In acute traumatic cases, the loose body may be a well-demarcated chondral or osteochondral fragment with a clear donor site. In these cases, repair the fragment to its origin when possible.
  ○ In chronic cases the loose bodies are typically well rounded and smooth, and are generally easy to remove arthroscopically (**Fig. 24**).[7]

Anterior ankle impingement (soft tissue)

Anterior ankle pain can occur from impingement of the ankle joint by a soft-tissue formation at the anterior aspect of the distal tibia and talar neck (**Fig. 25**). This condition can result from direct trauma (impaction force) or repetitive ankle dorsiflexion and plantarflexion (producing both impaction and traction forces). The anterolateral aspect of the ankle is a common location for impinging soft tissue after an ATFL tear caused by scarring (**Fig. 26**).[8,24,25]

- Anterior soft-tissue ankle impingement is commonly seen in jumping and kicking athletes.
- Symptoms include chronic ankle pain, swelling, and limitation of ankle dorsiflexion.
- It may arise from arthrofibrosis after ankle sprains and other traumatic ankle injuries.
- It may occur from scar formation after surgical intervention.[24]
- Conventional MRI can demonstrate the location and extent of soft-tissue impingement lesions.
  ○ T1 and proton density axial MRI are the most useful sequences in diagnosing anterolateral impingement of the ankle.
  ○ Thickened synovium in the anterior or anterolateral ankle joint is frequently associated with soft-tissue impingement (see **Fig. 25**).
  ○ MR arthrography has very high sensitivity (96%), specificity (100%), and accuracy (100%) in the assessment of soft-tissue impingement.[26]

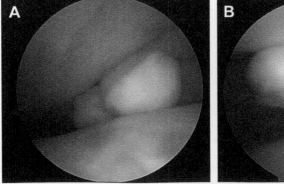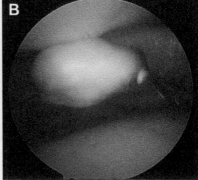

Fig. 24. (*A*, *B*) Arthroscopic images illustrating osteochondral loose bodies in the ankle joint.

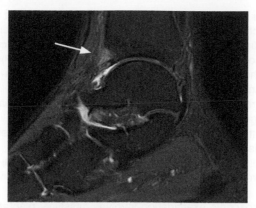

Fig. 25. Proton density–weighted fat-suppressed image of the ankle demonstrates ill-defined soft-tissue edema and scar tissue anterior to the tibial talar joint (*arrow*).

- Synovitis or scar tissue will impinge with dorsiflexion on dynamic examination.
- Bassett ligament, the distal AITFL fascicles, is a normal anatomic structure, but may thicken and cause symptomatic impingement in some patients (see **Fig. 4**).[8]
- Arthroscopic removal of impinging soft-tissue structures has demonstrated good results in more than 90% of patients.[27]

Anterior ankle impingement (bony)

Anterior bony impingement of the ankle results from osteophytes impinging tissue between the anterior rim of the tibia and the neck of the talus. This condition may be related to chronic ankle instability, a forceful dorsiflexion injury of the ankle joint, or repetitive force resulting in impaction or traction-related microtrauma of the anterior margin of the tibiotalar joint. Over time, the body's attempt to repair this microtrauma can lead to formation of osteophytes that may cause contact between opposing bone or entrap capsule or other soft tissue. Osteophytes often increase in size and may eventually break off into the joint, forming a loose body.

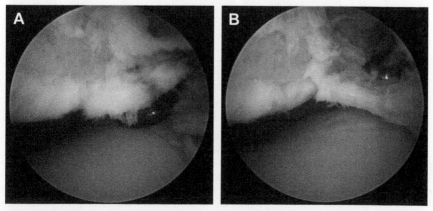

Fig. 26. (*A, B*) Arthroscopic images demonstrating scar tissue and inflamed synovium in the anterolateral tibiotalar space leading to soft-tissue impingement and anterior ankle pain.

- Tibial and talar osteophytes are usually located within the joint and away from the capsular attachment.
- Both plain radiography and conventional MR imaging can accurately detect and localize anterior osteophytes and associated lesions (**Fig. 27**).
  - MRI is also helpful in differentiating extra-articular from intra-articular causes of ankle impingement.
  - MR arthrography does not provide much additional information in diagnosing bony impingement.[28]
- The typical arthroscopic features of bony anterior impingement are:
  - Anterior tibial osteophyte (**Fig. 28**)
  - Corresponding dorsal talar neck/body osteophyte (**Fig. 29**)
  - May be more subtle with loss of normal talar neck sulcus or cam impingement lesion[29]
- Dynamic arthroscopic examination involves passively plantarflexing and dorsiflexing the ankle joint without joint distraction, allowing direct visualization of impingement (see **Fig. 29**).[30]

Lateral ankle ligaments

The ATFL and calcaneofibular ligament (CFL) are the primary ligamentous stabilizers of the lateral ankle. The ATFL can often be identified on arthroscopy.[31] The ATFL and CFL are typically disrupted with an inversion injury while the foot is in a plantarflexed position, resulting in varying degrees of injury to one or both ligaments.[32] Chronic instability can result in the need for surgical repair.

- Because of the high incidence of intra-articular injury with ankle instability,[23] arthroscopy can be a useful adjunct to ligament reconstruction techniques.
- An ATFL injury can often be identified on arthroscopy (**Fig. 30**).
  - An acutely torn ATFL will appear as injected, frayed ligament.

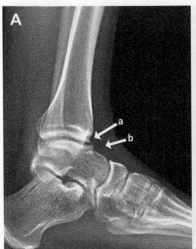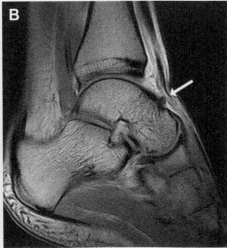

Fig. 27. (*A*) Lateral radiograph of the ankle demonstrates a 4-mm bony prominence of the talus at the tibiotalar joint anteriorly (*arrow* a). There is also a smaller bony prominence of the tibia at the tibiotalar joint anteriorly (*arrow* b). (*B*) Sagittal T1-weighted image of the ankle demonstrates a corresponding hypointense bony prominence along the dorsal aspect of the anterior talus, which likely results in anterior impingement of the ankle during dorsiflexion (*arrow*).

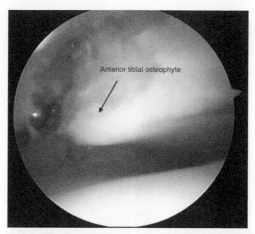

Fig. 28. Arthroscopic image demonstrating an anterior tibial osteophyte (*arrow*).

- ○ A chronic tear, as seen in chronic ankle instability, will resemble a mass of thickened, retracted scar tissue in the anterolateral region inferior to the AITFL.[31]
- ATFL injuries can be easily identified on MRI as well (**Fig. 31**).
- Arthroscopic-assisted ATFL repair has been described, with mixed results.[33]

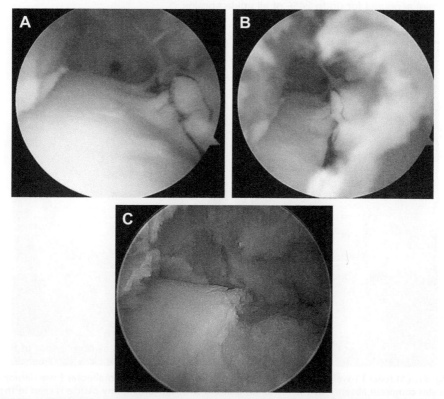

Fig. 29. Arthroscopic image illustrating a dynamic examination after resection of the anterior tibial osteophyte (*A, B*), after resection of the talar osteophyte (*C*).

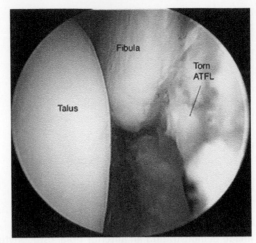

Fig. 30. Arthroscopic image demonstrating an anterior talofibular ligament (ATFL) tear, with avulsion of the ligament off of its fibular origin (*arrow*).

Syndesmosis injury

Syndesmosis injuries are typically associated with an ankle fracture, but may be an isolated ligamentous injury. Isolated syndesmosis ligamentous injury (ie, high ankle sprain) accounts for up to 24% of all ankle sprains.[34]

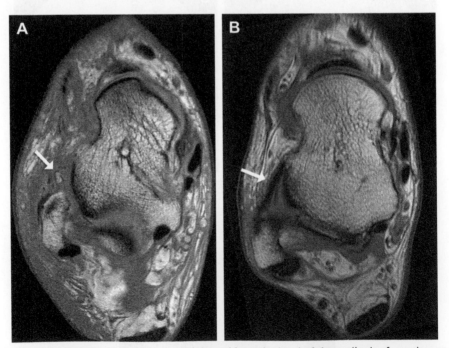

Fig. 31. (*A*) Axial T1-weighted image of the ankle at the level of the malleolar fossa demonstrates complete absence of the ATFL, compatible with rupture. A tiny ossicle is seen in the ligament space, suggestive of bony avulsion (*arrow*). (*B*) Axial T1-weighted image of the ankle at the level of the malleolar fossa demonstrates a normal, intact ATFL (*arrow*).

- Diagnosis may be made clinically and with stress radiographs, although syndesmotic injuries are frequently missed.
- Dynamic fluoroscopic and arthroscopic examination allows for direct visualization of syndesmotic instability.[35]
- MRI can be useful in diagnosing syndesmosis injury (**Fig. 32**), but arthroscopy is the most sensitive and accurate means of diagnosis.[36]
- Arthroscopic evaluation of an unstable syndesmosis demonstrates diastasis between the tibia and fibula.
  - In chronic syndesmosis instability, the syndesmosis is easily accessible.
  - The diagnosis can be confirmed by advancing the 3-mm transverse end of a probe into the syndesmosis and rotating it around its longitudinal axis (**Fig. 33**).
- Partial or complete tearing of the posterior inferior tibiofibular ligament may also be noted on both MRI and arthroscopy.[35]
- Evaluation of injury associated with anterior and posterior ligaments should be included.

Injuries Involving the Posterior Ankle and Subtalar Joint

Posterior impingement (Stieda process and os trigonum)

- The posterolateral and posteromedial portals allow excellent visualization of retrocalcaneal space, posterior tibiotalar joint, and the FHL tendon.
- The Stieda process is an elongation of the posterior process of the talus. Though considered a normal anatomic variant, it may be responsible for posterior impingement symptoms (**Figs. 34** and **35**).[37]
- An os trigonum is an accessory bone found posterior to the talus, and can be found in 3% to 14% of asymptomatic patients.

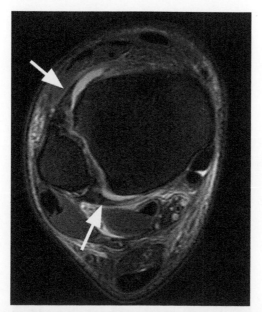

Fig. 32. Axial T2-weighted fat-suppressed image of the ankle at the level of the distal tibial fibular syndesmosis shows detachment of the anterior and posterior tibiofibular ligaments, compatible with syndesmosis disruption (*arrows*).

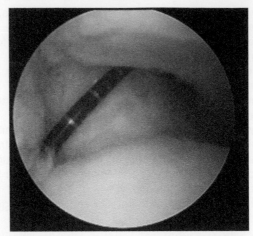

Fig. 33. During arthroscopic evaluation of the syndesmosis a probe is easily passed into the incisura, indicating syndesmosis diastasis. Rotating the 3-mm end of the probe within the syndesmosis confirms instability.

- It is thought to be a nonunited portion of the lateral tubercle of the talus.
- It is typically seen clearly both on lateral foot radiograph and sagittal MRI (**Fig. 36**).
- In some patients, an os trigonum can create impingement of the posterior capsular tissues and tenosynovitis of the FHL.[38]
- Although data are limited, arthroscopic removal of symptomatic os trigonum has reported success rates of up to 100% (**Fig. 37**).[27]

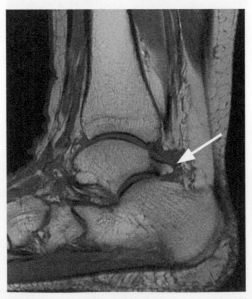

Fig. 34. Sagittal T1-weighted image of the ankle shows an elongated lateral tubercle of the talus, also known as a Stieda process (*arrow*).

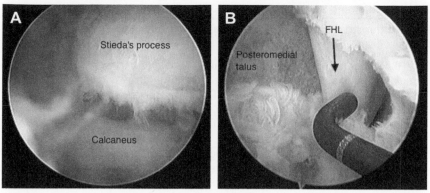

Fig. 35. (*A*) Stieda process of the talus causing posterior impingement. After arthroscopic resection of a Stieda process and debridement of synovium, the flexor hallucis longus (FHL) tendon can be visualized and assessed for tenosynovitis. This FHL tendon appears healthy (*B*).

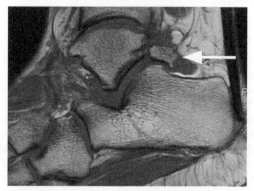

Fig. 36. Sagittal T1-weighted image of the ankle shows an ossicle posterior to the talus compatible with an os trigonum (*arrow*).

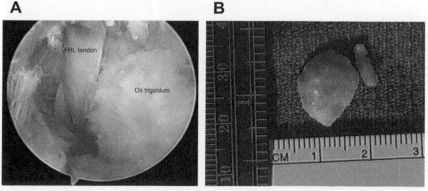

Fig. 37. (*A*) Arthroscopic image of an os trigonum viewed from the posteromedial portal. (*B*) After removal.

Hallux MTP Joint and Sesamoids

Although arthroscopic techniques for the hallux MTP joint are relatively new,[14] several indications exist.

- MRI can be useful for evaluation of the MTP joint complex, including the sesamoids, cartilage surfaces, and plantar plate (**Fig. 38**).
- Arthroscopic evaluation of the first MTP joint affords excellent visualization of the MT head, fibular and tibial sesamoids, and proximal phalangeal base.[14]
- Loose bodies, small dorsal osteophytes, small cartilage injuries, and synovitis can be addressed arthroscopically.
- A probe can be used to assess the integrity of the plantar plate with respect to the sesamoids (**Fig. 39**). Separation of the soft tissue from the sesamoid is consistent with a plantar plate injury.

Tendon Injuries

Although endoscopic treatment of tendon injuries has been described, these injuries remain most commonly treated by open means. Common injuries include Achilles tendinopathy, Achilles rupture, peroneal tendon tears, and FHL tenosynovitis or rupture.

Insertional Achilles tendinopathy and Haglund deformity

- Insertional Achilles tendinopathy is typically associated with a Haglund deformity, and usually involves some degree of retrocalcaneal bursitis.
  - It is most commonly seen in running athletes and those involved in hill running and interval training.[39]
- Clinically, complaints include pain at the bone-tendon interface and retrocalcaneal space, limited dorsiflexion, and thickening of the Achilles insertion.[40]
- Imaging, including plain radiography and MRI, are useful in defining the extent of tendon involvement and the degree of calcification present (**Fig. 40**).
- If conservative therapy fails, surgical treatment is recommended.

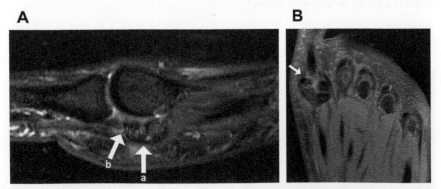

Fig. 38. (*A*) Sagittal short-tau inversion recovery (STIR) image of the first metatarsophalangeal joint demonstrates bone marrow edema and cystic change in a bipartite medial sesamoid bone, compatible with sesamoiditis (*arrow* a). There is also increased signal intensity along the anterior aspect of the sesamoid bone, consistent with a partial plantar plate tear (*arrow* b). (*B*) Coronal fat-suppressed proton density image shows partial disruption of the partial plantar plate tear (*arrow*).

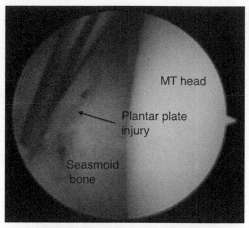

Fig. 39. An arthroscopic view of a plantar plate injury in a collegiate tennis player (*arrow*).

- ○ Surgery generally includes resection of the Haglund deformity, debridement of the inflamed retrocalcaneal bursa, debridement of diseased Achilles tendon, and repair of the tendon to calcaneus, often with suture anchors (**Fig. 41**).
- ○ Grossly, Achilles tendinosis has a classic "crab-meat" appearance, and is usually easily distinguished from the white, shiny longitudinal collagen fibers of healthy tendon.
- ○ Calcifications within the tendon may be encountered and should be debrided.

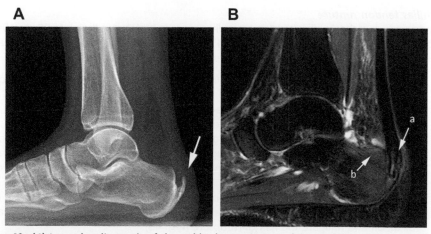

Fig. 40. (*A*) Lateral radiograph of the ankle demonstrates a large Achilles calcaneal enthesophyte with tiny calcific densities along the course of the Achilles tendon insertion (*arrow*). (*B*) Sagittal T2-weighted image of the ankle demonstrates diffuse thickening of the Achilles tendon at its insertion on the calcaneus with areas of linear increased signal intensity (*arrow* a), compatible with moderate tendinopathy and interstitial tearing. There is also calcaneal enthesopathy and bone marrow edema as well as a small retrocalcaneal bursitis (*arrow* b), compatible with Haglund syndrome.

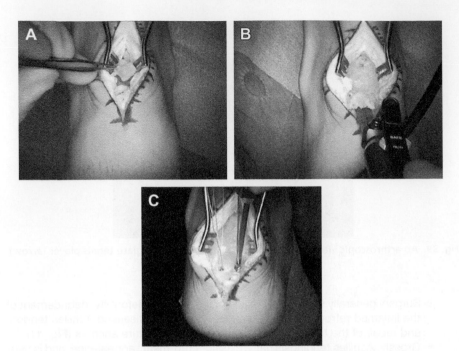

Fig. 41. Removal of retrocalcaneal fibrosis (*A*), removal of the Haglund deformity (*B*), and tendon repair with suture anchors (*C*).

- In less active individuals older than 50 years, the repair can be augmented with an FHL tendon transfer.[41]
  - FHL transfer is not recommended for young athletes.

Achilles tendon rupture

Acute rupture of the Achilles tendon typically occurs in athletes in their late 20s to 40s, most commonly at the watershed region 4 to 6 cm above its insertion on the calcaneus. Tear patterns are variable, and the rupture may be partial or complete.

- In a partial rupture there is significant intersubstance disruption with redundancy of fibers at the level of the tear.
- In complete and chronic ruptures the proximal segment may retract, making it initially difficult to identify without careful clinical evaluation or imaging.
- Physical examination findings are generally sufficient to diagnose Achilles rupture with high accuracy,[42] although MRI can be helpful in confirming the extent and location of injury, thus minimizing the surgical incision and extent of soft-tissue dissection (**Fig. 42**).
- Although nonoperative management can be successful for Achilles rupture, it is generally accepted that athletes undergo surgical treatment to accelerate rehabilitation and mitigate the risk of rerupture (**Fig. 43**).[43]
- Endoscopic techniques have been described,[44] but are not yet widely adopted in the athlete population.

Peroneal tendon tears

- Longitudinal split tears of the peroneus brevis or longus are associated with ankle sprains, chronic ankle instability, and varus hindfoot.

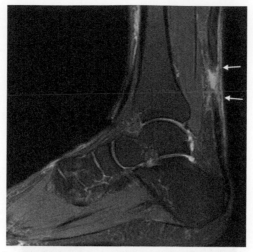

Fig. 42. Sagittal T2 fat-suppressed image of the ankle shows a complete rupture of the Achilles tendon with a gap outlined by the arrows.

- MRI can confirm the diagnosis of peroneal tendon abnormality (**Fig. 44**).
- Peroneal tears are easily visualized during surgery (**Fig. 45**).
  - Tears may be repaired if possible (**Fig. 46**), or debrided if the split is small or the tendon substance is of poor quality.
  - Tenosynovitis, presenting as hypertrophic injected-appearing synovium within the sheath, should also be debrided.[45]

Flexor hallucis longus rupture

Though an uncommon occurrence, the FHL tendon may be ruptured or lacerated. Physical examination is important in determining complete versus partial rupture and whether there is an associated injury of the flexor hallucis brevis tendon.

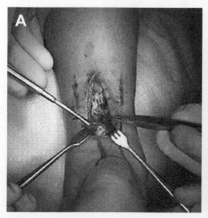
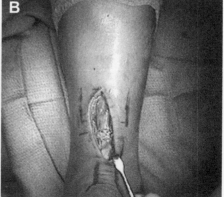

Fig. 43. Acute Achilles tendon rupture with identification of proximal and distal ends (*A*), and after primary end-to-end repair (*B*).

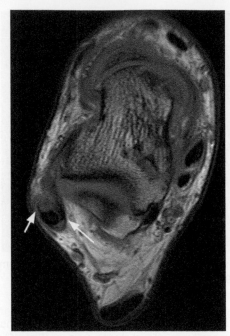

Fig. 44. Axial T1-weighted image of the ankle shows a longitudinal split of the peroneus brevis tendon with 2 fragments on either side of the intact peroneal longus tendon (*arrow*).

- FHL rupture occurs at various anatomic locations, including posterior to the talus and at the knot of Henry. FHL is vulnerable to rupture or laceration as it traverses the medial plantar foot.
- Rupture is uncommon in healthy young athletes. The most common mechanism of rupture is direct trauma.[46]

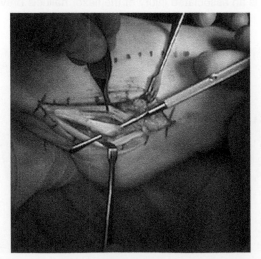

Fig. 45. A longitudinal split tear in the peroneus brevis tendon; note also the abnormal marked thickening of the tendon.

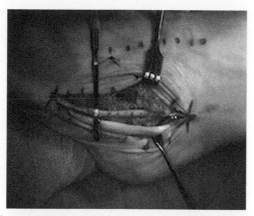

Fig. 46. After debridement and repair of the peroneus brevis tendon.

- MRI can confirm the diagnosis and rule out other tissue injuries (**Fig. 47**).
  - MRI can help determine the size and location of the surgical incision to minimize soft-tissue dissection.
- Decision for surgical repair depends on patient age, location and chronicity, deficits on physical examination, and functional status of the patient.
- Repair is recommended in sprinting and jumping athletes (**Fig. 48**).

Cysts and soft-tissue masses

The majority of soft-tissue masses in the foot and ankle are benign neoplasms and tumor-like lesions. Malignant tumors are rare, but can occur. To avoid misdiagnosis, particularly in young individuals with unspecific or long-standing clinical symptoms, MRI is the diagnostic method of choice in the evaluation of foot tumors.[47]

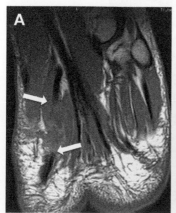
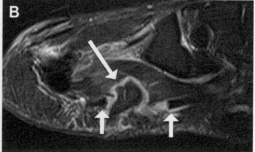

Fig. 47. (*A, B*) STIR images of the forefoot demonstrate a focal rupture of the distal flexor hallucis longus tendon (*short arrows*) with a 2.5-cm gap containing hemorrhage (*long arrow*).

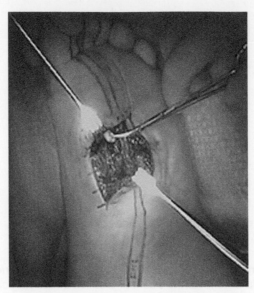

Fig. 48. Complete laceration of the FHL tendon in an adolescent before primary end-to-end repair.

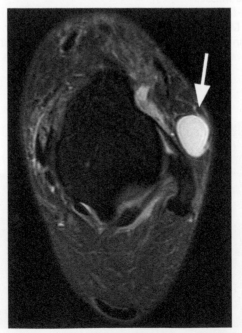

Fig. 49. Axial T2 fat-suppressed image of the ankle shows a well-defined T2 hyperintensity along the superficial surface of the anterior talofibular ligament, compatible with a ganglion cyst (*arrow*).

A B

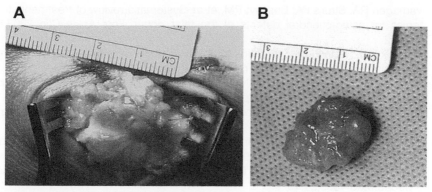

Fig. 50. (A, B) Removal of a ganglion cyst.

- Ganglion cysts are among the most common soft-tissue lesions (**Fig. 49**).
- Ganglion cysts can be symptomatic, tender masses, or produce neurologic symptoms or nerve or tendon entrapment (**Fig. 50**).

REFERENCES

1. Waterman BR, Owens BD, Davey S, et al. The epidemiology of ankle sprains in the United States. J Bone Joint Surg Am 2010;92(13):2279–84.
2. Waterman BR, Belmont PJ Jr, Cameron KL, et al. Epidemiology of ankle sprain at the United States Military Academy. Am J Sports Med 2010;38(4):797–803.
3. de Leeuw PA, van Sterkenburg MN, van Dijk CN. Arthroscopy and endoscopy of the ankle and hindfoot. Sports Med Arthrosc 2009;17:175–84.
4. Pena F. Gross Anatomy of the Ankle Joint. In: Amendola N, Stone WJ, editors. AANA Advanced Arthroscopy: The Foot and Ankle. Philadephia: Saunders; 2010. p. 1–11.
5. van Dijk CN, Scholten PE, Krips R. A 2-portal endoscopic approach for diagnosis and treatment of posterior ankle pathology. Arthroscopy 2000;16:871–6.
6. Ferkel RD. Arthroscopic surgery: the foot and ankle. Philadelphia: Lippincott-Raven; 1996.
7. Stetson WB, Ferkel RD. Ankle arthroscopy: II. Indications and results. J Am Acad Orthop Surg 1996;4:24–34.
8. Bassett FH III, Gates HS III, Billys JB, et al. Talar impingement by anteroinferior tibiofibular ligament: a cause of chronic pain in the ankle after inversion sprain. J Bone Joint Surg Am 1990;72:55–9.
9. Frey C, Gasser S, Feder K. Arthroscopy of the subtalar joint. Foot Ankle Int 1994; 15(8):424–8.
10. Parisien JS. Current techniques in arthroscopy. 3rd edition. New York: Thieme; 1998. p. 161–8.
11. Carreira DS. Arthroscopy of the hallux. Foot Ankle Clin 2009;14(1):105–14.
12. Lui TH. Arthroscopy and endoscopy of the foot and ankle: indications for new techniques. Arthroscopy 2007;23(8):889–902.
13. van Dijk CN, Veenstra KM, Nuesch BC. Arthroscopic surgery of the metatarsophalangeal first joint. Arthroscopy 1998;14(8):851–5.
14. Debnath UK, Hemmady MV, Hariharan K. Indications for and technique of first metatarsophalangeal joint arthroscopy. Foot Ankle Int 2006;27(12): 1049–54.

15. Verhagen RA, Struijs PA, Bossuyt PM, et al. Systematic review of treatment strategies for osteo-chondral defects of the talar dome. Foot Ankle Clin 2003;8: 233–42.
16. van Dijk CN, Reiling ML, Zengerlink M, et al. Osteochondral defects in the ankle: why painful? Knee Surg Sports Traumatol Arthrosc 2010;18(5):570–80.
17. Zengerink M, Struijs PA, van Dijk CN. Treatment of osteochondral lesions of the talus: a systematic review. Knee Surg Sports Traumatol Arthrosc 2010;18(2):238–46.
18. Ferkel RD, Scranton PE Jr. Arthroscopy of the ankle and foot. J Bone Joint Surg Am 1993;75:1233–42.
19. Berndt AL, Harty M. Transchondral fractures (osteochondritis dissecans) of the talus. J Bone Joint Surg Am 1959;41:988–1020.
20. Loomer R, Fisher C, Lloyd-Smith R, et al. Osteochondral lesions of the talus. Am J Sports Med 1993;21:13–9.
21. Guo QW, Hu YL, Jiao C, et al. Arthroscopic treatment for osteochondral lesions of the talus: analysis of outcome predictors. Chin Med J (Engl) 2010;123:296–300.
22. Hunt KJ, Lee AT, Lindsey DP, et al. Osteochondral lesions of the talus: effect of defect size and plantarflexion angle on joint stresses. Am J Sports Med 2012; 40(4):895–901.
23. Hua Y, Chen S, Li Y, et al. Combination of modified Broström procedure with ankle arthroscopy for chronic ankle instability accompanied by intra-articular symptoms. Arthroscopy 2010;26(4):524–8.
24. Ferkel RD. Soft tissue pathology of the ankle. In: McGinty JB, editor. Operative arthroscopy. New York: Raven Press; 1991. p. 713–25.
25. Ferkel RD, Karzel RP, Del Pizzo W, et al. Arthroscopic treatment of anterolateral impingement of the ankle. Am J Sports Med 1991;19:440–6.
26. Cerezal L, Llopis E, Canga A, et al. MR arthrography of the ankle: indications and technique. Radiol Clin North Am 2008;46:973–94.
27. Glazebrook MA, Ganapathy V, Bridge MA, et al. Evidence-based indications for ankle arthroscopy. Arthroscopy 2009;25(12):1478–90.
28. Haller J, Bernt R, Seeger T. MR-imaging of anterior tibiotalar impingement syndrome: agreement, sensitivity and specificity of MR-imaging and indirect MR-arthrography. Eur J Radiol 2006;58:450–60.
29. Vaseenon T, Amendola A. Update on anterior ankle impingement. Curr Rev Musculoskelet Med 2012;5(2):145–50.
30. Scranton PE Jr, McDermott JE. Anterior tibiotalar spurs: a comparison of open versus arthroscopic debridement. Foot Ankle 1992;13:125–9.
31. Komenda GA, Ferkel RD. Arthroscopic findings associated with the unstable ankle. Foot Ankle Int 1999;20:708–13.
32. Hertel J. Functional anatomy, pathomechanics, and pathophysiology of lateral ankle instability. J Athl Train 2002;37:364–75.
33. Nery C, Raduan F. Arthroscopic-assisted Brostrom-Gould for chronic ankle instability: a long-term follow-up. Am J Sports Med 2011;39(11):2381–8.
34. Hunt KJ, George E, Harris AH, et al. Epidemiology of syndesmosis injuries in intercollegiate football: incidence and risk factors from National Collegiate Athletic Association Injury Surveillance System Data from 2004-2005 to 2008-2009. Clin J Sport Med 2013 Jan 21. [Epub ahead of print].
35. Bonasia DE, Rossi R, Saltzman CL, et al. The role of arthroscopy in the management of fractures about the ankle. J Am Acad Orthop Surg 2011;19:226–35.
36. Wagener ML, Beumer A, Swierstra BA. Chronic instability of the anterior tibiofibular syndesmosis of the ankle. Arthroscopic findings and results of anatomical reconstruction. BMC Musculoskelet Disord 2011;12:21.

37. Yilmaz C, Eskandari MM. Arthroscopic excision of the talar Stieda's process. Arthroscopy 2006;22(2):225.e1–3.
38. van Dijk CN, van Bergen CA. Advancements in ankle arthroscopy. J Am Acad Orthop Surg 2008;16:635–46.
39. Schepsis AA, Jones H, Haas AL. Achilles tendon disorders in athletes. Am J Sports Med 2002;30:287–305.
40. Reddy SS, Pedowitz DI, Parekh SG, et al. Surgical treatment for chronic disease and disorders of the Achilles tendon. J Am Acad Orthop Surg 2009;17:3–14.
41. Schon LC, Shores LJ, Faro FD, et al. Flexor hallucis longus tendon transfer in treatment of Achilles tendinosis. J Bone Joint Surg Am 2013;95(1):54–60.
42. Maffulli N. The clinical diagnosis of subcutaneous tear of the Achilles tendon. A prospective study in 174 patients. Am J Sports Med 1998;26(2):266–70.
43. Maffulli N, Longo UG, Maffulli GD, et al. Achilles tendon ruptures in elite athletes. Foot Ankle Int 2011;32(1):9–15.
44. Phisitkul P. Endoscopic surgery of the Achilles tendon. Curr Rev Musculoskelet Med 2012;5(2):156–63.
45. Philbin TM, Landis GS, Smith B. Peroneal tendon injuries. J Am Acad Orthop Surg 2009;17:306–17.
46. Scaduto AA, Cracchiolo A. Lacerations and ruptures of the flexor or extensor hallucis longus tendons. Foot Ankle Clin 2000;5:725–36.
47. Woertler K. Soft tissue masses in the foot and ankle: characteristics on MR Imaging. Semin Musculoskelet Radiol 2005;9(3):227–42.

Dilemmas in Distinguishing Between Tumor and the Posttraumatic Lesion with Surgical or Pathologic Correlation

Eric Walker, MD[a,b,*], Pam Brian, MD[a], Victor Longo, DO[a],
Edward J. Fox, MD[c], Elizabeth E. Frauenhoffer, MD[d],
Mark Murphey, MD[b,e,f]

KEYWORDS

- Bone tumor • Soft tissue tumor • Sports injury • Hemorrhagic soft tissue sarcoma
- Myositis ossificans • Hematoma

KEY POINTS

- Prolonged and atypical swelling of soft tissue, even in combination with a previous traumatic lesion, may be an indication of underlying malignancy, and proper imaging studies should be obtained before surgery or arthroscopy.
- A history of spontaneous fracture or fracture with minor trauma should raise suspicion for underlying disorder as the cause. MR imaging is often useful to show marrow abnormality and the accompanying soft tissue mass often associated with a pathologic fracture.
- Traumatic hematomas commonly develop under an area of subcutaneous ecchymosis, and the absence of this finding should raise the suspicion of tumor-associated hemorrhage. The absence of edema surrounding a large, round hematoma on imaging also suggests tumor.
- Healing avulsion injuries may show lytic and destructive imaging characteristics mimicking osteomyelitis or aggressive tumor.
- The earlier stages of myositis ossificans are likely to mimic a soft tissue neoplasm. Follow up radiograph or CT will demonstrate the typical peripheral calcification pattern.

Disclosure: E. Walker is a consultant for Medical Metrics. E.J. Fox is a speaker for Eli Lilly and his spouse works for GlaxoSmithKline.
[a] Department of Radiology, Penn State Milton S. Hershey Medical Center, 500 University Drive, Hershey, PA 17033, USA; [b] American Institute for Radiologic Pathology, 1010 Wayne Avenue, Suite 320, Silver Spring, MD 20910, USA; [c] Department of Orthopaedics, Penn State Hershey Bone and Joint Institute, 30 Hope Drive, Building B, Suite 2400, Hershey, PA 17033, USA; [d] Department of Pathology and Laboratory Medicine, Penn State Milton S. Hershey Medical Center, 500 University Drive, Hershey, PA 17033, USA; [e] Department of Radiology, Walter Reed National Military Medical Center, 8901 Wisconsin Avenue, Bethesda, MD 20889, USA; [f] Department of Radiology and Nuclear Medicine, Uniformed Services University of the Health Sciences, 4301 Jones Bridge Road, Bethesda, MD 20814, USA
* Corresponding author. Department of Radiology (H066), Penn State Milton S. Hershey Medical Center, 500 University Drive, Hershey, PA 17033, USA.
E-mail address: ewalker@hmc.psu.edu

INTRODUCTION

A bone or soft tissue tumor occasionally presents clinically or by imaging with characteristics suggesting a traumatic injury. The opposite is also true, because posttraumatic lesions may be confused with soft tissue or bone tumor at presentation. Both joint-related tumors and sports injuries often afflict young active patients and the symptoms may display significant overlap. To add to the diagnostic dilemma, the lower extremity is the most frequent location for sports injuries as well as for the development of osseous or soft tissue neoplasms.[1] Without adequate imaging studies, there may be a significant delay in diagnosis or an inappropriate arthroscopic procedure may ensue. For the sports physician, it is crucial to realize that prolonged and atypical swelling of soft tissue, even in combination with a previous traumatic lesion, may be an indication of underlying malignancy.

PART I. TUMORS THAT PRESENT AS SPORTS INJURY OR OTHER TRAUMA
Bone Tumors that Mimic Traumatic Lesions

An osseous lesion may occasionally be misdiagnosed as a sports-related injury on clinical grounds. When a patient presents with a trauma-related complaint that does not respond to treatment, the possibility of underlying malignancy should be considered and appropriate imaging studies obtained. Delay in diagnosis is the most frequent complication in this scenario, but an arthroscopy may be erroneously performed if the proper imaging studies have not been obtained to allow accurate diagnosis. In the literature, arthroscopy has been reported to cause seeding of a tumor into a joint or the adjacent soft tissues.[2–4] For persistent knee pain, a radiographic series should be sufficient in identifying most osseous lesions, but is not as effective for identifying soft tissue masses. The most frequent bone tumors to be confused with trauma on clinical presentation in the literature include giant cell tumor (GCT), osteosarcoma, chondroblastoma, osteoid osteoma, and Ewing sarcoma.[2,4,5] If a lesion arising from the bone is encountered during an arthroscopic procedure, it must not be biopsied by transsynovial approach, but through a separate extracapsular procedure, with the biopsy path discussed with the orthopedic oncologist or treating surgeon before the procedure. Tumors of bone do not often invade joints, because the articular capsule and synovial tissues present a barrier to tumor invasion. Violation of the synovial lining to obtain a biopsy specimen may result in seeding of the joint by tumor and preclude the possibility of limb sparing procedure.[4] Diagnostic errors that may contribute to performance of an inappropriate arthroscopy of a bone tumor include failure to obtain presurgical radiographs, obtaining the radiographs too close to the scheduling of an arthroscopy, or failure to recognize the lesion on radiographs.[6]

GCT of Bone

GCT of bone is a benign lytic, periarticular lesion centered at the metaepiphasis usually with subchondral involvement.[7,8] The knee is the site of almost 50% of GCTs, with the distal femur affected more often than the proximal tibia.[8] A GCT is usually accompanied by pain, local swelling, mechanical symptoms, and occasionally pathologic fracture, and approximately 80% occur in patients between 20 and 50 years of age.[8] The prevalence of this lesion at the knee of young adults can lead to GCT being confused with several sports-related injuries, resulting in a delay in diagnosis.

Osteosarcoma (Conventional Intramedullary Subtype)

Osteosarcoma is the most common primary malignant tumor of bone to afflict children and adolescents. The conventional intramedullary subtype is most frequently recognized as an intramedullary lesion with prominent osteoid matrix (90%) and lytic destruction with a robust periosteal reaction at radiology (**Fig. 1**). The osteoid matrix may be misdiagnosed as callus about a healing fracture if the lesion morphology is not emphasized. Callus should show linear morphology along a fracture plane as opposed to round and oval osteoid associated with tumor. Pathologic fracture is present in approximately 15% to 20% of cases, either at presentation or during therapy. Aggressive Codman triangle and sunburst periosteal reaction patterns are classically associated with osteosarcoma. The long bones are involved in 70% to 80% of cases. In order of frequency of involvement, the distal femur, the proximal tibia, and the proximal humerus are the most common lesion locations.[9] Persistent pain occurring after an innoxious sports-related injury involving the knee or shoulder is a common presentation of osteosarcoma.[6]

Chondroblastoma

Chondroblastoma should be considered in teenagers or young adults with a lesion located in the epiphysis or apophysis. The proximal humerus is the most common

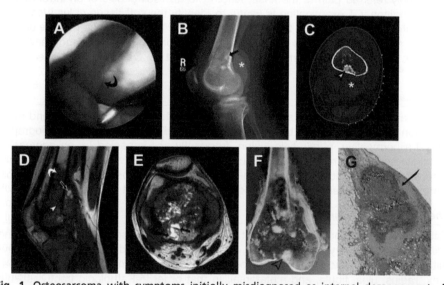

Fig. 1. Osteosarcoma with symptoms initially misdiagnosed as internal derangement. A 19-year-old man presents with joint pain and knee swelling and a vague history of trauma to the knee while playing with the family dog. An arthroscopy was performed before any imaging was obtained. (*A*) Arthroscopy reveals an inflammatory mass within the joint space at the intracondylar notch (*arrow*). Osteosarcoma was not discovered during the arthroscopy. (*B*) Lateral radiograph reveals osteoid matrix (*arrow*) within the distal metaphysis and soft tissue mass (*asterisk*) posterior to the metaphysis. (*C*) Axial computed tomography (CT) shows bone lysis and osteoid matrix within the metaphysis (*arrowhead*) and soft tissue mass dorsal to the femur (*asterisk*). (*D*) Sagittal T1-weighted image (TR447/TE11) shows marrow replacement (*curved arrow*), hemorrhagic soft tissue mass (*arrow*), and foci of osteoid (*arrowhead*). (*E*) Axial T2-weighted sequence (TR6900/TE72) shows cystic change within the lesion with multiple fluid levels (*arrows*). (*F*) Cross section of distal femur gross specimen shows extension of osteosarcoma to articular surface at intercondylar notch (*arrowhead*). (*G*) Focus of osteosarcoma (*arrow*) within synovium (hematoxylin and eosin [H&E], low power). This patient was featured in a recent case report. (*Data from* Sielatycki JF, Fox EJ, Frauenhoffer, EE. Arthroscopy-associated complications in osteosarcoma: a case report and review of the literature. JBJS Case Connector 2012;2(4):1–4.)

location.[10] Patients typically have aching, intermittent pain, decreased motion, and swelling of the adjacent joint.[6] Computed tomography (CT) scan often reveals a well-demarcated lesion, frequently with punctate calcifications within the lesion. A chondroblastoma usually appears on magnetic resonance (MR) as low intensity on a T1-weighted sequence and variable intensity on a T2-weighted sequence (but often low signal). A T2-weighted image also commonly shows significant perilesional bone marrow edema[11] that may simulate a reactive, traumatic, or inflammatory process if not recognized as a component of chondroblastoma.

Osteoid Osteoma

Osteoid osteoma is a benign, usually painful lesion found in children and young adults. The common presentation is night pain relieved by salicylates. Intraarticular lesions often cause reactive synovitis and joint dysfunction without the typical extensive periosteal and endosteal reactive bone formation causing marked cortical thickening. These lesions most frequently simulate an inflammatory or traumatic process. In the proximal femur, which is the most common location, osteoid osteoma may cause only referred pain to the knee, leading to a misdiagnosis of an intraarticular knee condition. CT examination is useful to identify the soft tissue nidus with small punctuate calcifications (**Fig. 2**). MR imaging usually reveals intense marrow edema on fluid-sensitive sequences that can be misinterpreted as malignancy and may obscure the nidus. The current optimal treatment is CT-guided radiofrequency ablation.[6,11]

Ewing Sarcoma

Ewing sarcoma is one of the small, round, blue-cell tumors, and is the second most common primary malignant bone tumor in the pediatric population. Radiographs reveal a permeative, purely lytic lesion, frequently accompanied by an aggressive lamellated periosteal reaction in an onion-skin appearance. Ewing sarcoma is usually diaphyseal and the most common long-bone location is the proximal femur. The only symptom may be referred pain to the knee, which may result in delay in diagnosis.[6]

The Pathologic Fracture

Pathologic fractures occur in bones that are weakened by a disease process, including primary and secondary bone neoplasm, a variety of metabolic disorders, and osteomyelitis. The most common sites of pathologic fracture are the femur, humerus, tibia, phalanx, radius, ulna, fibula, and metatarsal, in that order.[12] Pathologic fractures from tumors metastatic to bone are usually treated with internal fixation or joint arthroplasty as a means of surgical stabilization. The goal is pain relief with rapid mobilization and ambulation.[13,14] In patients with pathologic fractures through a primary bone tumor, a planned resection with adjuvant or neoadjuvant radiation and chemotherapy needs to be considered so as not to seed the adjacent bone and soft tissues with tumor. In some cases, immediate amputation may be considered necessary because the locally developed hematoma may facilitate dissemination of the malignancy.[15] Inadvertent fixation of a presumed bone metastasis, which is a primary bone tumor, may result in the contamination of the surrounding bone and soft tissues, an increased risk of local recurrence, and possibly limb amputation or patient demise. If the tumor type cannot be determined by imaging alone, a biopsy should be performed before internal fixation.

Radiographs comprise the first step of fracture imaging evaluation. Some bone tumors with a highly permeative pattern or an invisible margin, such as Ewing sarcoma, malignant fibrous histiocytoma (MFH), or lymphoma, may be difficult to appreciate as the cause of a fracture. MFH has the highest misdiagnosis rate.[12] Fracture margins

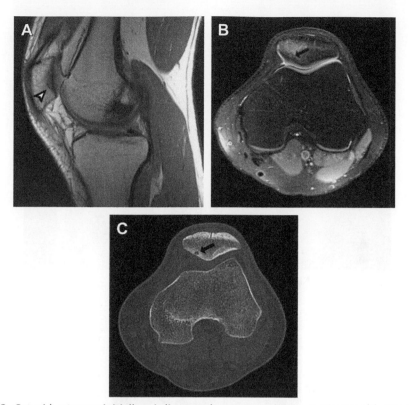

Fig. 2. Osteoid osteoma initially misdiagnosed as a sports injury. A 19-year-old man with symptoms of tightness around the knee after a season of lacrosse. Radiographs (not shown) were normal. After 3 months of conservative therapy the patient returned to his physician with persistent patellar pain that was worse at night, and often awakened him during sleep. The process was thought to be patellofemoral syndrome or an articular cartilage injury and MR imaging was obtained. (*A*) Sagittal proton density (TR2160/TE14) shows a possible nidus (*arrowhead*) in the subchondral patella. (*B*) Axial T2-weighted sequence with fat saturation (TR1620/TE31) again reveals the subchondral nidus (*arrow*) with significant surrounding edema within the patella. CT 14 days later (*C*) was performed to verify the presence of a nidus (*arrow*). Note the minute punctate calcification within the nidus.

should be assessed carefully for abnormal lucency (lucency that cannot be accounted for by the fracture alone) (**Fig. 3**), sclerosis, or periosteal reaction because these findings may indicate an underlying abnormality.[16] History of spontaneous fracture or fracture with minor trauma should also raise suspicion for an underlying disorder as the cause. MR imaging is often useful to show marrow abnormality and the accompanying soft tissue mass often associated with a pathologic fracture.

Intraarticular Lesions Causing Mechanical Symptoms

Intraarticular lesions such as pigmented villonodular synovitis, synovial chondromatosis, and lipoma arborescens may cause mechanical symptoms that can be confused with a sports injury. This article does not discuss intraarticular processes because they are extensively reviewed in "Arthritis Mimicking Sports-Related Injuries" by Flemming and Bernard, a separate article elsewhere in this issue.

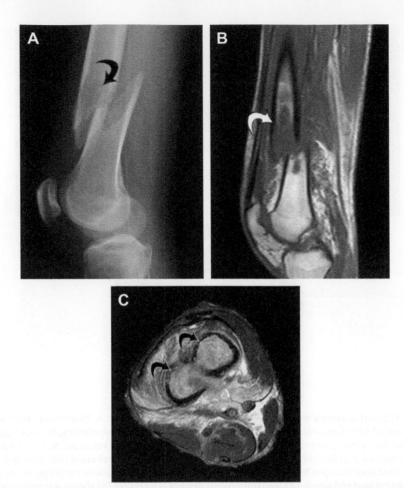

Fig. 3. Pathologic fracture. A 47-year-old man with a history of non–small cell lung carcinoma undergoing chemotherapy and radiation. While taking an evening walk, he fell and injured his right leg. (*A*) On close examination, the diaphysis above the fracture site shows a subtle permeative lytic destruction (*curved arrow*) and deep endosteal scalloping representing metastatic disease. (*B*) Sagittal T1-weighted sequence (TR425/TE7) reveals marrow replacement above (*curved arrow*) and to a lesser extent below the fracture. (*C*) Axial T2-weighted sequence (TR2825/TE25) with fat saturation shows deep endosteal scalloping and marrow replacement (*curved arrows*) along with surrounding soft tissue edema.

Soft Tissue Tumors that May Present as Trauma

Soft issue malignancies may occasionally present clinically as sports injuries. The eight soft tissue malignant neoplasms most frequently confused with sport injury include synovial sarcoma, extraosseous Ewing sarcoma, fibrosarcoma, undifferentiated sarcoma, and juxtacortical chondroma.[5]

Synovial Sarcoma

Synovial sarcoma may be the most clinically important soft tissue sarcoma with which an orthopedic surgeon should be familiar because they most often affect the extremities (80%–95% of cases), usually arising adjacent to (but rarely involving) a joint, particularly the popliteal fossa at the knee. Most patients with synovial sarcoma are between the ages of 15 and 40 years.[17] Two features of this lesion that may lead to the false assumption of a benign process are the slow growth (average time to diagnosis is often 2–4 years) and small lesion size (<5 cm at initial presentation). Distinguishing imaging characteristics for synovial sarcoma include the presence of calcifications (**Fig. 4**) on radiograph or CT in 30% of cases and significant lesion heterogeneity on MR imaging leading to the triple sign or bowl-of-grapes sign on fluid-sensitive sequences.[17–19]

Myxoid sarcomas (such as myxofibrosarcoma, myxoid liposarcoma [**Fig. 5**], and myxoid chondrosarcoma) and occasionally a synovial sarcoma with high water content (**Fig. 6**) adjacent to a joint may mimic a ganglion on MR imaging. For large lesions appearing to have high water content adjacent to a joint it is important to identify a connection neck attaching the presumed ganglion to the capsule or an adjacent tendon sheath. A mass with high water content with atypical location for ganglion or synovial cyst should receive further imaging with contrast-enhanced MR or sonography to exclude a cyst mimicker such as a myxoid neoplasm. It may be useful to do both precontrast and postcontrast T1-weighted fat-saturation sequences to distinguish true lesion enhancement from high T1-weighted signal fluid, such as can result from hemorrhagic or increased proteinaceous fluid.

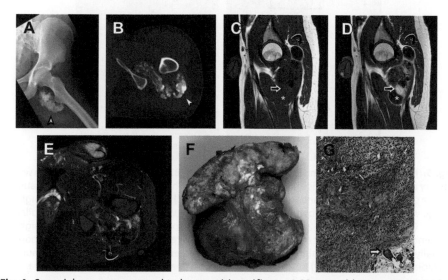

Fig. 4. Synovial sarcoma assumed to be myositis ossificans. A 23-year-old man with posterior thigh pain and mass for 4 years that has recently worsened. The mass was stable in size over 4 years. The prior surgeon thought the lesion to be myositis ossificans because of the dense mineralization, and chose to follow it. The patient started seeing a new orthopedic oncologist who was concerned with the lesion appearance and the worsening pain and ordered a biopsy. (A) Frog leg lateral radiograph reveals a highly mineralized soft tissue lesion adjacent to the lesser trochanter (*arrowhead*). (B) Axial CT shows extensive mineralization throughout the lesion (*arrowhead*). Sagittal T1-weighted sequence (TR621/TE7) before (C) and after (D) contrast administration shows extensive low signal intensity mineralization (*curved arrows*), a focus of nodular enhancement (*arrows*), and a cystic or necrotic area caudally (*asterisks*). (E) Axial T2-weighted sequence (TR2500/TE70) with fat saturation also shows extensive mineralization throughout the lesion (*curved arrow*). (F) Resected gross specimen of right thigh synovial sarcoma with areas of calcification. (G) Photomicrograph of synovial sarcoma with spindle cells and foci of calcification (*arrow*) (H&E, low power).

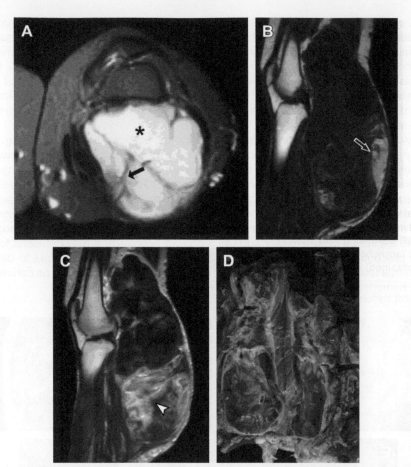

Fig. 5. Myxoid liposarcoma misdiagnosed as a popliteal (Baker) cyst. A 63-year-old man with a history of rheumatoid arthritis and posterior knee mass. This popliteal fossa mass was assumed to be a popliteal (Baker) cyst and was followed for 10 years before biopsy. (*A*) Axial T2-weighted image with fat saturation shows a large popliteal lesion with signal characteristics similar to water (*asterisk*). Thickened septae are noted posteriorly (*arrow*). Sagittal T1-weighted sequence before (*B*) and after (*C*) contrast administration reveals a prominent fatty component dorsally (*arrow*) and a nodular focus of avid contrast enhancement (*arrowhead*) caudally excluding a popliteal cyst. (*D*) Resected, bivalved gross specimen of myxoid liposarcoma.

The Hemorrhagic Soft Tissue Sarcoma Mimicking a Hematoma

Soft tissue tumors may initially be misdiagnosed as simple hematoma.[20–22] The soft tissue sarcoma with intratumoral hemorrhage is an infrequently described entity, usually mistaken for intramuscular hematoma. The necrosis and/or hemorrhage may be so extensive that a large blood-filled cavity results with only a small cuff of viable tumor tissue present, usually at the periphery. The most common location for this presentation is in the thigh. Soft tissue tumors most commonly associated with hematoma formation are undifferentiated pleomorphic sarcoma (formerly known as MFH),[20,22] synovial sarcoma,[17] extraskeletal Ewing sarcoma,[23] myxoid or pleomorphic liposarcoma,[24] leiomyosarcoma,[20] and angiosarcoma.[25]

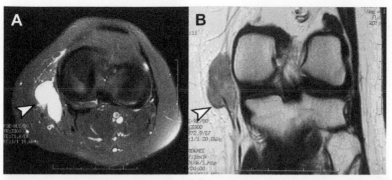

Fig. 6. Myxoid liposarcoma mimicking a meniscal cyst. A 27-year-old woman with history of medial knee mass. (*A*) Axial T2-weighted fat (TR3300/TE71.8) saturation sequence shows high-signal medial knee lesion (*arrowhead*) with an appearance and location mimicking a meniscal cyst. (*B*) Coronal T2-weighted (TR3300/TE72.9) sequences reveals heterogeneity within the lesion (*arrowhead*) not appreciated in the fat-saturation sequence. Contrast administration (not obtained) would have helped by showing diffuse enhancement of the lesion.

A soft tissue tumor presenting as hematoma should be suspected in the following circumstances: (1) if there is a spontaneous intramuscular hematoma, and there is no clear history of trauma, bleeding disorder (hemophilia, liver insufficiency), or antico-agulation/antiplatelet medication, that could justify bleeding predisposition. However, a history of trauma or a bleeding disorder does not rule out the possibility of an under-lying malignancy. (2) When the mechanism of injury does not justify the clinically detected severity of the injury, based on the extent of swelling, ecchymosis, pain, and functional disability. (3) If the lesion does not follow the expected clinical course of resolution after initial conservative treatment. (4) If the hematoma recurs, continues to expand, or does not regress, and if pain progressively increases or the supposed muscle strain easily recurs.[26]

The following guidelines from the literature may be used to help identify the hemor-rhagic soft tissue sarcoma. Traumatic hematomas commonly develop under an area of subcutaneous ecchymosis, and the absence of this finding should raise the suspi-cion of tumor-associated hemorrhage.[21] The absence of edema surrounding a large, round hematoma on imaging also suggests tumor.[22] After gadolinium administration, the viable sarcomatous portion of the lesion enhances (**Fig. 7**) and 55% of these le-sions have well-defined tumor nodules within the wall of the hematoma.[22] The walls of a hemorrhagic sarcoma have also been noted to be more irregular and thicker than those of hematomas[20] (although in our experience, unsupported by data, hema-toma often has thicker walls than tumor pseudocapsule). Identification of hemosiderin in the lesion wall also suggests hematoma and not hemorrhagic tumor.

PART II. POSTTRAUMATIC LESIONS THAT MAY MIMIC A MALIGNANCY
Avulsion Fractures

Avulsion injuries of the pelvis occur most frequently in the adolescent athlete, usually resulting in displacement of an unfused apophysis at the site of tendon attachment. Healing avulsions may show lytic and destructive characteristics mimicking osteomy-elitis or Ewing sarcoma.[27] In addition, healing with osteoid formation may simulate conventional osteosarcoma or parosteal osteosarcoma. A thorough knowledge of the various tendon attachments about the pelvis helps to avoid misinterpreting an old or healing avulsion injury as a more aggressive lesion.[28]

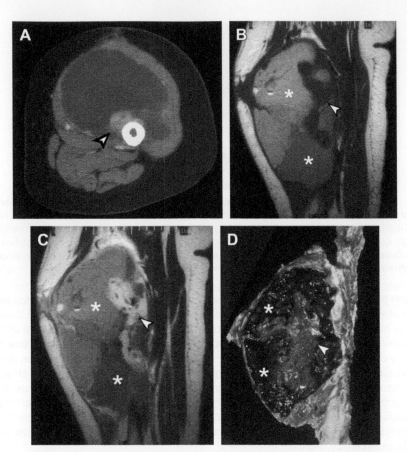

Fig. 7. Undifferentiated pleomorphic sarcoma (previously known as MFH) presenting as a hematoma. A 58-year-old woman with a spontaneous hematoma. (*A*) Axial CT shows an anterior thigh mass that is largely fluid attenuation. Close inspection reveals a small focus of enhancement anterior to the femur (*arrowhead*). Sagittal T1-weighted sequence before (*B*) and after (*C*) contrast administration shows a large heterogeneous fluid collection with intermediate and high-signal components (*asterisks*). An enhancing solid component is noted at the dorsal aspect of the lesion (*arrowheads*). (*D*) Resected, sagittally sectioned gross specimen containing hemorrhagic (*asterisks*) and solid components (*arrowhead*).

The ischial tuberosity is the most common location for apophyseal injury in the pelvis. It is the site of origin of the semimembranosus, semitendinosus, adductor magnus, and the long head of the biceps femoris tendons. Enlargement or prominence of the ischial tuberosity (**Fig. 8**) is a radiographic finding related to remote avulsion injury. Other common avulsion injuries of the pelvis include the anterior superior iliac spine and the anterior inferior iliac spine. The anterior superior iliac spine is the site of origin of the sartorius tendon and tensor fascia lata. The anterior inferior iliac spine is the site of origin of the rectus femoris tendon.

Myositis Ossificans

Myositis ossificans is the most common bone-forming lesion of soft tissue. The anterior musculature of the thigh and arm are most frequently involved.[29] A significant minority of patients (40%) have no history of trauma, and the diagnosis may not be

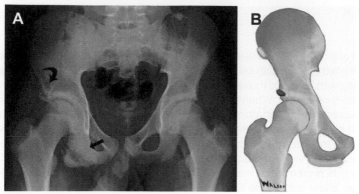

Fig. 8. Ischial tuberosity avulsion potentially misdiagnosed as periosteal osteosarcoma. A 14-year-old boy with an injury occurring during the football season. The patient was referred to Hershey Medical Center for a second opinion regarding a right inferior pubic ramus lesion noted on radiograph. (*A*) anteroposterior (AP) radiograph of the pelvis shows hypertrophy and irregularity of the ischial tuberosity (*arrow*), which may be confused with tumor. Also note the heterotopic ossification at the anterior inferior iliac spine (*curved arrow*) representing sequelae of avulsion at the rectus femoris origin. (*B*) Common areas for avulsion in the pelvis, which may be confused with a neoplastic lesion: the ischial tuberosity (aqua), the anterior superior iliac spine (yellow), and the anterior inferior iliac spine (pink).

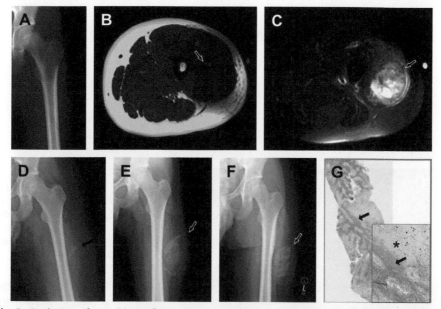

Fig. 9. Evolution of myositis ossificans. A 16-year-old boy presents to the orthopedic oncology clinic with increasing soft tissue mass of the left thigh for the last several weeks, which was painful to palpation. He is unable to give any specific history of trauma. An outside radiograph performed 11 days earlier (*A*) reveals no mineralization. (*B*) Axial T1-weighted (TR500/TE14) and (*C*) T2-weighted sequence (TR4700/TE85) with fat saturation obtained 8 days after the initial radiograph shows an ill-defined mass (*arrows*) with surrounding soft tissue edema. Faint lower signal border of the lesion on T2-weighted sequence may represent early mineral deposition. Serial radiographs performed 11 days (*D*), 22 days (*E*), and 8 months (*F*) after the initial radiograph show progressive increase in peripheral ossification (*arrows*) in a classic zonal phenomena distribution. (*G*) Irregular bone trabeculae (*arrow*) formed by osteoblasts, arising in a loose spindled stroma, and adjacent chondroid matrix, with zones of transition, characteristic of myositis ossificans. (H&E, low power). Inset: chondroid matrix (*asterisk*) transitioning to woven bone (*arrow*) (H&E, high power).

suspected clinically.[30] When questioning a patient and the family, it may be valuable to expand on what the clinician considers to be trauma. One of the authors recalls a 12-year-old boy with a triceps mass for 4 months. The patient and his family insisted there was no history of trauma. When the boy's shirt was removed for the biopsy procedure, several bruises were noted about his trunk. When questioned about the injuries, the patient and his parents recounted a dog bite and a fall down the stairs, but no trauma (they equated trauma with a motor vehicle accident). The moniker heterotopic ossification is a broader term, because it describes the process in extramuscular locations as well, and is preferred by many to the term myositis ossificans. The initial radiographs may show soft tissue fullness without calcification. Peripheral calcifications can be recognized on plain radiographs by the third week (**Figs. 9** and **10**), although their appearance may vary from 11 days to 6 weeks.[31] The time to identification depends on patient age, with young patients forming calcification earlier than those who are older. Calcification is also present in some soft tissue tumors (soft tissue osteosarcoma, soft tissue chondrosarcoma, synovial sarcoma) but is noted diffusely throughout the lesion and in most cases is distinguished from the typical peripheral

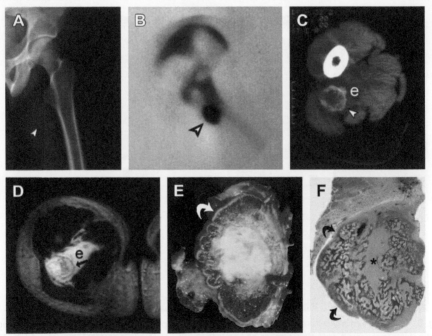

Fig. 10. Myositis ossificans misdiagnosed as soft tissue sarcoma. A 20-year-old woman with a 6-week history of lump in the right thigh and no recollection of prior injury. AP radiograph (*A*) reveals soft tissue lesion with subtle peripheral calcification (*arrowhead*). Nuclear medicine bone scan (*B*) shows marked radionuclide uptake in the lesion (*arrowhead*) greater than the iliac spines. Axial CT image (*C*) shows a well-defined peripheral rim of calcification (*arrowhead*) and surrounding muscle edema (*e*) causing lower attenuation. (*D*) Axial T2-weighted image (TR2200/TE70) reveals a mass with thin border of lower signal intensity (*arrow*) secondary to calcium deposition and significant surrounding edema (*e*). Resected gross specimen (*E*) and histologic macrosection (H&E, low power) (*F*) show a well-defined border of cortex (*curved arrows*) and trabeculation and more immature tissue centrally (*asterisk*) representing the zonal phenomenon.

pattern of calcification that becomes more evident as heterotopic ossification matures.[32] The ossifications in myositis ossificans are described as peripheral and centripetal, whereas, in the typical soft tissue osteosarcoma, they are central and centrifugal.[33] The zone phenomena has been described histologically with the lesion separated into central, middle, and outer zones. The outer zone consists of well-formed bone, which is seen on radiographs about the third week. The middle zone contains oriented osteoid, and the central zone features an extreme variation of cells and mitotic figures,[34] which are not atypical.[35] CT is more sensitive than radiography at detecting early mineralization and, in atypical cases, it may be useful because of its ability to show the peripheral calcified ring and the central low attenuation zone.[36–38] The earlier stages of myositis ossificans are likely to mimic a soft tissue neoplasm on MR, showing heterogeneous low signal intensity on T1-weighted images, heterogeneous high signal intensity on T2-weighted images, and enhancement after intravenous gadolinium administration. The significant soft tissue edema surrounding myositis ossificans during the early stages tends to be prominent on CT and MR and is a key to discriminating this lesion from soft tissue tumors, which usually have little or no surrounding edema.[39] It is important not to consider the surrounding edema as a component of the mass because this may lead to the erroneous diagnosis of

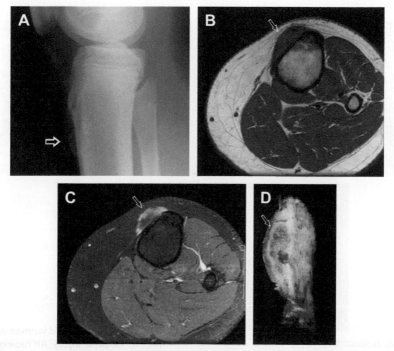

Fig. 11. Juxtacortical heterotopic ossification initially diagnosed as osteochondroma. A 14-year-old boy with a pretibial mass and pain with no history of trauma. Initial radiograph with pretibial lesion interpreted as osteochondroma versus myositis ossificans. Later diagnosed as periosteal osteosarcoma on MR examination at an outside institution. Radiograph (*A*) shows a juxtacortical lesion (*arrow*) beneath the tibial tubercle with a thin rim of peripheral calcification. Axial T1-weighted sequence before (TR466/TE10) (*B*) and after (TR416/TE10) contrast administration (*C*) shows an intermediate lesion with T1 signal intensity (*arrows*) with irregular peripheral enhancement. Resected gross specimen (*D*) shows a well-corticated mass (*arrow*) adherent to the tibial cortex.

aggressive infiltrative malignancy. During the subacute phase, a rim of low signal intensity is noted on MR, which corresponds with peripheral ossification.[29] Biopsy of myositis ossificans may seem aggressive histologically and be confused with malignancy when obtained from the central zone of the lesion.[34] When heterotopic ossification occurs in a subperiosteal or juxtacortical location, it may be confused with a surface osteosarcoma or a periosteal chondroid lesion (**Figs. 11** and **12**).

Hematoma

Although hematomas are more common than soft tissue sarcomas, they both have a high propensity to occur in the extremities, and usually the lower extremity.[35] Frequent locations of hematoma include the thigh, particularly proximally and distally, and the lumbosacral area.[40] Subcutaneous ecchymosis is frequently present with an underlying hematoma.[29] The characteristic behavior of a soft tissue neoplasm is to increase in size. In contrast, hematomas initially expand, but most stop growing when clotting occurs. The classic MR signal characteristics of hematoma are clearly described in the literature. Acute hematomas (0–2 days) contain intracellular deoxyhemoglobin, which causes an isointense signal intensity on T1-weighted sequences and a hypointense signal intensity on T2 weighting. The early subacute hematoma (2–7 days) has

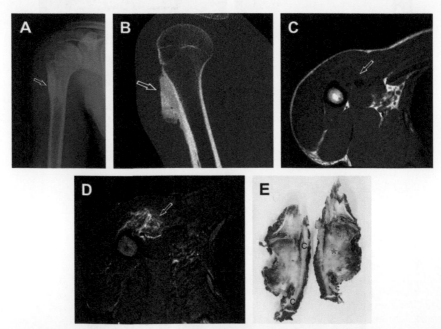

Fig. 12. Juxtacortical heterotopic ossification related to pectoral attachment avulsion initially misinterpreted as osteosarcoma. A 15-year-old boy presents with a painful mass in the right upper arm. The mass was first noticed 1 year earlier after a twisting injury during a wrestling match. AP radiograph (*A*) reveals a calcified lesion (*arrow*) anterior to the humeral metaphysis. CT coronal reconstruction (*B*) image shows a densely mineralized, irregular periosteal mass (*arrow*) adherent to the anterior humeral cortex. Axial T1-weighted sequence (*C*) shows a heterogeneous mass with intermediate signal intensity (*arrow*) with several low-signal foci. Axial T2-weighted sequence with fat saturation (*D*) shows an irregular, heterogeneous lesion with surrounding edema (*arrow*). (*E*) Resected, sectioned gross specimen (*asterisk*) adherent to the humeral metaphysis cortex (*c*).

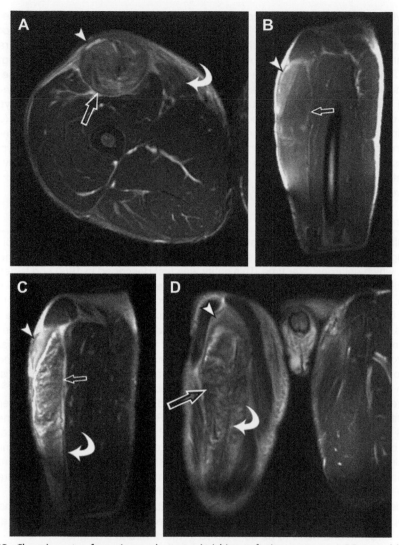

Fig. 13. Chronic rectus femoris muscle tear mimicking soft tissue tumor. A 26-year-old male soldier with mild anterior thigh pain and mass without recollection of prior trauma. (*A*) Axial T2-weighted sequence reveals replacement of the rectus femoris muscle with heterogeneous mass with intermediate to high signal (*arrow*). A small high-signal fluid level is noted anteriorly (*arrowhead*) and edema is present in the adjacent sartorius muscle (*curved arrow*). Sagittal T1-weighted (*B*) and T2-weighted (*C*) images show intermediate T1 and intermediate to high T2 signal with a disorganized, heterogeneous appearance to the rectus femoris (*arrows*) secondary to torn muscle fibers, which may be confused with tumor. High T1 and T2 signal fluid level is present at the anterior superior aspect (*arrowheads*) of the lesion. Feathery edema is present in the more caudal fibers of the rectus femoris (*curved arrow*). Coronal T2-weighted sequence (*D*) with disorganized muscle fibers (*arrow*) and small superior fluid level (*arrowhead*). Note the central tendon slip (*curved arrow*) passing through the lesion. The key to recognizing this as injury rather than tumor is the significant perilesional edema, fluid, long extent, and maintained muscle texture on T1 weighting.

deoxyhemoglobin transforming to intracellular methemoglobin, usually peripherally, and this results in a rim of high T1-weighted signal and low signal intensity on T2 weighting. In the late subacute phase (1–4 weeks), methemoglobin becomes extracellular and the hematoma then displays peripheral high signal intensity on T1-weighted and T2-weighted MR images. As the hematoma evolves into the chronic phase, the final degradation product, hemosiderin, is formed peripherally, and this displays low signal intensity on all pulse sequences.[41] However, in the musculoskeletal system these elements are typically admixed, resulting in heterogeneous signal with foci (often curvilinear) of high signal on T1 and T2 weighting, and fluid levels may be seen. Peripheral enhancement with lack of central enhancement on CT and MR imaging is typical. Perilesional edema is common in the acute and subacute stages, but this resolves in the later stages.[37] To exercise caution, a hematoma should be followed until it resolves clinically or radiologically.

Chronic Hematoma

The blood in a hematoma is usually broken down into its components and resorbed, leaving little to no residua. An exception is the less common chronic expanding hematoma, which enlarges over time. This entity was first described in 1980 and is defined as a hematoma that continues to enlarge for more than a month after initial hemorrhage. It is thought that the continued bleeding occurs because of the irritant effects of the blood and its byproducts, causing repeated exudation or bleeding from the capillaries in the granulation tissue.[42] Another proposed mechanism is that the vessels on the inner wall of the hematoma rupture because of the wall expansion and propagate the process. The increase in lesion size over time may cause concern for sarcoma. To add to the confusion, chronic hematoma may contain organizing fibrovascular tissue, which has been noted in the literature to display nodular internal enhancement.[43] This feature is extremely rare, both in the literature and in our experience. Characteristic features of chronic expanding hematoma on MR imaging include heterogeneous signal intensity on both T1-weighted and T2-weighted images, reflecting the central zone of fluid collection caused by fresh and altered blood, and a peripheral rim of low signal intensity representing a wall of collagenous fibrous tissue,[44] which may be thick and often contains hemosiderin. Sedimentation may occur, with separation of the cellular and fluid components resulting in a fluid level.

Other posttraumatic lesions, such as Morel-Lavallee lesion,[45] pseudotumor of hemophilia,[24,46] and chronic rectus femoris muscle tear (**Fig. 13**),[47] can mimic a soft tissue sarcoma and need to be considered in the differential diagnosis.

SUMMARY

Tumors may present mimicking a sports injury and vice versa. It is important to consider the mechanism of injury and obtain appropriate imaging studies to identify key imaging features in an attempt to distinguish these lesions. It may be necessary to obtain follow-up imaging or to perform a biopsy to obtain a definitive diagnosis.

REFERENCES

1. Kelm J, Ahlhelm F, Engel C, et al. Synovial sarcoma diagnosed after a sports injury. Am J Sports Med 2001;29(3):367–9.
2. Muscolo DL, Ayerza MA, Makino A, et al. Tumors about the knee misdiagnosed as athletic injuries. J Bone Joint Surg Am 2003;85(7):1209–14.

3. Sielatycki JF, Fox EJ, Frauenhoffer EE. Arthroscopy-associated complications in osteosarcoma: a case report and review of the literature. JBJS Case Connector 2012;2(4):1–4.
4. Joyce MJ, Mankin HJ. Caveat arthroscopos: extra-articular lesions of bone simulating intra-articular pathology of the knee. J Bone Joint Surg Am 1983;65(3): 289–92.
5. Lewis MM, Reilly JF. Sports tumors. Am J Sports Med 1987;15(4):362–5.
6. Damron TA, Morris C, Rougraff B, et al. Diagnosis and treatment of joint-related tumors that mimic sports-related injuries. Instr Course Lect 2009;58:833–47.
7. Campanacci M, Gluntini A, Olmi R. Giant cell tumour of bone: a study of 209 cases with long term follow-up in 130 cases. Ital J Orthop Traumatol 1975;1:249–77.
8. Murphey MD, Nomikos GC, Flemming DJ, et al. From the archives of AFIP. Imaging of giant cell tumor and giant cell reparative granuloma of bone: radiologic-pathologic correlation. Radiographics 2001;21(5):1283–309.
9. Murphey MD, Robbin MR, McRae GA, et al. The many faces of osteosarcoma. Radiographics 1997;17(5):1205–31.
10. Lin PP, Thenappan A, Deavers MT, et al. Treatment and prognosis of chondroblastoma. Clin Orthop Relat Res 2005;438:103–9.
11. Stacy GS, Heck RK, Peabody TD, et al. Neoplastic and tumorlike lesions detected on MR imaging of the knee in patients with suspected internal derangement: part I, intraosseous entities. AJR Am J Roentgenol 2002;178(3):589–94.
12. Hu YC, Lun DX, Wang H. Clinical features of neoplastic pathological fracture in long bones. Chin Med J (Engl) 2012;125(17):3127–32.
13. Harrington KD. Orthopedic surgical management of skeletal complications of malignancy. Cancer 1997;80(Suppl 8):1614–27.
14. Peabody T. The rodded metastasis is a sarcoma: strategies to prevent inadvertent surgical procedures on primary bone malignancies. Instr Course Lect 2004;53:657–61.
15. Finn HA, Simon MA. Limb-salvage surgery in the treatment of osteosarcoma in skeletally immature individuals. Clin Orthop Relat Res 1991;(262):108–18.
16. Muchantef K, Pollock AN. Osteosarcoma of the lower extremity presenting as a pathologic fracture. Pediatr Emerg Care 2012;28(9):936–7.
17. Murphey MD, Gibson MS, Jennings BT, et al. From the archives of the AFIP: imaging of synovial sarcoma with radiologic-pathologic correlation. Radiographics 2006;26(5):1543–65.
18. Walker EA, Salesky JS, Fenton ME, et al. Magnetic resonance imaging of malignant soft tissue neoplasms in the adult. Radiol Clin North Am 2011;49(6):1219–34, vi.
19. Walker EA, Song AJ, Murphey MD. Magnetic resonance imaging of soft-tissue masses. Semin Roentgenol 2010;45(4):277–97.
20. Imaizumi S, Morita T, Ogose A, et al. Soft tissue sarcoma mimicking chronic hematoma: value of magnetic resonance imaging in differential diagnosis. J Orthop Sci 2002;7(1):33–7.
21. Ward WG Sr, Rougraff B, Quinn R, et al. Tumors masquerading as hematomas. Clin Orthop Relat Res 2007;465:232–40.
22. Sternheim A, Jin X, Shmookler B, et al. 'Telangiectatic' transformation in soft tissue sarcomas. A clinicopathology analysis of an aggressive feature of high-grade sarcomas. Ann Surg Oncol 2008;15(1):345–54.
23. Ogose A, Hotta T, Yamamura S, et al. Extraskeletal Ewing's sarcoma mimicking traumatic hematoma. Arch Orthop Trauma Surg 1998;118(3):172–3.
24. Allen DJ, Goddard NJ, Mann HA, et al. Primary malignancies mistaken for pseudotumours in haemophilic patients. Haemophilia 2007;13(4):383–6.

25. Weiss SW, Goldblum JR, editors. Enzinger and Weiss' soft tissue tumors. 5th edition. Philadelphia: Mosby Elsevier; 2008.
26. Kontogeorgakos VA, Martinez S, Dodd L, et al. Extremity soft tissue sarcomas presented as hematomas. Arch Orthop Trauma Surg 2010;130(10):1209–14.
27. Stevens MA, El-Khoury GY, Kathol MH, et al. Imaging features of avulsion injuries. Radiographics 1999;19(3):655–72.
28. Sanders TG, Zlatkin MB. Avulsion injuries of the pelvis. Semin Musculoskelet Radiol 2008;12(1):42–53.
29. Stacy GS, Kapur A. Mimics of bone and soft tissue neoplasms. Radiol Clin North Am 2011;49(6):1261–86, vii.
30. Parikh J, Hyare H, Saifuddin A. The imaging features of post-traumatic myositis ossificans, with emphasis on MRI. Clin Radiol 2002;57(12):1058–66.
31. Norman A, Dorfman HD. Juxtacortical circumscribed myositis ossificans: evolution and radiographic features. Radiology 1970;96(2):301–6.
32. van Vliet M, Kliffen M, Krestin GP, et al. Soft tissue sarcomas at a glance: clinical, histological, and MR imaging features of malignant extremity soft tissue tumors. Eur Radiol 2009;19(6):1499–511.
33. Mirra JM, Picci P, Gold RH. Bone tumors: clinical, radiologic, and pathologic correlations. Philadelphia: Lea & Febiger; 1989.
34. Ackerman LV. Extra-osseous localized non-neoplastic bone and cartilage formation (so-called myositis ossificans): clinical and pathological confusion with malignant neoplasms. J Bone Joint Surg Am 1958;40(2):279–98.
35. Fletcher CD, UK, Mertens F. Pathology and genetics of tumours of soft tissue and bone (IARC WHO classification of tumours). 3rd edition. 2006.
36. Hanquinet S, Ngo L, Anooshiravani M, et al. Magnetic resonance imaging helps in the early diagnosis of myositis ossificans in children. Pediatr Surg Int 1999;15(3–4):287–9.
37. McKenzie G, Raby N, Ritchie D. Pictorial review: non-neoplastic soft-tissue masses. Br J Radiol 2009;82(981):775–85.
38. Amendola MA, Glazer GM, Agha FP, et al. Myositis ossificans circumscripta: computed tomographic diagnosis. Radiology 1983;149(3):775–9.
39. Stein-Wexler R. MR imaging of soft tissue masses in children. Magn Reson Imaging Clin N Am 2009;17(3):489–507, vi.
40. Sreenivas M, Nihal A, Ettles DF. Chronic haematoma or soft-tissue neoplasm? A diagnostic dilemma. Arch Orthop Trauma Surg 2004;124(7):495–7.
41. Bush CH. The magnetic resonance imaging of musculoskeletal hemorrhage. Skeletal Radiol 2000;29(1):1–9.
42. Reid JD, Kommareddi S, Lankerani M, et al. Chronic expanding hematomas. A clinicopathologic entity. JAMA 1980;244(21):2441–2.
43. Liu PT, Leslie KO, Beauchamp CP, et al. Chronic expanding hematoma of the thigh simulating neoplasm on gadolinium-enhanced MRI. Skeletal Radiol 2006;35(4):254–7.
44. Aoki T, Nakata H, Watanabe H, et al. The radiological findings in chronic expanding hematoma. Skeletal Radiol 1999;28(7):396–401.
45. Mellado JM, Perez del Palomar L, Diaz L, et al. Long-standing Morel-Lavallee lesions of the trochanteric region and proximal thigh: MRI features in five patients. AJR Am J Roentgenol 2004;182(5):1289–94.
46. Hatzipantelis ES, Athanassiou-Metaxa M, Koussi A, et al. Tibial pseudotumor in a child with hemophilia. Pediatr Hematol Oncol 2007;24(8):623–30.
47. Temple HT, Kuklo TR, Sweet DE, et al. Rectus femoris muscle tear appearing as a pseudotumor. Am J Sports Med 1998;26(4):544–8.

Arthritis Mimicking Sports-Related Injuries

Donald J. Flemming, MD, Stephanie A. Bernard, MD

KEYWORDS

- Arthritis • Sports injury • Diagnostic error

KEY POINTS

- Arthritis can be confused with sports injury, leading to unnecessary surgery or delay in diagnosis.
- Careful history should be obtained in all patients presenting with joint pain. Inflammatory joint pain and/or lack of history of trauma should alert the physician that an arthritis may explain the patients symptoms.
- Orthopedic surgeons and sports physicians should be aware of the common clinical presentations of and diagnostic criteria for common arthropathies.
- Laboratory and imaging may be required to establish the diagnosis of a specific arthritis.

INTRODUCTION

Joint pain is the initial presentation for many orthopedic conditions and the initial assumption may be that the symptoms may be related to a surgically amenable internal derangement. On occasion, however, the presentation of chronic or acute arthritis can mimic a sports-related injury and lead to a referral to an orthopedic surgeon.[1] The purpose of this article is to review the clinical and radiographic presentation of arthropathies that can produce diagnostic confusion. The conditions that will be discussed include inflammatory arthritis, crystal deposition disease, and masslike synovial proliferative disorders.

The evaluating physician must be diligent in their clinical approach to distinguish arthritis from mechanical internal derangement. Clues in the history may be swollen joints, morning stiffness, and progression of symptoms despite rest or change in activity. Concern for a nonmechanical diagnosis should always be considered when there is no history of trauma or the mechanism of injury does not fit the clinical presentation. Appropriate radiologic and laboratory investigation should be initiated in these cases because early diagnosis and treatment may minimize joint damage and allow the athlete to return to normal physical activity.

Radiology, Penn State Milton S. Hershey Medical Center, 500 University Drive, Hershey, PA 17033, USA
E-mail address: dflemming@hmc.psu.edu

Clin Sports Med 32 (2013) 577–597
http://dx.doi.org/10.1016/j.csm.2013.03.003
0278-5919/13/$ – see front matter © 2013 Elsevier Inc. All rights reserved.
sportsmed.theclinics.com

INFLAMMATORY ARTHRITIS

The major inflammatory arthropathies that are encountered in clinical practice are rheumatoid arthritis, psoriatic arthropathy, reactive arthritis, and ankylosing spondylitis. The first 3 most commonly present with peripheral disease affecting multiple joints. Ankylosing spondylitis, however, typically affects the axial skeleton with low back pain being the most common early presentation. Radiographically, they all share features of synovitis, erosions, and uniform loss of articular cartilage but the distribution and specific radiographic findings help differentiate between these entities.

Rheumatoid Arthritis

Rheumatoid arthritis (RA) is a relatively common disorder that is clinically diagnosed using history, physical examination, serologic tests, and radiographic imaging. Patients are typically young to middle-aged women that complain of morning stiffness in the peripheral joints in a bilateral and symmetric distribution. The classic presentation of RA is usually diagnosed with relative ease but the atypical and early presentations may result in delay of diagnosis. The clinical criteria for the establishment of the diagnosis of RA[2] are listed in **Box 1**.

The initial presentation of RA may be confused with internal derangement of a joint and overuse injury of a tendon.[3] Patients with RA may initially be diagnosed with meniscal tear and undergo arthroscopic surgery that reveals significant synovitis.[4] Tendon disease, including rotator cuff tear or Achilles tendonitis, may also be the first clinical complaint in patients with RA.[5] One of the earliest manifestations of RA is flexor tenosynovitis of the hands.[6]

Box 1
The 2010 American College of Rheumatology/European League Against Rheumatism classification criteria for RA

For patients:
  1. That have at least 1 joint with definite clinical synovitis (swelling)
  2. With synovitis that is not better explained by another disease

	Score
A. Joint involvement	
1 large joint	0
2–10 large joints	1
1–3 small joints (with or without involvement of large joints)	2
4–10 small joints (with or without involvement of large joints)	3
>10 joints (at least 1 small joint)	5
B. Serology (at least 1 test result is needed for classification)	
Negative RF and negative ACPA	0
Low-positive RF or low-positive ACPA	2
High-positive RF or high-positive ACPA	3
C. Acute-phase reactants (at least 1 test result is needed for classification)	
Normal CRP and normal ESR	0
Abnormal CRP or normal ESR	1
D. Duration of symptoms	
<6 weeks	0
≥6 weeks	1

A score of ≥6/10 is needed for classification of a patient as having definite RA.

Abbreviations: ACPA, anti-citrullinated protein autoantibody; CRP, C-reactive protein; ESR, erythrocyte sedimentation rate; RF, rheumatoid factor.

The radiographic presentation reflects the pathologic condition of the disease.[7] Soft tissue swelling and effusion represent synovitis. Uniform destruction of articular cartilage manifests as uniform narrowing of the involved joint (**Fig. 1**). Erosions without bone repair may be appreciated in the small joints of the hands and feet with a proximal distribution. Erosions and synovitis are more accurately and sensitively assessed on magnetic resonance imaging (MRI) and ultrasound. Distal interphalangeal joint involvement in RA is extremely rare. In large joints, erosions are uncommon and the predominant imaging feature is more commonly uniform joint space narrowing. Congruent narrowing of a joint without subchondral sclerosis or osteophyte formation should alert the interpreting physician that they are dealing with an inflammatory arthritis such as RA. Erosion of the humeral head in RA may lead to confusion with tumor because large lucent lesions may be seen in the proximal humerus (**Fig. 2**). Accompanying joint space narrowing in this situation provides confirmation that the lucencies represent a manifestation of erosive arthropathy rather than neoplasm.

Psoriatic Arthritis

Psoriatic arthritis (PsA) is an inflammatory arthritis in the family of spondyloarthropathies. The typical patient has a long-standing history of severe psoriasis and, in this setting, a clinical diagnosis is usually rapidly established. Arthritis may precede the onset of skin disease in up to 19% of patients.[8] Careful and thorough evaluation for rash should be performed in any patient with suspected inflammatory arthritis. It is important to understand that a patient need only have a family history of PsA and not have psoriatic skin disease themselves to help establish this diagnosis.[9] The current criteria for establishing a diagnosis of PsA are listed in **Box 2**.

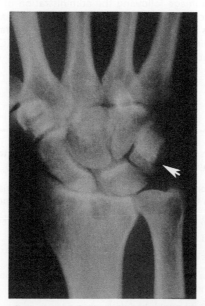

Fig. 1. A 25-year-old active duty man with wrist pain and rheumatoid arthritis that was clinically diagnosed as ligament tear. Posteroanterior radiograph of the wrist shows uniform joint space narrowing of radiocarpal joint without osteophyte formation (*arrowhead*). Pattern of joint space narrowing and erosion at the proximal aspect of the triquetrum are characteristic of inflammatory arthritis.

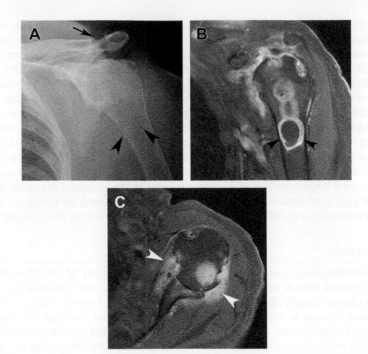

Fig. 2. A 48-year-old woman with rheumatoid arthritis and shoulder pain. AP radiograph of shoulder (*A*) shows lucent lesion in the proximal humeral diaphysis (*arrowheads*). Note erosive changes producing tapered appearance of distal clavicle (*black arrow*). Coronal fat-saturated T1-weighted image following the administration of intravenous gadolinium (*B*) shows rim-enhancing cyst (*arrowheads*) that extends from the subchondral surface of the humerus that accounts for lucency seen on radiography. Axial fat-saturated T1-weighted image following the administration of intravenous gadolinium (*C*) shows synovitis (*white arrowheads*), diffuse joint space narrowing, and erosions that are characteristic of an inflammatory arthritis.

Box 2
Classification criteria for Psoriatic Arthritis (CASPAR) classification criteria for psoriatic arthritis in patient inflammatory articular disease (joint, spine, or entheseal)

1. Evidence of current psoriasis (2 points), a personal history of psoriasis (1 point), or a family history of psoriasis in a first-degree or second-degree relative (1 point).

2. Psoriatic nail dystrophy, including onycholysis, pitting, and hyperkeratosis (1 point).

3. A negative rheumatoid factor test (1 point).

4. Either current dactylitis or a history of dactylitis (1 point).

5. Radiographic evidence of juxta-articular ill-defined new bone formation on plain radiographs of the hand or foot (1 point).

Diagnosis of psoriatic arthritis established with score ≥3.

Data from Taylor W, Gladman D, Helliwell P, et al. Classification criteria for psoriatic arthritis: development of new criteria from a large international study. Arthritis Rheum 2006;54(8):2665–73.

PsA can be confused with a sports injury when it presents as an effusion in an athlete.[10] Arthroscopy revealed synovitis in a National Football League player presenting in this manner.[10] A rheumatology consult was obtained after the patient's effusion recurred. This case highlights the importance of the need for heightened awareness of potential inflammatory arthritis in the setting of atraumatic joint pain. Early diagnosis can prevent significant joint damage since the development of anti-TNF- $\alpha1$ agents.

The radiographic manifestations of PsA are most dominant in the small joints of the hands and feet.[11,12] Erosive changes are identified in a bilateral and asymmetric distribution and the distal interphalangeal joints, which are typically spared in RA, can be involved in PsA. Erosive changes can lead to the classic presentation of pencil-in-cup deformity. The erosive disease is frequently associated with bone repair, including ill-defined bone formation adjacent to cortical interruption and periosteal reaction. Small joint disease may be accompanied by the enlargement of the entire affected digit (dactylitis) (**Fig. 3**).

Bone formation and joint space narrowing are the predominant findings in large joints as opposed to erosive changes. Bone formation presents as ill-defined enthesopathic changes at ligamentous and tendinous insertions.[13,14] Enthesitis on MRI is most commonly appreciated in the medial and lateral collateral ligaments as well as the patellar tendon. Ill-defined bone formation on conventional radiography is most commonly recognized at the medial epicondyle and patellar tendon insertion in the affected knee (**Fig. 4**). Erosive changes with accompanying bone formation at the calcaneal insertion of the Achilles tendon[15] and plantar fascia are commonly seen in PsA. Hip involvement is very uncommon but sacroiliac disease is seen in 30% to

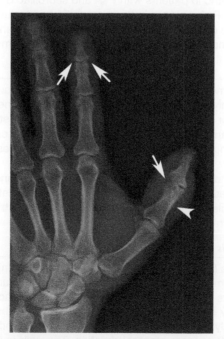

Fig. 3. A 38-year-old man with psoriatic arthritis. AP radiograph of the hand shows dactylitis of the thumb. Erosions are appreciated in the thumb interphalangeal joint and index finger distal interphalangeal joint (*arrows*). Note bone production that accompanies the erosions and periosteal new bone involving the radial aspect of the thumb metacarpal (*arrowhead*).

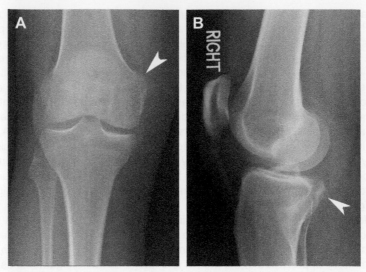

Fig. 4. (*A, B*) A 48-year-old man with psoriatic arthritis and knee pain. AP radiographs of the knee show bone formation (enthesopathy) at the medial epicondyle insertion of the medial collateral ligament (*arrowhead*).

50% of patients with PsA. The erosive changes and bone formation can be bilateral asymmetric or symmetric in patients with PsA and sacroiliac disease.

The MRI findings of PsA are frequently nonspecific and include effusion, synovitis, and tenosynovitis. The diagnosis should be considered when enthesopathic changes manifesting as bone marrow edema are a component of the imaging findings.[16]

Reactive Arthritis

Reactive arthritis, formerly known as Reiter disease, is a spondyloarthropathy that occurs more commonly in male patients after an infectious illness, typically sexually transmitted disease or diarrheal illness. This disorder has a strong predilection for the lower extremities and, like many arthopathies, it too can be confused with a sports injury.[17] It is self-limiting in two-thirds of patients but can progress to severe disabling disease.

The radiographic findings are almost identical to PsA but tend to be limited to the lower extremities.[12] Reactive arthritis is more commonly associated with periosteal reaction and juxta-articular osteoporosis, both of which may contribute to misdiagnosis of infection or stress fracture (**Fig. 5**).

Ankylosing Spondylitis

Ankylosing spondylitis (AS) is a spondyloarthropathy that is clinically associated with axial skeletal symptoms more commonly than small joints, unlike PsA or reactive arthritis.[12] Patients are typically men that complain of low back pain and stiffness. Low back pain is very common in athletes but, unlike in mechanical low back pain, AS patients are usually less than 40 years of age and have inflammatory-type back pain and stiffness of 3 or more months' duration. The pain is worse in the morning and improves with activity but is not relieved by rest.[18] Most patients (90%) are HLA-B27-positive. Sacroiliac disease is one of the hallmarks of this disorder but not all patients will develop radiographically identifiable sacroiliitis and this is particularly

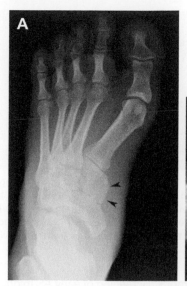
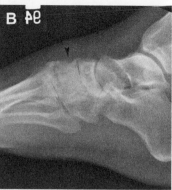

Fig. 5. A 33-year-old man with midfoot pain and reactive arthritis. AP (*A*) and lateral (*B*) radiograph of the foot shows marked medial soft tissue swelling, midfoot joint space narrowing, and bone formation (*arrowheads*).

true in women.[19] More recent studies have suggested that the earliest manifestations of AS actually are demonstrated in the thoracic and lumbar spine on MRI.[20] The symptoms of ankylosing arthritis may also be seen in patients with inflammatory bowel disease and so a careful history to assess for diarrhea, weight loss, and abdominal pain should be performed.

Radiographically, the diagnosis of AS is considered when bilateral symmetric sacroiliitis is appreciated on pelvic or lumbar spine radiographs. Erosive changes are detected in the synovial portion of the joint (anterior inferior two-thirds) and the erosive disease is accompanied by sclerosis and repair. The sacroiliac joint may eventually completely ankylose. These findings can be easily overlooked and so the sacroiliac joint should always be carefully evaluated on any pelvis, hip, or lumbar spine examination (**Fig. 6**). It is also important not to confuse bilateral sacroiliitis with osteitis condensans illi that also presents with subchondral sclerosis at the inferior half of the sacroiliac joints.[21] Patients with osteitis condensans illi have pubic instability (multiparous women, rugby players, sports hernia patients) and they develop subchondral sclerosis in a sail-shaped configuration that is wider inferiorly than superiorly (**Fig. 7**).[22] Unlike AS, osteitis condensans is not associated with erosive disease.

Lumbar spine findings on radiographs include the shiny corner sign on lateral radiographs early in the disease. Erosive changes are accompanied by reparative sclerosis at the superior and inferior anterior aspect of involved vertebral bodies (**Fig. 8**). Patients may also develop ossification in the Sharpey fibers of disks that will present as thin vertically oriented bone spanning the disk space on lateral or anteroposterior (AP) radiographs of the spine. An easily overlooked pattern of bone formation is loss of normal anterior concavity of lumbar vertebral bodies that may be accompanied by squaring of vertebral bodies at the superior and inferior margins.

Early diagnosis of axial spondyloarthropathy is best achieved by MRI and serum assay for HLA-B27 positivity.[23] Early disease of the sacroiliac joints on MRI manifests as erosion with accompanying bone marrow edema and these changes may be

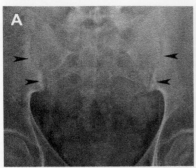
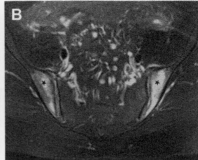

Fig. 6. A 27-year-old man with hip pain that led to performance of MRI arthrogram for possible internal derangement. AP radiograph of the pelvis (*A*) shows sacroiliitis that was missed on initial interpretation. Erosions (*arrowheads*) and sclerosis are seen in a bilateral symmetric pattern. Coronal oblique fat-saturated T2-weighted image (*B*) shows subchondral bone marrow edema (*stars*) and widening of the bilateral sacroiliac joint. Following MRI, diagnosis of AS was established.

appreciated in the setting of normal radiographs. Screening of early AS might be best achieved though by assessing the thoracic spine because recent literature suggests that this is where the disease is actually first identifiable on MRI.[24]

CRYSTAL DEPOSITION DISEASE
Gout

Gout is a disease well described in the literature since ancient times. The classic presentation is the abrupt onset of symptoms of intense pain, redness, and swelling over a 2- to 6-hour period in the great toe of a middle-aged male patient. The patient will typically demonstrate hyperuricemia on serum testing and acute symptoms resolve over 7 to 10 days. In this setting, the diagnosis is relatively straightforward. The prevalence of gout is increasing in developed countries in part because of metabolic syndrome and in part because of medications such as diuretics.[25] The increasing number of patients with gout has increased the likelihood of unusual presentations, including the growing number of women developing the disease. Gout should be in the differential for the acute onset of any monoarticular arthropathy even in young adult men.

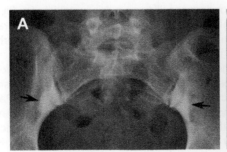
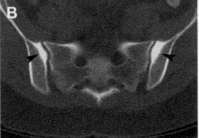

Fig. 7. A 36-year-old multiparous woman with low back pain. Features of osteitis condensans ilii are appreciated on AP view of the pelvis (*A*). Note the sail-shaped sclerosis in the bilateral ilium at the inferior aspect of the sacroiliac joints (*arrows*). Axial CT scan (*B*) through sacroiliac joints again shows sclerosis limited to the iliac side of the joint (*arrowheads*). Note the lack of erosions or joint space narrowing.

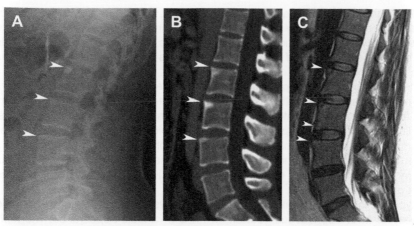

Fig. 8. A 35-year-old man with AS and low back pain. Lateral view of the lumbar spine (A) and sagittal CT reconstruction (B) demonstrate focal sclerosis (*arrowheads*) at the anterior superior endplate of L2, L3, and L4, producing the "shiny corner sign." sagittal fat-suppressed T2-weighted image of the lumbar spine (C) shows subtle faint increased T2 signal at the anterior endplate of L2 through L4 (*arrowheads*) indicating active inflammation.

Gout can present in a sports medicine practice in some unexpected ways. Intra-articular tophus can lead to clicking that is confused with meniscal tear on clinical assessment.[26] Gout can infiltrate the patellar tendon and produce masslike enlargement that may be confused with tumor[27] or degenerative tendinopathy.[28] Tendon involvement may be associated with erosion of the patella and, when this erosive process is extensive, it may lead to fracture as the initial presentation of the disorder (**Fig. 9**).[29] Interestingly, patients with patellar tendon disease often have no other clinically apparent joint disease.[30] Gout also has a peculiar predilection for involving the

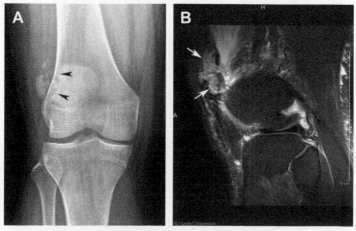

Fig. 9. A 54-year-old man with gout and pathologic fracture of the patella. AP view of the knee (A) shows scalloped well-corticated marginated erosion (*arrowheads*) in the lateral patella typical of tophus. Sagittal fat-suppressed proton density image of the knee (B) shows nonspecific increased signal of tophus (*arrows*) replacing the marrow of the patella.

popliteal tendon and the lateral capsule of the knee.[27] Masslike infiltration of the cruciate ligaments may also be seen on imaging and arthroscopy (**Fig. 10**).[31] Other tendons that may be involved include the flexor tendons of the ankle, the Achilles tendon, and the extensor tendons of the wrist. Tenosynovitis may also rarely be the dominant initial clinical presentation.

The radiographic evaluation of gout tends to be very specific but not sensitive.[32,33] When findings are present, they usually are appreciated in the small joints of the hands and feet as well as corticated periarticular erosions adjacent to lumpy soft tissue swelling that represents a tophus. Erosive gout is typically seen in patients with at least a 7-year history of symptoms. Computed tomography (CT), MRI, and ultrasound are much more sensitive for the detection of early manifestations of gout.[34–36] Dual-energy CT has been shown to be particularly effective for the detection and assessment of tophus burden.[35–37]

Atypical clinical or masslike presentation on physical examination may lead to a request for MRI. Tophaceous gout on MRI has a variable appearance. The tophus will be appreciated as a rounded mass with intermediate to low signal on T1-weighted images and may range from high to very low signal on T2-weighted sequences.[38,39] This low-signal presentation on T2-weighted sequences can lead to an erroneous diagnosis of pigmented villonodular synovitis (PVNS) (**Fig. 11**). Tophus has a more amorphous appearance on T2 images than the more well-defined lobular growth pattern of PVNS. Contrast enhancement is variable, ranging from little to marked increased signal following the administration of intravenous gadolinium. Tendon involvement is appreciated as enlargement of the tendon and this may be accompanied by erosion of the adjacent bone.

Gout is appreciated as white crystalline material on arthroscopy that may be visualized in a masslike distribution[26,27,31,39] or diffusely cover the articular cartilage.[40,41] Cloaking of the articular cartilage is appreciated as the double contour sign on ultrasound of a joint affected by gout.[42,43] It is important for the arthroscopist to submit

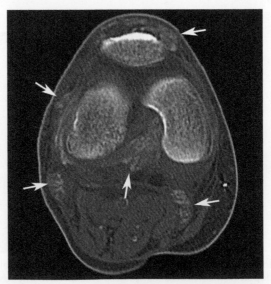

Fig. 10. Axial CT scan shows high-attenuation gout crystal deposition (*arrows*) in the posterior cruciate ligament, lateral capsule, posterior soft tissues, and prepatellar bursa.

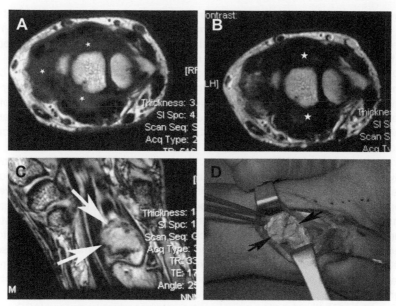

Fig. 11. A 42-year-old man with wrist swelling and gout. Axial T1 (*A*) and axial fast spin-echo T2-weighted (*B*) images of the wrist show intermediate T1 and predominantly low T2 signal in tophus involving the volar, ulnar, and dorsal wrist (*stars*). Preoperative diagnosis of PVNS was rendered based on low T2 signal. Note high signal of tophus (*arrows*) on gradient echo image through the volar wrist (*C*) rather than expected low signal of PVNS. Typical appearance of tophus (*arrows*) in volar incision of wrist appreciated at surgery (*D*).

biopsy material of gout crystal in alcohol rather than formalin.[41] The crystals can dissolve in formalin, preventing the detection of the classic strongly negative birefringent crystals on polarized light microscopy. Surprisingly, joint aspiration may be negative for crystal despite extensive covering of the articular cartilage at arthroscopy.[44] In addition, false negatives on joint aspiration can be secondary to suboptimal laboratory quality control, so the diagnosis of gout cannot be entirely excluded based on lack of crystals on joint aspiration.[45] Repeat aspiration should be considered whenever joint aspiration is normal despite a classic presentation.

Hydroxyapatite Deposition Disease

Hydroxyapatite deposition disease (HADD), commonly known as calcific tendinopathy, is frequently seen in clinical practice. In a study performed in 1941 on 12,222 shoulders, 3% of the study participants demonstrated calcific deposits about the shoulder.[46] The deposits were most commonly appreciated in women 20 to 40 years of age. Only one-third of the study population was symptomatic at the time of evaluation. In practice, patients typically present to clinical attention with complaints of acute onset of pain in the involved joint. The most common articulations affected are the shoulder, hips, elbow, wrist, hands, and ankle in decreasing order of frequency.

Uncommonly, HADD may be clinically confused with fracture, infection,[47] or neoplasm.[48] Misdiagnosis of HADD in the hand and wrist at initial presentation can be seen in up to 75% of cases with acute onset of redness and swelling leading to erroneous diagnosis of infectious tenosynovitis, septic joint, cellulitis, abscess, inflammatory arthritis, gout, pseudogout, and tendonitis. Up to one-third of patients report antecedent trauma that leads to improper diagnosis of fracture (**Fig. 12**).[47] Involvement of the popliteus tendon may be associated with symptoms of "locked knee" that can be confused with meniscal injury or loose body.[49]

HADD is usually easily detected on radiography and CT. The concretions are ovoid or comet-shaped and can be smoothly marginated and homogeneously dense or may demonstrate shaggy margins and heterogenous density. Shaggy or poorly defined concretions are typically those that are undergoing resorption. On CT, the concretions may be associated with perilesional soft tissue edema in patients that are acutely symptomatic.

MRI manifestations of HADD are variable. The concretion will usually be low in signal on T1-weighted and T2-weighted images. Small concretions may escape detection on routine sequences because both the calcific deposit and the involved tendon are low in signal. Improved detection on MRI of deposits of hydroxyapatite crystals is possible when the concretion is surrounded by increased signal on T2 (edema) or on postcontrast or gradient echo sequences. Periconcretional soft tissue edema may lead to the erroneous diagnosis of muscle strain, ligamentous injury, hematoma, or abscess (**Fig. 13**). It is imperative to review conventional radiographs whenever interpreting MRI images because even subtle concretions are readily appreciated on conventional radiography despite sometimes causing diagnostic confusion on MRI.

Review of conventional radiographs is extremely important because HADD can be confused with tumor particularly when it is associated with cortical erosion or extension into the underlying bone marrow (**Fig. 14**).[48] This unusual presentation is most commonly seen in the anterior humerus adjacent to the insertion of the pectoralis major tendon; in the lesser or greater tuberosity of the proximal humerus; and along the linea aspera of the posterior proximal femur. The MRI findings may be confusing but clues to the nonneoplastic nature of HADD include perilesional edema and lack

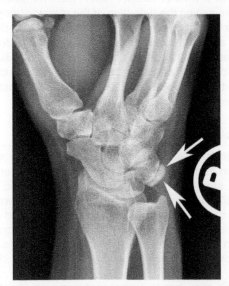

Fig. 12. A 38-year-old woman with dorsal wrist pain after a fall on her outstretched hand and HADD. Incorrect original diagnosis was triquetral fracture. Note the typical amorphous cloudlike appearance typical of calcium deposition dorsal to triquetrum (*arrows*) and lack of ossification that would be expected in a fracture fragment.

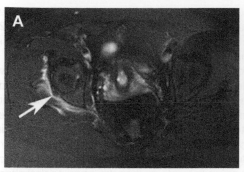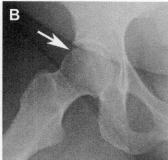

Fig. 13. A 48-year-old woman with acute right hip pain and HADD. Axial fat-suppressed T2-weighted image (*A*) through the hips shows subtle small focus of low signal (*arrow*) surrounded by marked edema in adjacent soft tissues. Original diagnosis was muscle strain. Review of conventional radiograph (*B*) of right hip shows amorphous calcification of HADD in the tendon of the reflected head of the rectus femoris (*arrow*).

of soft tissue mass associated with the calcification. Review of conventional radiographs typically demonstrates typical findings of calcific tendinopathy in the adjacent tendon.

Calcium Pyrophosphate Deposition Disease

Calcium pyrophosphate deposition disease (CPPD) is commonly seen in clinical practice. Most patients are clinically asymptomatic and the diagnosis is recognized as chondrocalcinosis on conventional radiography. Chondrocalcinosis in and of itself is not sufficient to establish a diagnosis of CPPD[50] because more than one joint must be involved and chondrocalcinosis can be seen in a single joint following injury or surgery.

Multiarticular chondrocalcinosis is unusual in patients less than 50 years of age and if encountered the patient should be evaluated for possible hypomagnesemia, familial

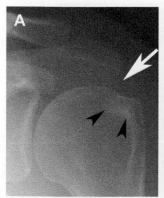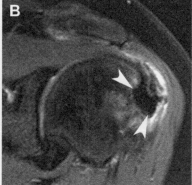

Fig. 14. A 52-year-old man with left shoulder pain and HADD. Grashey view of shoulder (*A*) shows faint calcification in supraspinatus tendon (*arrow*) and sclerosis in the adjacent greater tuberosity (*arrowheads*). Coronal oblique fat-suppressed T2-weighted image of the shoulder (*B*) demonstrates low signal in the marrow of the greater tuberosity (*arrowheads*) secondary to intraosseous extension of HADD with faint edema in adjacent marrow. Note subacromial subdeltoid bursitis and heterogeneous appearance of supraspinatus tendon secondary to crystal deposition.

chondrocalcinosis, hemochromatosis, and hyperparathyroidism,[51] which are rare diagnoses but the fact that their initial presentation may be joint-related pain cannot be overemphasized.

Delayed diagnosis of hemochromatosis is particularly common with patients on average seeking medical attention for 10 years before establishing the diagnosis.[52] One of the challenges is that hemochromatosis presents as osteoarthritis that is indistinguishable from routine osteoarthritis other than distribution and age of presentation. Although hemochromatosis is considered a rare disease, homozygosity for the gene responsible for primary hemochromatosis is found in 1 of every 200 patients of Northern European decent.[53] The penetrance of the genetic disorder is variable and arthritis may be the sole presentation. Hemochromatosis should be considered in the differential diagnosis of early onset osteoarthritis regardless of whether chondrocalcinosis is present.[54] Early diagnosis is important to avoid the end organ damage of cirrhosis of the liver, cardiomyopathy, and diabetes. Suspicion for hemochromatosis should be heightened in a young patient with atraumatic osteoarthritis in the metacarpal phalangeal, ankle, or wrist articulations particularly when there is a family history of early-onset osteoarthritis (**Fig. 15**).[55] Screening for the diagnosis is accomplished with assay for serum iron/transferrin saturation ratio. If the ratio is higher than 45%, the patient should be referred for further evaluation and genetic counseling.[53]

Acute calcium pyrophosphate arthritis (formerly known as pseudogout) is a term that should be reserved for the presentation of acute arthritis secondary to calcium pyrophosphate in the joint.[56,57] This presentation is much more common in elderly people and can be confused with septic arthritis or gout. Patients may or may not demonstrate chondrocalcinosis on radiography. A search for crystals should be part of the clinical assessment of any patient presenting with acute monoarticular arthritis.

A rare presentation of CPPD is tophaceous pseudogout. Patients will present with a calcified mass that may raise concern for neoplasm or loose body (**Fig. 16**).[58,59] Interestingly, these patients do not have multiarticular chondrocalcinosis but typically present with pain and limited range of motion. Most commonly affected joints are the

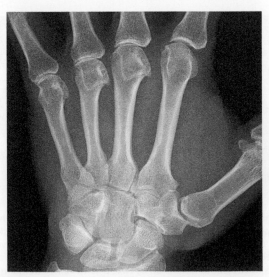

Fig. 15. Osteoarthritis of the metacarpal phalangeal joint in a patient with hemochromatosis-associated arthropathy.

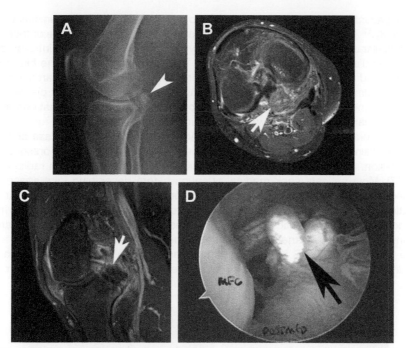

Fig. 16. A 50-year-old man with tophaceous pseudogout of the knee presented with pain-less lack of flexion of the knee. Lateral view of the knee (*A*) shows amorphous calcification posterior to the joint line (*arrowhead*). Axial fat-suppressed proton density image (*B*) shows intermediate to low signal of mass posterior to cruciate ligament (*arrow*) with extension posterior to medial femoral condyle. Fat-suppressed T1-weighted image (*C*) through the knee shows mild peripheral but no central enhancement of tophus (*arrow*). Arthroscopic image in posteromedial knee (*D*) shows white crystal in tophus (*arrow*).

temperomandibular joints, cervical spine, and wrist. Imaging will demonstrate amor-phous calcification on conventional radiography or CT that may erode the adjacent bone. On MRI, the mass will show low to intermediate signal on T2-weighted images but will not enhance with gadolinium administration. The intra-articular tophus may be resected with arthroscopy at which time the chalky nature of crystal deposition will be appreciated.

MASSLIKE ARTHROPATHY

The masslike arthropathies are neoplastic disorders of the synovium that lead to pain, swelling, and mechanical symptoms. The conditions in this category of arthritis are pigmented villonodular synovitis and synovial chondromatosis. These diseases typi-cally affect large joints but almost any joint or tendon sheath can be affected. Despite being relatively rare, both PVNS and synovial chondromatosis are seen by orthopedic surgeons dealing with athletes.

Pigmented Villonodular Synovitis

PVNS is a benign neoplastic proliferative disorder of the synovium that involves male and female patients equally.[60] Patients typically present with complaints of swelling and pain.[61] A history of trauma may be elicited in ~50% of cases.[60] Mechanical symptoms may be appreciated in 26% of patients with the diffuse disease and in

90% of patients with focal disease, leading to a clinical diagnosis of meniscal tear or loose body.[62] The distribution of disease depends on whether it is diffuse or focal and intra-articular or extra-articular. PVNS is rarely polyarticular. The diffuse intra-articular form of the disease is most commonly seen in the knee followed by the hip, ankle, shoulder, and elbow in decreasing order of frequency. The focal intra-articular form of PVNS is almost exclusively diagnosed in the knee. The extra-articular presentation of PVNS (formerly known as giant cell tumor of the tendon sheath) is most commonly seen in the hand and wrist followed by the foot and ankle.

The radiographic presentation varies based on the form of the disease and joint involved. Plain films are commonly normal in the focal intra-articular presentation. On occasion, a soft tissue mass may be seen in the Hoffa fat pad on radiography (**Fig. 17**). Most patients seek medical attention before developing joint space loss and secondary osteoarthritis. Erosions may accompany the diffuse intra-articular presentation in 2% to 18% of cases that involve the knee.[61,62] Erosions are more commonly seen in extra-articular PVNS of the hands and feet. It is extremely rare to see any mineralization in the soft tissue component of PVNS.

The diagnosis of PVNS is most commonly established clinically on MRI. In this modality, PVNS presents as diffuse involvement or focal mass arising from the

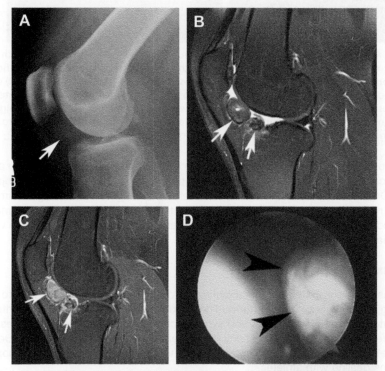

Fig. 17. A 31-year-old man with focal PVNS and knee locking. Original clinical diagnosis was meniscal tear. Lateral view of the knee (*A*) shows subtle density in Hoffa fat pad (*B*). Sagittal fat-suppressed T2-weighted image through the knee shows low signal mass in the posterior aspect of Hoffa fat pad (*arrows*). Enhancement of the mass (*arrows*) is shown on the following intravenous gadolinium administration on sagittal fat-suppressed T1-weighted image (*C*). Arthroscopic image (*D*) shows rust color of mass (*arrowheads*) that is typical of PVNS.

synovium or tendon sheath. The masses of PVNS will have intermediate to low signal on T1-weighted and T2-weighted images and will be accompanied by effusion in most cases.[60] The hemosiderin that is seen pathologically in this disorder results in marked loss of signal on T2-weighted images and the unusually low signal on this sequence will lead to radiologic diagnosis of PVNS in most cases. However, low signal in the synovium on T2-weighted images can also be seen in other diseases, including amyloidosis, gout, mineralized synovial chondromatosis, chronic rheumatoid arthritls, and chronic bleeding in the joint because of bleeding diathesis (hemophilia, anticoagulation) or intra-articular neoplasm (synovial hemangioma). Thorough review of patient history and conventional radiographs should be performed before assuming that low T2 signal in the synovium is secondary to PVNS.

Synovial Chondromatosis

Synovial chondromatosis is a benign neoplastic condition that arises from the synovium. Patients typically present with pain, swelling, and limited range of motion. It can be confused with internal derangement of the joint[63–65] but careful history will usually establish an insidious onset of complaints with 5 years of clinical symptoms on average before diagnosis. On a rare occasion, synovial chondromatosis will be diagnosed after an acute sports injury.[66] Men are more commonly affected than women and the disease is most commonly encountered in patients in the third to fifth decade of life. Any articulation may be involved but the knee, followed by hip, shoulder, elbow, and ankle are most commonly affected. The disorder may be rarely encountered in an extra-articular location particularly in tendon sheaths or bursae.[67]

Radiography shows mineralized rounded or ovoid bodies in the involved joint in most cases. The ossific opacities tend to be small and numerous as opposed to the large loose bodies that are often appreciated in osteoarthritis (so-called secondary chondromatosis). The calcific opacities can be very subtle (**Fig. 18**). Erosion of adjacent bone may be seen in up to 30% of cases.[68] Joint space narrowing and osteoarthritis may be appreciated on initial presentation, causing confusion with secondary chondromatosis.

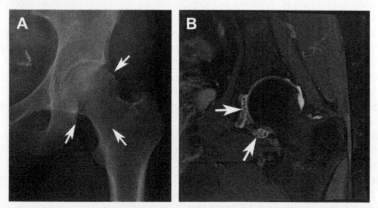

Fig. 18. A 42-year-old woman with left hip pain and synovial chondromatosis. AP view of the left hip (*A*) shows subtle rounded or ovoid calcifications (*arrows*) in the left hip joint. Coronal fat-suppressed T1-weighted image (*B*) following intra-articular injection of gadolinium shows rounded low signal intra-articular chondral bodies (*arrows*) typical of synovial chondromatosis.

MRI is the preferred modality for the evaluation and diagnosis of synovial chondromatosis. The appearance of the disease on MRI depends on the extent of mineralization in it.[69] On T1-weighted images, synovial chondromatosis may range from high to low signal. On T2-weighted sequences, the unmineralized components will be intermediate to very high in signal secondary to the high water content of hyaline cartilage tissue that is seen pathologically in this disease. In fact, it may be difficult to separate synovial chondromatosis from fluid in some cases.[63] Mineralized components may be low in signal on T2-weighted images, causing potential confusion with PVNS if the MRI is not reviewed with conventional radiographs (see **Fig. 18**).

SUMMARY

Most patients presenting to an orthopedist complaining of joint pain and swelling have an internal derangement that explains the symptoms. However, uncommonly arthropathies can present in a way that mimics sports injury and the astute clinician must carefully evaluate for clues that separate these entities from typical internal derangement, particularly in the setting of a monoarticular arthropathy. Lack of history of trauma, inflammatory joint pain, and radiologic findings may allow for an accurate early diagnosis to be rendered that may prevent joint damage through surgical and/or medical intervention.

REFERENCES

1. Jennings F, Lambert E, Fredericson M. Rheumatic diseases presenting as sports-related injuries. Sports Med 2008;38(11):917–30.
2. Aletaha D, Neogi T, Silman AJ, et al. 2010 Rheumatoid arthritis classification criteria: an American College of Rheumatology/European League Against Rheumatism collaborative initiative. Ann Rheum Dis 2010;69(9):1580–8.
3. Kuechle DK, Stuart MJ. Isolated rupture of the patellar tendon in athletes. Am J Sports Med 1994;22(5):692–5.
4. Jari S, Noble J. Meniscal tearing and rheumatoid arthritis. Knee 2001;8(2):157–8.
5. Suzuki T, Ishihara K. Achilles paratendonitis as the initial manifestation of rheumatoid arthritis. Mod Rheumatol 2010;21(2):219–22.
6. Eshed I, Feist E, Althoff CE, et al. Tenosynovitis of the flexor tendons of the hand detected by MRI: an early indicator of rheumatoid arthritis. Rheumatology 2009;48(8):887–91.
7. Tan YK, Conaghan PG. Imaging in rheumatoid arthritis. Best Pract Res Clin Rheumatol 2011;25(4):569–84.
8. Scarpa R, Oriente P, Pucino A, et al. Psoriatic arthritis in psoriatic patients. Br J Rheumatol 1984;23(4):246–50.
9. Taylor W, Gladman D, Helliwell P, et al. Classification criteria for psoriatic arthritis: development of new criteria from a large international study. Arthritis Rheum 2006;54(8):2665–73.
10. Brophy RH, MacKenzie CR, Gamradt SC, et al. The diagnosis and management of psoriatic arthritis in a professional football player presenting with a knee effusion: a case report. Clin J Sport Med 2008;18(4):369–71.
11. Day MS, Nam D, Goodman S, et al. Psoriatic arthritis. J Am Acad Orthop Surg 2012;20(1):28–37.
12. Amrami KK. Imaging of the seronegative spondyloarthopathies. Radiol Clin North Am 2012;50(4):841–54.

13. Emad Y, Ragab Y, Bassyouni I, et al. Enthesitis and related changes in the knees in seronegative spondyloarthropathies and skin psoriasis: magnetic resonance imaging case-control study. J Rheumatol 2010;37(8):1709–17.

14. Yasser R, Yasser E, Hanan D, et al. Enthesitis in seronegative spondyloarthropathies with special attention to the knee joint by MRI: a step forward toward understanding disease pathogenesis. Clin Rheumatol 2011;30(3):313–22.

15. Yedon DF, Howitt S. Heel pain due to psoriatic arthritis in a 50 year old recreational male athlete: case report. J Can Chiropr Assoc 2011;55(4): 288–93.

16. Spira D, Kotter I, Henes J, et al. MRI findings in psoriatic arthritis of the hands. Am J Roentgenol 2010;195(5):1187–93.

17. Hart RS, Detro JF. A case of reactive arthritis in a Ranger Indoctrination Program (RIP) student. J Spec Oper Med 2009;9(2):22–8.

18. Sieper J, van der Heijde D, Landewé R, et al. New criteria for inflammatory back pain in patients with chronic back pain: a real patient exercise by experts from the Assessment of SpondyloArthritis international Society (ASAS). Ann Rheum Dis 2009;68(6):784.

19. van Tubergen A, Weber U. Diagnosis and classification in spondyloarthritis: identifying a chameleon. Nat Rev Rheumatol 2012;8(5):253–61.

20. Bennett AN, Rehman A, Hensor EM, et al. Evaluation of the diagnostic utility of spinal magnetic resonance imaging in axial spondylarthritis. Arthritis Rheum 2009;60(5):1331–41.

21. Canella C, Schau B, Ribeiro E, et al. MRI in seronegative spondyloarthritis: imaging features and differential diagnosis in the spine and sacroiliac joints. Am J Roentgenol 2012;200(1):149–57.

22. Mitra R. Osteitis condensans Ilii. Rheumatol Int 2009;30(3):293–6.

23. Rudwaleit M, Sieper J. Referral strategies for early diagnosis of axial spondyloarthritis. Nat Rev Rheumatol 2012;8(5):262–8.

24. Konca Ş, Keskin D, Cılız D, et al. Spinal inflammation by magnetic resonance imaging in patients with ankylosing spondylitis: association with disease activity and outcome parameters. Rheumatol Int 2012;32(12):3765–70 Springer-Verlag.

25. Pascual E, Pedraz T. Gout. Curr Opin Rheumatol 2004;16(3):282–6.

26. Espejo-Baena A, Coretti SM, Fernandez JM, et al. Knee locking due to a single gouty tophus. J Rheumatol 2006;33(1):193–5.

27. Li TJ, Lue KH, Lin ZI, et al. Arthroscopic treatment for gouty tophi mimicking an intra-articular synovial tumor of the knee. Arthroscopy 2006;22(8):910.e1–3.

28. Rodas G, Pedret C, Català J, et al. Intratendinous gouty tophus mimics patellar tendonitis in an athlete. J Clin Ultrasound 2012;41(3):178–82.

29. Price MD, Padera RF, Harris MB, et al. Case reports: pathologic fracture of the patella from a gouty tophus. Clin Orthop Relat Res 2006;445:250–3.

30. Recht MP, Seragini F, Kramer J, et al. Isolated or dominant lesions of the patella in gout: a report of seven patients. Skeletal Radiol 1994;23(2):113–6.

31. Melloni P, Valls R, Yuguero M, et al. An unusual case of tophaceous gout involving the anterior cruciate ligament. Arthroscopy 2004;20(9):e117–21.

32. Perez-Ruiz F, Dalbeth N, Urresola A, et al. Imaging of gout: findings and utility. Arthritis Res Ther 2009;11(3):232.

33. Dalbeth N, Doyle A, McQueen FM. Imaging in gout. Curr Opin Rheumatol 2012; 24:132–8.

34. Carter JD, Kedar RP, Anderson SR, et al. An analysis of MRI and ultrasound imaging in patients with gout who have normal plain radiographs. Rheumatology 2009;48(11):1442–6.

35. Choi HK, Burns LC, Shojania K, et al. Dual energy CT in gout: a prospective validation study. Ann Rheum Dis 2012;71(9):1466–71.
36. Glazebrook KN, Guimaraes LS, Murthy NS, et al. Identification of intraarticular and periarticular uric acid crystals with dual-energy CT: initial evaluation. Radiology 2011;261(2):516–24.
37. Desai MA, Peterson JJ, Garner HW, et al. Clinical utility of dual-energy CT for evaluation of tophaceous gout. Radiographics 2011;31(5):1365–75.
38. Yu JS, Chung C, Recht M, et al. MR imaging of tophaceous gout. AJR Am J Roentgenol 1997;168(2):523–7.
39. Chen CK, Yeh LR, Pan HB, et al. Intra-articular gouty tophi of the knee: CT and MR imaging in 12 patients. Skeletal Radiol 1999;28(2):75–80.
40. Baker JF, Synnott KA. Clinical images: gout revealed on arthroscopy after minor injury. Arthritis Rheum 2010;62(3):895.
41. Wilczynski MC, Gelberman RH, Adams A, et al. Arthroscopic findings in gout of the wrist. J Hand Surg Am 2009;34(2):244–50.
42. Ávila Fernandes E, Kubota ES, Sandim GB, et al. Ultrasound features of tophi in chronic tophaceous gout. Skeletal Radiol 2010;40(3):309–15.
43. Thiele RG. Role of ultrasound and other advanced imaging in the diagnosis and management of gout. Curr Rheumatol Rep 2011;13(2):146–53.
44. Kennedy TD, Higgens CS, Woodrow DF, et al. Crystal deposition in the knee and great toe joints of asymptomatic gout patients. J R Soc Med 1984;77(9):747–50.
45. Essen von R, Hölttä AM, Pikkarainen R. Quality control of synovial fluid crystal identification. Ann Rheum Dis 1998;57(2):107–9.
46. Bosworth BM. Calcium deposits in the shoulder and subacromial bursitisa survey of 12,122 shoulders. JAMA 1941;116(22):2477–82.
47. Doumas C, Vazirani RM, Clifford PD, et al. Acute calcific periarthritis of the hand and wrist: a series and review of the literature. Emerg Radiol 2007;14(4):199–203.
48. Flemming DJ, Murphey MD, Shekitka KM, et al. Osseous involvement in calcific tendinitis: a retrospective review of 50 cases. AJR Am J Roentgenol 2003;181(4):965–72.
49. Tibrewal SB. Acute calcific tendinitis of the popliteus tendon–an unusual site and clinical syndrome. Ann R Coll Surg Engl 2002;84(5):338–41.
50. Rosenthal AK, Ryan LM. Crystal arthritis: calcium pyrophosphate deposition—nothing "pseudo" about it! Nat Rev Rheumatol 2011;7(5):257–8.
51. Richette P, Bardin T, Doherty M. An update on the epidemiology of calcium pyrophosphate dihydrate crystal deposition disease. Rheumatology 2009;48(7):711–5.
52. McDonnell SM, Preston BL, Jewell SA, et al. A survey of 2,851 patients with hemochromatosis: symptoms and response to treatment. Am J Med 1999;106(6):619–24.
53. Alexander J, Kowdley KV. HFE-associated hereditary hemochromatosis. Genet Med 2009;11(5):307–13.
54. Carlsson Å. Hereditary hemochromatosis: a neglected diagnosis in orthopedics. Acta Orthop 2009;80(3):371–4.
55. Sahinbegovic E, Dallos T, Aigner E, et al. Musculoskeletal disease burden of hereditary hemochromatosis. Arthritis Rheum 2010;62(12):3792–8.
56. Zhang W, Doherty M, Bardin T, et al. European league against rheumatism recommendations for calcium pyrophosphate deposition. Part I: terminology and diagnosis. Ann Rheum Dis 2011;70(4):563–70.

57. Fam AG, Topp JR, Stein HB, et al. Clinical and roentgenographic aspects of pseudogout: a study of 50 cases and a review. Can Med Assoc J 1981; 124(5):545–51.
58. Kato H, Nishimoto K, Yoshikawa T, et al. Tophaceous pseudogout in the knee joint mimicking a soft-tissue tumour: a case report. J Orthop Surg (Hong Kong) 2010;18(1):118–21.
59. LaPrade RF, Burnett QM. Localized chondrocalcinosis of the lateral tibial condyle presenting as a loose body in a young athlete. Arthroscopy 1992; 8(2):258–61.
60. Murphey MD, Rhee JH, Lewis RB, et al. Pigmented villonodular synovitis: radiologic-pathologic correlation. Radiographics 2008;28(5):1493–518.
61. Ottaviani S, Ayral X, Dougados M, et al. Pigmented villonodular synovitis: a retrospective single-center study of 122 cases and review of the literature. Semin Arthritis Rheum 2011;40(6):539–46.
62. Myers BW, Masi AT. Pigmented villonodular synovitis and tenosynovitis: a clinical epidemiologic study of 166 cases and literature review. Medicine (Baltimore) 1980;59(3):223–38.
63. Lin RC, Lue KH, Lin ZI, et al. Primary synovial chondromatosis mimicking medial meniscal tear in a young man. Arthroscopy 2006;22(7):803.e1–3.
64. Doward DA, Troxell ML, Fredericson M. Synovial chondromatosis in an elite cyclist: a case report. Arch Phys Med Rehabil 2006;87(6):860–5.
65. Chou PH, Huang TF, Lin SC, et al. Synovial chondromatosis presented as knocking sensation of the knee in a 14-year-old girl. Arch Orthop Trauma Surg 2006; 127(4):293–7.
66. Wong CK, Restel BH. Unusual cause of knee pain mimicking meniscal pathology in a 14-year-old baseball player. Clin J Sport Med 2000;10(2):146–7.
67. Walker EA, Murphey MD, Fetsch JF. Imaging characteristics of tenosynovial and bursal chondromatosis. Skeletal Radiol 2010;40(3):317–25.
68. Norman A, Steiner GC. Bone erosion in synovial chondromatosis. Radiology 1986;161(3):749–52.
69. Kramer J, Recht M, Deely DM, et al. MR appearance of idiopathic synovial osteochondromatosis. J Comput Assist Tomogr 1993;17(5):772–6.

Index

Note: Page numbers of article titles are in **boldface** type.

A

ABER position (abduction external rotation), 378
Accessory flexor tendons, injuries to, 443–444
Acetabular labrum, normal, 413–414
Achilles tendinopathy, insertional, and Haglund deformity, 548–550
Achilles tendon, rupture of, 550, 551
Adductor injury, 437–439, 440
Adductor longus, and rectus abdominis, in biomechanics of pelvic core atability, 430–431
Adhesive capsulitis, 356–357
Ankle, and foot, MRI techniques for, 526–527
    anterior impingement of (bony), 541–542, 543
    anterior impingement of (soft tissue), 540–541
    cysts and soft-tissue masses of, 553–555
    lateral ligaments of, injury to, 542–543, 544
    ligamentous structures of, 527–529
    loose bodies in, 538–540
    posterior, and subtalar joint, injuries involving, 545–547
        impingement of, 545–547
    posterior structures of, 527–529
    sports injuries in, 535–553
    syndesmosis of, 530–532
        injury to, 544–545
    synovitis of, 537–538
    tendon injuries of, 548–553
Ankle and foot injuries, in sport, **525–557**
    MRI correlations with anatomy, 527–535
Ankle joint, anatomy of, 527
Ankylosing spondylitis, 582–584, 585
Anterior labroligamentous periosteal sleeve avulsion, 351, 372–373
Apophysitis, 444–445
Arthritis, inflammatory, 578–594
    mimicking sports-related injuries, **577–597**
    psoriatic, 579–582
    reactive, 582, 583
    rheumatoid, 578–579, 580
Arthrography, intra-articular, of hip, 412
    magnetic resonance, and magnetic resonance imaging, studies of labral lesions using, 377–379
Arthropathy, masslike, 591–594
Arthroscopy, and magnetic resonance imaging appearance of menisci of knee, **449–475**

Clin Sports Med 32 (2013) 599–605
http://dx.doi.org/10.1016/S0278-5919(13)00039-2
0278-5919/13/$ – see front matter © 2013 Elsevier Inc. All rights reserved.

sportsmed.theclinics.com

Athletic pubalgia, and core muscle injuries, as pelvic musculoskeletal injuries, 427–428
     imaging of, **427–447**
     patterns of, with MRI findings, 431–441

B

Bankart lesion, 350–354, 371
     reverse, 352–353
Basal cystic degeneration, after anterior cruciate ligament reconstruction, 492–493, 494
Biceps pulley, 370
     lesions of, 380
Biceps tendon, long head of, pathology of, 355
          subluxation patterns of, 355–356
     normal anatomy of, 354–355
Bone, giant cell tumor of, 560
Bone tumors, mimicking traumatic lesions, 560
Buford complex, 362–354

C

Calcium hydroxyapatite deposition disease, 346, 347
Calcium pyrophosphate deposition disease, 589–591
Capsular anatomy, and normal labrum, 348
Cartilage, acute injury of, with patellar dislocation, 483–484
     and osteochondral injuries, imaging of, **477–505**
          technical considerations for, 478–481
     impaction injury, chronic, 484–487, 488
     in chondral delamination, 487–491
     injury of, patterns of, 482–503
     normal, structure and MRI appearance of, 481–482
Children, elbow injury in, 491–492
     knee pain in, 493–495, 496, 497
Chondral delamination, cartilage in, 487–491
Chondroblastoma, 561–562
Chondrocalcinosis, 589–590
     confused with meniscal tear, 468
Chondromatosis, synovial, 593–594
Computed tomography, for evaluation of shoulder, 340, 379
Coracohumeral ligament, 369–370
Core muscle injuries, and athletic pubalgia, as pelvic musculoskeletal injuries, 427–428
     imaging of, **427–447**
     patterns of, with MRI findings, 431–441
Cruciate ligament, anterior, injury of, 508–511
          arthroscopic findings in, 509–511
          MRI findings in, 508–509, 510
     reconstruction of, basal cystic degeneration after, 492–493, 494
     posterior, injury of, arthroscopic findings in, 513
          MRI features of, 511–512, 513
Crystal deposition disease, 584
Cysts, and soft tissue masses, of ankle, 553–555
     of foot, 553–555
     paralabral, 375–377

E

Elbow injury, pediatric, 491–492
Ewing sarcoma, 562

F

Femoral head cartilage, normal, 414
Femoroacetabular impingement, assessment of, structures to identify in, 412
    bony structures in, 412
    case examples of, 416–424
    evaluation of cartilage in, 412–413
    MRI pathologic anatomy associated with, 414–416
Flexor hallucis longus, rupture of, 551–553, 554
Foot, and ankle, MRI techniques for, 526–527
    cysts and soft tissue masses of, 553–555
Foot and ankle injuries, in sport, **525–557**
    MRI correlations with anatomy, 527–535
Fractures, avulsion, 567–568, 569
    pathologic, 562–563, 564
    stress, 443
Frozen shoulder, 356–357

G

Giant cell tumor of bone, 560
Glenohumeral instability, 346–354
    lesions not associated with, 373
    lesions of, 349–350
    traumatic, lesions associated with, 370–373
Glenohumeral ligament(s), anatomy of, 363, 367–369
    humeral avulsion of, 352
    inferior, 368–369
    middle, 368
    superior, 367–368, 370
Glenoid labrum, anatomy of, 362, 363
        variants and pitfalls of, 362–367
    lesions of, imaging of, **361–390**
Glenolabral articular disruption lesion, 351–352, 374–375, 377
Gout, 584–587

H

Haglund deformity, and insertional Achilles tendinopathy, 548–550
Hallux, aand sesamoids, metatarsophalangeal joint of, injury of, 548, 549
Hematoma, 572–574
    chronic, 573, 574
    hemorrhagic soft tissue sarcoma mimicking, 566–567, 568
Hemochromatosis, 590
Hip, disorders of, and activity-related groin pain, 442
        pubic symphysis and, 442–445

Hip (*continued*)
    intra-articular arthrography of, 412
    MRI normal anatomy of, 412–413
    MRI techniques for, 411–412
Hip-femoral acetabular impingement, **409–425**
    cam impingement, 410, 414, 415, 416, 417
    combined impingement, 411, 421–424
    MRI technical considerations in, 411–412
    pincer impingement, 410–411, 415–416, 417
Hydroxyapatite deposition disease, 587–589

I

Inguinal hernia, 441
Intraarticular lesions, causing mechanical symptoms, 563

K

Knee, menisci of. See *Meniscus(i)*.
    MRI of, with arthroscopic correlation, **507–523**
    posterolateral corner of, injury of, arthroscopic findings in, 514, 515
        MRI features of, 514, 515
      structures of, 513
Knee pain, microfracture repair in, 495–498, 499
    pediatric, 493–495, 496, 497
Kocher-Lorenz osteochondral fracture, 491–492

L

Labral disease, 370–380
Labral lesions, MRI and MR arthrography studies of, 377–379
Labrum, acetabular, normal, 413–414
    and capsule, normal anatomic variants of, 348–349
    normal, and capsular anatomy, 348
Liposarcoma, myxoid, 565, 566, 567
Long head biceps tendon, 370
    lesions of, 379–380

M

Magnetic resonance imaging, and arthroscopic appearance of menisci of knee, **449–475**
    and magnetic resonance arthrography, studies of labral lesions using, 377–379
    for evaluation of shoulder complaints, 341–342
    of knee, with arthroscopic correlation, **507–523**
    technical considerations, in hip-femoral acetabular impingement, 411–412
Malignancy, posttraumatic lesions mimicking, 567–574
Masslike arthropathy, 591–594
Medial collateral ligament injury, 516–517
    MRI features of, 517–518
    surgical findings in, 518
Meniscal flounce, confused with meniscal tear, 468

Meniscal ligament, transverse, confused with meniscal tear, 465–467
Meniscal roots, striations of, confused with meniscal tear, 468
Meniscal variants, anterior horn medial, confused with meniscal tear, 472
Meniscofemoral ligaments, confused with meniscal tear, 467
Meniscoidlike superior labrum, 364
Meniscomeniscal ligament, oblique, confused with meniscal tear, 471–472
Meniscus(i), bucket handle tear of, 456–458
    arthroscopic findings in, 519
    MRI features of, 518–519
  discoid, confused with meniscal tear, 468–470
  magnetic resonance imaging and arthroscopic appearance of, **449–475**
  normal, 450–453, 454, 455
  ring, confused with meniscal tear, 470
  tears of, bucket-handle, 456–458, 518–519
    complex, 462, 463
    horizontal, 458, 459
    horizontal flap, 460–462
    longitudinal-vertical, 455–456
    MRI of, 453–455
    patterns of, 455–463
    pitfalls and normal variants of, 465–472
    radial, 458, 460
    root, 462–463, 464
    secondary MRI signs of, 463–465, 466
    vertical flap, 459, 461
    with displaced fragment, arthroscopic findings in, 519–520
      MRI findings in, 519, 520
Metatarsophalangeal joint, first, anatomy of, 533–535
  of hallux and sesamoids, injury of, 58, 549
Microfracture repair, in knee pain, 495–498, 499
Musculoskeletal core, anatomy of, 429–430
Myositis ossificans, 568–572
Myxoid liposarcoma, 565, 566, 567

O

Osteitis pubis, 434–438
Osteoarticular transfer system evaluation, 498, 500, 501
Osteochondral allograft repair, 500–503
Osteochondral defect, arthroscopic findings in, 521–522
  MRI features of, 520, 521
Osteochondral injuries, and cartilage, imaging of, **477–505**
    technical considerations for, 478–481
Osteoid osteoma, 562, 563
Osteosarcoma (conventional intramedullary subtype), 560–561
Ostrigonum, and Stieda process, posterior impingement of, 545–547

P

Paralabral cysts, 375–377
Patella, dislocation of, acute cartilage injury with, 483–484

Patella (*continued*)
    dislocation/subluxation of, transient, 514–515
        arthroscopic findings in, 516, 517
        MRI features of, 515–516, 517
Pelvic core stability, rectus abdominis and adductor longus in biomechanics of, 430–431
Peroneal tendon, teas of, 550–551, 552, 553
Perthes lesion, 350, 351, 373
Posttraumatic lesion(s), and tumor, dilemmas in distinguishing between, **559–576**
    mimicking malignancy, 567–574
Pseudogout, tophaceous, 590–591
Psoriatic arthritis, 579–562
Pubic symphysis, hip disorders and, 442–445

R

Radiography, for evaluation of shoulder complaints, 340
Rectus abdominis, and adductor longus, in biomechanics of pelvic core atability, 430–431
    strain of, 439–441
Rectus abdominis/adductor aponeurosis injury, unilateral or bilateral, 431–432, 433–434
Rectus abdominis/adductor aponeurosis tic plate injury, midline, 432–434, 435, 436
Rheumatoid arthritis, 578–579, 580
Rotator cuff, complete tear of, 345
    evaluation of, ultrasound for, 392
    full thickness tear of, 345
    injuries to, patterns of, 401–404
    normal, appearance of, 342, 343, 392–394
    pathology of, MRI appearance of, 344–346, 347
    sonographic evaluation of, pitfalls in, 404
    tendinosis of, 394–395, 396
    tendon tears, 396–401
    ultrasound appearance of, 343–344
Rotator interval, 369
    lesions of, 379

S

Sesamoids, and hallux, metatarsophalangeal joint of, injury of, 548, 549
Shouder pain, as common complaint, 339
Shoulder, anterior superior internal impingement of, 402
    CT in evaluation of, 379
    imaging of, with arthroscopic correlation, **339–359**
    posterosuperior internal impingement of, 401–402
    subacromial impingement of, 402–404
    ultrasonography of, with arthroscopic correlation, **391–408**
Shoulder complaints, evaluation of, CT for, 340
        MRI for, 341–342
        radiography for, 340
        ultrasound for, 340–341
SLAP lesion, 348–350, 353, 354, 355, 373–374, 375, 376
Soft tissue masses, and cysts, of foot, 553–555
    cysts and, of foot, 553–555

Soft tissue sarcoma, hemorrhagic, mimicking hematoma, 566–567, 568
Sports-related injuries, arthritis mimicking, **577–597**
Stieda process, and ostrigonum, posterior impingement of, 545–547
Stress fractures, 443
Subacromial impingement, 342–346
Subacromial spur, MRI evaluation of, 346
Sublabral foramen, 366–367
Sublabral recess, 364–365
Subscapularis tendon, tears of, 345
Subtalar joint, anatomy of, 533, 534
    and posterior ankle, injuries involving, 545–547
Superior labral from anterior to posterior lesion. See *SLAP lesion*.
Supra-acetablar fossa, 414
Supraspinatus tendon, full-thickness tears of, 395–397, 398
    partial-thickness tears of, 398–401
Synovial chondromatosis, 593–594
Synovial sarcoma, 564–565, 566, 567
Synovitis, villonudular pigmented, 591–593

T

Talus, osteochondral lesions of, 535–536, 537
Tendinosis, of rotator cuff, 394–395, 396
Tophaceous pseudogout, 590–591
Tumor(s), and posttraumatic lesion, dilemmas in distinguishing between, **559–576**
    presenting as sports injury or other trauma, 560–567, 568
    soft-tissue, presenting as trauma, 564

U

Ultrasound, for evaluation of rotator cuff, 392
    for evaluation of shoulder complaints, 340–341
    of shoulder, with arthroscopic correlation, **391–408**

V

Villonodular synovitis, pigmented, 591–593

Moving?

Make sure your subscription moves with you!

To notify us of your new address, find your **Clinics Account Number** (located on your mailing label above your name), and contact customer service at:

Email: journalscustomerservice-usa@elsevier.com

800-654-2452 (subscribers in the U.S. & Canada)
314-447-8871 (subscribers outside of the U.S. & Canada)

Fax number: 314-447-8029

Elsevier Health Sciences Division
Subscription Customer Service
3251 Riverport Lane
Maryland Heights, MO 63043

*To ensure uninterrupted delivery of your subscription, please notify us at least 4 weeks in advance of move.

Printed and bound by CPI Group (UK) Ltd, Croydon, CR0 4YY

03/10/2024

01040431-0006